Treat Yourself!

with

Nutritional Therapy

Linda Lazarides

WATERFALL 2000

London

Other books by Linda Lazarides

Principles of Nutritional Therapy
Nutritional Health Bible
The Waterfall Diet
HIV Self-Help Manual
Gourmet Nutritional Therapy Cookbook
Facts of Health Factsheets
Amino Acid Report

This book is not a substitute for medical advice.
Always consult your doctor if you have a persistent health problem.

© 2002 Linda Lazarides
First published in 2002 by
Waterfall 2000
BCM Waterfall
London WC1N 3XX
United Kingdom
www.waterfall2000.com

Linda Lazarides asserts the moral right to be identified as the author of this work.

ISBN 0-9538046-3-1

Clipart by GSP (Global SoftwarePublishing) Ltd, Huntingdon, UK
and Microsoft Corporation (Publisher 2000)

Printed and bound in Great Britain by Anthony Rowe Ltd, Eastbourne

CONTENTS

Part III: A-Z of health problems

Part IV: Preparing food

Part V: Gourmet recipes 139

Appendices

How to use this book

You can use this book both to prevent health problems and to treat them. The recipes in Part V are delicious enough for anyone to use every day, even for entertaining guests. When they were first published in the *Gourmet Nutritional Therapy Cookbook* the author received positive feedback from all quarters about the high quality and simplicity of the recipes, and the book became a favourite cookbook for many people.

If you have a specific health problem to treat, you will need to start with the Nutritional Therapy Questionnaire on pages 21-22. Depending on your scores, you will be directed to further information and to one of the specific health programmes on pages 41, 46-47 or 61, all of which are supported by the recipes. This approach can be used by anyone with a chronic (long-term) health problem. Your body is its own best healer—all it needs is your help with:

- Avoiding the foods and other substances which hinder its internal processes,
- Getting enough of the raw materials it needs delivered to the cells which carry out these processes.

Parts I and II also provide plenty of information to help you understand the health programmes and to get motivated with the sometimes difficult task of changing your eating habits.

Much research has also been carried out using special diets and food supplements against ailments and illnesses. Part III summarizes some of that research, which suggests more specific ways of helping yourself fight these problems.

Part IV is about cooking techniques, helping you get the most out of your food and helping you to find substitutes for foods you have cut out.

Wishing you good health!

Linda Lazarides

A note for doctors

To all general practitioners; this book could revolutionize your practice, and provide improvements in cost-effectiveness of which the Government can only dream. Linda Lazarides provides first-line strategies for patients to start taking control of their own health. Dr Hugh Cox, who recently died, applied these principles in his single-handed general practice for many years, and achieved one of the lowest prescribing costs in the country. There is every reason why you should be able to do the same.

Treat Yourself with Nutritional Therapy provides a crash course in the basics of self-help. The three-year experiment described in Chapter 1 documents the fact that these measures enable more than 50 per cent of patients to sort themselves out without recourse to prescription medicines or other medical interventions. The added advantage for patients is that they gain autonomy over their own bodies; the advantage for their doctors is that they achieve this without consuming medical time and expense.

Those of us who take a specific interest in nutritional and environmental medicine will recognize that Ms Lazarides does not lead patients into areas where they would be out of their depth. The large majority of people who come to see me have already attempted some of what is covered in this book, but have done it badly. If they follow the instructions in the next 300 pages they will certainly do themselves no harm, and have a better than even chance of really helping themselves. I therefore recommend to all doctors with an open mind that you go further than simply buying this book; buy several and leave them in your waiting-room. Then see how many of the patients who came through the front door make it as far as your office!

Dr Damien Downing MB BS
Nutritional Medicine Specialist
Senior Editor, *Journal of Nutritional and Environmental Medicine*

Part I

The Basics

Start to look and feel better
Right now!

Nutrition used to be a boring old subject. Gone are the days when all we worried about was fats, carbohydrate and protein. Modern nutrition covers everything from the cancer-protective effects of broccoli to the health benefits of oily fish and the humble bacteria found in yoghurt.

In the old days, the only diet we heard of was a "balanced" diet. Now there are books everywhere about cleansing diets, food combining diets, elimination diets, low carbohydrate diets, rotation diets, and even the macrobiotic diet which originated in Japan.

Food supplements have also undergone a revolution. We no longer worry simply about whether we need B vitamins or iron. We are now faced with choices about hundreds of different combinations and doses. Should we buy vitamin E or "mixed tocopherols"? Zinc citrate or zinc picolinate? Is the refrigerated Acidophilus superior to the one on the shelf?

Treat Yourself with Nutritional Therapy puts an end to all these worries, for one main reason. It is not a book of theories. You are not reading it to find out more about diets or supplements so that you can choose one which might (if you are lucky) help you. You are reading it to get well—now!

Is that really possible? Don't take my word for it—take a look at the charts opposite. These show the results achieved in one of the rare GP practices which know how to spot food-related problems. The patients were all those referred to a nutritional therapist from 1990-1993, who complied well with the health programmes they were given.

The chances are that your doctor's surgery does not yet employ a nutritional therapist, so at present you probably won't get on the NHS the kind of treatment advice you will find in this book. Your doctor cannot be expected to look for links between your symptoms and what you eat. He or she is primarily trained to prescribe pharmaceutical medicines (drugs). While dieticians and some practice nurses are very knowledgeable about nutrition, their training likewise does not cover very much of the material you will find in this book. *Treat Yourself with Nutritional Therapy* could save you years of expensive experimenting with your health while getting nowhere.

This situation is changing as new, forward-thinking academics are emerging at universities such as the University of Westminster and the University of Surrey. Soon there will be more NHS staff qualified in nutritional therapy, and the face of medicine will change forever.

Figure I: Results achieved with nutritional therapy in a GP practice

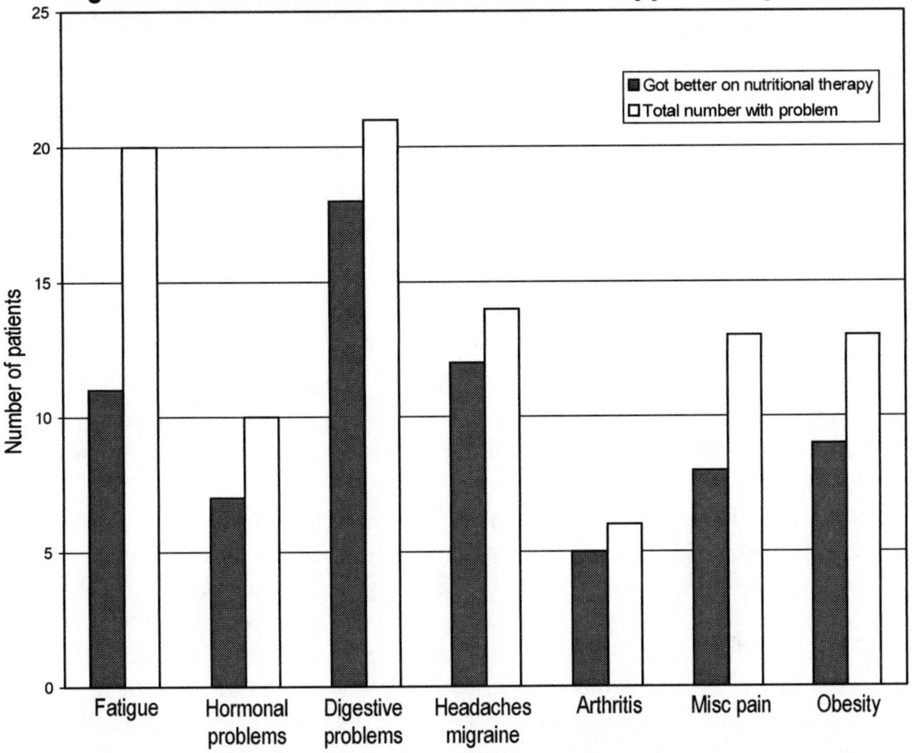

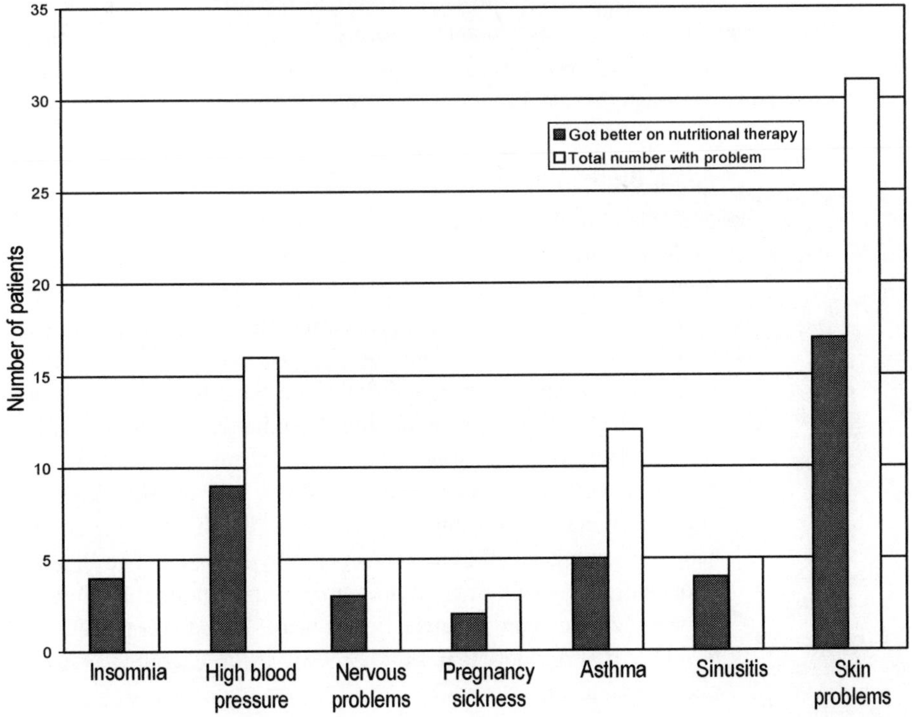

Linda Lazarides 1993

In the meantime, you can administer your own nutritional therapy using this book. It cannot cure everybody, but you can get an idea of your chances by looking at Figure I on page 11. The good news is that in some cases nutritional therapy can work very fast indeed—sometimes within days. So by this time next week you could feel and look like a new person.

What is nutritional therapy and how does it work?

How well you feel depends on how efficiently your body produces essential enzymes, hormones and other substances, and gets rid of wastes and toxins that could interfere with your internal chemistry. Nutritional therapy involves assessing what *you* need to get these jobs done better.

Nutritional therapy is *not* about giving the same treatment to everyone—for example vitamin B6 pills for everyone with premenstrual syndrome (PMS). Although some research studies have used this approach with moderate success, it is not the most effective way to treat PMS because not all women with PMS have a vitamin B6 deficiency. In nutritional therapy *we find out* which vitamins and food combinations you do need to help you feel better. We also find out whether any particular foods are disagreeing with you and contributing to your symptoms.

Two people with identical symptoms can have entirely different needs since everyone is genetically unique, has a history of eating different foods and lives in a different environment. This is why each person has to be individually assessed and given their own nutritional therapy programme based on these findings.

Period pains heavy periods PMS

Low immunity low fertility

Nervous problems stress, mood swings depression weight gain

Bad skin and nails, lifeless hair, dandruff, split ends

Food, digestion, absorption, assimilation

Nutritional deficiencies occur when you do not consume enough foods rich in vitamins, minerals, essential fatty acids and other important ingredients. Deficiencies can affect every system in your body, from your skin to your immune system, nerve cells, bones and hormones. Your tissues lose their strength and hormones become weaker and fail to do their job. Your nerves jangle, fertility wanes, skin and hair become dry and lifeless. As the deficiency progresses, your moods are affected, sleep becomes difficult, or chronic tiredness develops. Women experience period pains, heavy periods and PMS; adolescents get acne and younger children may become hyperactive. The longer your immune system goes without proper nourishment, the lower your protection against cancers. Even heart disease can be caused by B vitamin deficiencies, because they encourage high cholesterol levels.

Many people eat such a poor diet that they live permanently with these problems and take them for granted. When you go to the doctor with various ailments he/she does not ask you what you eat. Instead he hands out antidepressants, tranquillizers, sleeping pills, painkillers, antibiotics, and offers hysterectomies and coronary bypass operations. Of course none of these are really cures. The lives of millions of people could be changed within weeks if they switched to wholemeal bread and brown rice, ate fruit and vegetables every day, consumed nuts, fish and olive oil regularly, and drastically reduced sugary and convenience foods and alcohol.

The vast majority of people don't need any complicated nutritional treatments, they just need a little knowledge. On the other hand there are thousands who already eat an excellent diet, yet still suffer from nutritional deficiency symptoms. Their problem is food absorption.

When food is digested, it should be broken down to individual nutrients, which should then pass through the wall of your small intestine into your blood. The blood is simply a transport system which takes oxygen, vitamins, minerals and other nutrients to your organs, glands and other tissues. Here, the individual cells assimilate what they need for their various tasks.

Complicated mechanisms are involved in absorption and assimilation. There are many stages where things can go wrong, allowing valuable vitamins and minerals to pass out of your body through your stools, or to float uselessly around in your blood without getting into your cells. We will take a closer look at this in later chapters. Nutritional therapy reverses nutritional deficiencies caused by this type of problem, which cannot be treated simply by eating a better diet.

Food intolerances

**Headaches
migraine**

**lirritable bowel
syndrome
colitis**

Arthritis

**Sinus
congestion
catarrh**

**Eczema
asthma**

Weight gain

One of the first steps in nutritional therapy is always to check whether any particular foods are disagreeing with you and causing your symptoms. Many symptoms can be due to a food "intolerance" - otherwise known as an allergy. It is not an allergy in the strict sense of the word. Food intolerances do not cause life-threatening reactions like a peanut allergy for instance. Food intolerances can come out of the blue—sometimes after a period of stress when your digestion is weaker. Particles of a food which you are not digesting completely come into contact with white cells in your blood, resulting in histamine being produced in one or more areas of your body. Histamine is the body chemical responsible for swellings after an insect bite, and for the redness and sneezing associated with hay fever, so you can imagine what symptoms it can cause when produced in your organs and internal blood vessels.

- Migraine and headaches
- Congested sinuses
- Catarrh
- Wheezing and breathing difficulties
- Eczema and rashes
- Bloating
- Severe constipation
- Diarrhoea and colitis
- Swollen, painful joints

Imagine also what happens if you eat the offending food several times every day! Lots of people eat toast for breakfast, sandwiches for lunch and pasta for dinner, not to mention biscuits or cake in between. If your problem food is wheat, then you could have one of these symptoms practically all the time. If wheat is not removed from your diet to give your body the chance to recover, you may never know that your arthritis, for instance, has anything to do with what you are eating!

The same applies if you develop an intolerance to milk and dairy products. Just a few spoonfuls of milk in tea or coffee several times a day, plus the occasional portion of cheese or yoghurt, can keep your symptoms going forever. But you won't feel particularly worse just after consuming the problem food. Symptoms usually come and go with no particular pattern. Migraine sufferers may get a migraine once every few days, or only when they are under stress. But take the problem food away, and stress on its own no longer brings on a migraine.

Doctors who specialize in nutritional therapy say that up to one third of all people who consult a GP for long-term health problems could be cured within a week by removing the foods they are allergic to[33]. This book will show you how to test yourself for food intolerances. It also gives you lots of really delicious recipes which help you easily to live without staples like wheat and dairy products if you find that you have to cut them out.

Giving your liver a helping hand

Lethargy, exhaustion, tired all the time, can't concentrate, frequent nagging headaches

Sallow skin, psoriasis

Arthritis, fluid retention allergies, chronic degenerative diseases

Much ill health is caused by an overloaded liver. Toxins in the form of

- Environmental pollutants: pesticides, lead, vehicle exhausts, factory emissions etc.
- Fumes in the home from sprays, paint, fabrics, artificial air fresheners, cigarette smoke, cleaning fluids etc.
- Artificial food additives
- Prescribed and over-the-counter medicines

- Wastes produced in your body: ammonia, formaldehyde, uric acid etc.
- Toxins produced by the resident bacteria in your intestines

All must be dealt with by your liver. The harder it has to work, the better it needs to be nourished. If your liver does not get enough nutrients to make its essential enzymes then it cannot process toxins properly. A vicious circle results: as toxins build up your liver becomes poisoned and less and less efficient. The result is known as a toxic overload. The symptoms of this are difficult to pinpoint because they take the form of increasing allergies and sensitivity to even small amounts of chemicals. Just one whiff of diesel fumes, or even sitting next to someone wearing strong perfume, and you could find yourself feeling suddenly drained and exhausted, or feeling faint, your muscles unable to work properly. Nagging headaches or liver pains are common, yellowish skin or eyes, and skin reactions or drowsiness after meals.

Nutritional therapy for your liver consists of

- Helping to drain your liver of built-up toxins,
- Protecting its cells against damage from toxins,
- Giving it the nutrients it needs to do its job better.

As your liver improves, your symptoms can be gradually reversed. This aspect of nutritional therapy is also vital in helping to combat serious illnesses like Alzheimer's, cancers, parkinsonism, arthritis, lupus, motor neurone disease and multiple sclerosis. Research at Birmingham University suggests that several such diseases are caused or aggravated by a liver overload[1,2].

Time to change your diet?
It's not as hard as you think

By now you will have gathered that nutritional therapy usually requires a change in eating habits. If your eating habits are already good, this may only be a temporary change to allow repairs to your digestive system or to your tissues and organs. If your current eating habits leave something to be desired, you may need some help with motivating you to change them. Other people's successes are usually the best motivation. After all, if others have got rid of unpleasant health or skin problems, why not you?

The success rates on page 11 mainly represent people who decided to give nutritional therapy their best shot and were not half-hearted about following the advice they were given. But if you feel rather daunted at the thought of changing your eating habits, take a look at the comments of some people who have tried nutritional therapy. Like you, they assumed the worst before they started, but once they actually got going, they were pleasantly surprised.

Sue

I was dreading getting started. The thought of eating beans and rice instead of steak and chips made me feel depressed. But I'd got to the stage where I would do anything, absolutely anything, to get rid of my awful skin problem. Then came the magic—it worked! After that no-one could ever get me to return to my old ways again, even when Linda said I could indulge myself occasionally.

Fred

I had already made quite a few changes to my diet. I'd given up chocolate, biscuits and other sweet things, and I'd cut down on fried, fatty foods. I'd started eating a lot more white meat, salads and vegetables. So it wasn't really hard to stick to the nutritional therapy, but it did make all the difference to have a proper programme designed for me. From then on it only took two weeks to be free of my perpetual migraines—free of them forever, as long as I didn't eat the wrong foods.

Lizzie

What I think a lot of people don't realize when they start on nutritional therapy is that it's not a starvation diet. You can eat lots of really nice food. My problem was overweight, although I was only eating about 1,000 calories a day. Linda told me I could eat another 500 calories a day as long as I gave up two foods which she thought I could be allergic to. I did give them up and within three weeks I lost more than a stone in weight despite the extra calories. The food allergy had been making me retain fluid. I looked fat, but I wasn't actually fat at all—it was all water, and it stayed away as long as I stayed off my problem foods.

Alicia

I'm afraid I was addicted to chocolate, and giving it up was the hardest thing in my life—for about two weeks! After that I hardly missed it at all. There are lots of nice things like almonds, pecan nuts and dried fruit which have a naturally sweet taste, and I could still have foods and drinks flavoured with cocoa powder and vanilla, which anyway is what gives chocolate its taste. After I had finished the first stage of my nutritional therapy I was allowed to eat chocolate again occasionally, but I find I don't crave it much now. I am very glad I stayed the course because I no longer feel exhausted all the time.

All these people dreaded making changes to their diet. What kept them going was really, *really* wanting to be free of their problems. It generally took about two weeks to get into the swing of things; then the benefits they gained stopped them from slipping back into old habits.

Before we move on to the next section, where you will actually learn how to treat yourself, I would like to suggest some advice to follow if your doctor is offering you medication for your symptoms and you are not sure whether you need it or not.

Questions you should ask your doctor

You should always consult a doctor first of all if you have any persistent symptoms. Some medical treatments are essential for your own safety. There is no doubt that drugs can save lives, but at the same time most are really just crutches, and can lead to problems of their own. If you want to try to *reverse* a long-term health problem, you should not rely on drugs. An alternative medicine system such as nutritional therapy is different. It aims to encourage your body's functions to work better, hopefully allowing you to gradually wean yourself off any medication which you may need in the meantime.

For instance if you suffer from high blood pressure—an extremely common problem in later life—you will probably be given a prescription to control it. But this prescription will not cure your problem. It will not remove the blockages in your arteries which are causing the high blood pressure. As long as you take them the drugs just artificially reduce your heart's pumping power, which is a way around the problem. If you continue with the same eating and lifestyle habits, your blood pressure may continue to rise despite the medication, in time affecting your heart. Then the heart medicines start, but they are not a cure either. In exchange for giving you a few more years of life, heart and blood pressure drugs can cause impotence, coldness, depression and memory loss among other problems.

If, on the other hand, you begin a nutritional therapy programme as soon as your high blood pressure is diagnosed, you can hopefully start to clear out your arteries so that in time, and with your doctor's permission, you can become independent from medication.

Not all prescriptions are necessary for your safety. Some, such as steroid creams for eczema, or anti-inflammatories for osteoarthritis, are only for your comfort and pain control. So how can you tell the difference? The answer is that you can ask your doctor the following questions if he or she offers you a prescription:

- Will the medicine cure me?
- If it won't cure me, is it essential for my safety or will it just help me to feel better?
- Will my problem get worse despite the medicine?

You may be surprised at the answers. With the exception of antibiotics, doctors have very few cures and are rarely able to reverse illnesses. This is why so many people are on medication like blood pressure drugs for life.

How well you feel depends directly on how efficiently your body produces essential enzymes, hormones and other substances, and gets rid of wastes and toxins that interfere with your internal chemistry. These functions depend on nutrients.

Part II

How to Treat Yourself

Assessing your needs

Y ou are going to start by analyzing your symptoms to find out if you suffer from:

- Nutritional deficiencies
- Food intolerances
- Overloaded liver

If you have any of these three problems, our first priority is to treat them. This will help your body to repair itself, thus combating your main health problem—if you have one.

On the next two pages you will find a Nutritional Therapy Questionnaire. Take a look at the lists of symptoms. Consider them very carefully before you tick the boxes. You are looking for symptoms that are really noticeable or persistent. So if you get the odd spot on your chin only once a year or so, do not bother to tick "spotty skin". On the other hand, if you are perpetually troubled by spots, definitely do tick it. Similarly if you occasionally do not feel hungry at mealtimes, then do not tick "poor appetite". But if your desire to eat is abnormally low compared with other people, then definitely do tick it.

As you will gather, the aim is not to see how many boxes you can tick, but to identify anything definitely abnormal and unhealthy.

Once you have added up your score for each section, copy it into the box below:

Nutritional deficiency and dietary imbalance score	
Food intolerance score	
Liver overload score	

If your nutritional deficiency and dietary imbalance score is higher than three

Your health is probably being undermined by some nutritional deficiencies. The higher your score, the more deficiencies you have. Turn to page 23 now.

If your food intolerance score is two or more

It is quite likely that certain foods are not agreeing with you and are causing some of your symptoms. Turn to page 42 now.

If your liver overload score is two or more

Turn to page 53.

NUTRITIONAL THERAPY QUESTIONNAIRE

Part I: Symptoms of nutritional deficiency and dietary imbalance

Eyes

- ❑ Abnormally poor vision in bad light
- ❑ Eyes always sore, dry or bloodshot
- ❑ Very sensitive to bright lights

Skin and Fingernails

- ❑ Spotty skin (acne)
- ❑ Dry, flaky skin
- ❑ Persistent dandruff
- ❑ Puffy skin & fluid retention
- ❑ Itchy red patches
- ❑ Eczema
- ❑ Sore, raw tongue
- ❑ Sores that won't heal
- ❑ Split or brittle fingernails
- ❑ White-spotted fingernails

Immune System

- ❑ Frequent colds or infections
- ❑ Persistent thrush

Brain and Nervous System

- ❑ "Spaced-out" feeling
- ❑ Deteriorating co-ordination
- ❑ Increasing confusion
- ❑ Mood swings
- ❑ Poor concentration
- ❑ Tremors
- ❑ Easily startled

Muscles

- ❑ Cramps
- ❑ Muscles knotted—won't relax

Hormones

- ❑ Premenstrual symptoms
- ❑ Painful menstrual periods
- ❑ Enlarged prostate
- ❑ Adult-onset diabetes

Bones

- ❑ Pain and tenderness
- ❑ Brittleness (osteoporosis)

Miscellaneous

- ❑ Easy exhaustion
- ❑ Easy bruising
- ❑ Irregular heartbeats
- ❑ Palpitations
- ❑ Fainting or headaches if you miss a meal
- ❑ Poor appetite
- ❑ Poor sense of taste or smell
- ❑ Many symptoms of overloaded liver (see page 22)

Tick the boxes in the list above if the symptom is persistent or quite noticeable.
Now add up the ticks and write the total in the box below.

Total score for nutritional deficiency and dietary imbalance symptoms

21

Part II: Symptoms of food intolerance

- ❑ Chronic fatigue or unexplained daytime drowsiness
- ❑ Head feels "foggy"
- ❑ Sudden bouts of unusual aggression or depression
- ❑ Skin rashes
- ❑ Frequent severe headaches
- ❑ Diarrhoea or severe constipation or both (alternating)
- ❑ Griping tummy pains with or without mucus discharge
- ❑ Painful or swollen joints
- ❑ Frequently congested sinuses
- ❑ Fluid retention
- ❑ Chronic catarrh
- ❑ Wheezing and breathing difficulties
- ❑ Dark colour under your eyes
- ❑ Symptoms of poor digestion and absorption, e.g. frequently bloated, uncomfortable tummy with much gas or much undigested food in stools

Tick the boxes in the list above if the symptom is persistent or quite noticeable. Now add up the ticks and write the total in the box below.

Total score for food intolerance symptoms

Part III: Symptoms of an overloaded liver

- ❑ Many nagging headaches
- ❑ Head often feels "foggy"
- ❑ Often slightly nauseous
- ❑ Skin problems
- ❑ Great lethargy
- ❑ Bad reactions to chemicals
- ❑ Yellowish skin or eyes
- ❑ Feeling unwell after coffee or small amount of alcohol
- ❑ Tenderness under right-hand ribs
- ❑ Many food intolerance symptoms
- ❑ Premenstrual mood changes
- ❑ Cysts and tumours of breast and uterus, fibroids, endometriosis
- ❑ Have you been diagnosed with multiple sclerosis, rheumatoid arthritis, lupus, Parkinson's disease or Alzheimer's?
- ❑ Have you ever abused drugs or alcohol?

Tick the boxes in the list above if the symptom is persistent or quite noticeable. Now add up the ticks and write the total in the box below.

Total score for overloaded liver symptoms

Nutritional deficiencies

Your symptom score suggests that you may suffer from nutritional deficiencies. In this chapter we will look at the many causes of nutritional deficiencies and how to get better nourished. We will also explain why food supplements are often used in nutritional therapy. Try to read all the explanations if you can, since understanding what you are doing helps to motivate you. But if you want to go straight to self-treatment, then it is possible to skip to the summary on page 41.

Nutritional deficiency problems are caused by any of the following:
- Faulty eating habits, i.e. not enough nutrient-rich foods
- Faulty digestion and absorption
- Faulty assimilation, i.e. there is enough of the nutrient in your blood, but it is not getting into the cells that need it.

So it makes sense that to reverse health problems caused by these, you need
- To ensure that you eat a healthy, nutrient-rich diet
- To ensure that you digest and absorb your food well
- If necessary, to use techniques which get more nutrients into your cells straight away.

What is a healthy diet?

Do you think you know the answer? If you've said "lots of fresh fruit and veg" then yes, you're getting the idea, but protein is also important, and essential polyunsaturated oils as found in nuts and seeds. Getting enough good quality calories, i.e. calories accompanied by the whole symphony of vitamins, minerals and other "micro-nutrients" that your body needs, is another priority. It's not always easy to get it right. A lot of product advertising is confusing and attempts to make some foods seem healthy when they may be the last thing you need. Comprehensive official advice is sadly lacking. Take a look at the picture on page 26. This is the ideal balanced, healthy diet. Then take a look at some of the recipes in Part V. They show you how these foods can be combined together to make delicious meals. There is much more to cooking vegetables than boiling them!

Later in this chapter we will also be looking at how to identify signs that you are not digesting, absorbing or assimilating your food properly. Step-by-step instructions for addressing these problems are also given.

The politics of food

There is no greater confusion in today's world than over what constitutes a good diet. But the truth is that as modern convenience food grows in popularity, our health as a nation is deteriorating. More heart disease, more cancers, more degenerative diseases, allergies, asthma, weaker immune systems. Not so long ago we considered measles a virtually harmless illness which most children would get as part of their development. Now our immune systems are so weak and undernourished that we are told measles is a terrible killer disease that all children must be vaccinated against or else banned from their doctor's surgery.

Nutritional therapists blame the misuse of science for many of today's ills. The convenience food industry—and its cronies who sit on Government committees— uses science to deliberately obstruct common sense. People who warn of the dangers of overconsuming its fatty, salty, over-processed and nutrient-depleted products are mockingly asked to provide "scientific proof". But the scientific proof is strangely never good enough to persuade the Government and the National Health Service to start telling people to cut down on these foods. A clever scientist can run rings around the advocates of healthy eating with arguments about what constitutes "proper" proof. To those in the know, it is a game. The media, who don't know the rules of the game, are often bamboozled and confused. Articles on the health benefits of wholefood eating and vitamin supplements are relegated to women's pages and light magazines, not published as serious medical articles.

The food industry is extremely powerful and influential in government circles, universities where dieticians are trained, hospitals and research institutions. Like the drug industry, it gives research grants to encourage institutions not to do or say anything which it might disagree with—otherwise the grants may be taken away and people put out of work. Its employees can gain influential positions within these institutions. Leading "experts" who are not widely known to be in the industry's pay may be trotted out from time to time to make high-profile comments about particular products; for instance "Crisps are a highly nutritious food". Believe it or not, because fat is a nutrient, any food high in fat can scientifically be described as highly nutritious even if the words mean something entirely different to the average lay person. The "expert" simply leaves out the fact that the nutrient he/she is referring to is fat, and the press avidly take notes and write articles extolling the nutritional value of crisps. You in turn are relieved to be told that it is ok to go on eating exactly what you're eating.

It works the other way too. If a nutrition professor is being paid by a company which makes junk breakfast cereals, he can announce that eating muesli is unhealthy. Once again the media will jump on his words and treat them as pearls of wisdom because of his rank and position. Sales of junk cereals will quickly rise.

The food industry also distributes promotional literature to doctors' surgeries in the guise of health advice. When I worked for a GP I was surrounded with stacks of "patients' advice" leaflets that had never been ordered nor asked for, urging people to eat butter and meat. Naturally the sole purpose of these leaflets was to give these foods a healthier image after cholesterol and BSE scare stories in the media had damaged sales. Most people will believe that if they obtained a leaflet from a doctor's surgery then the leaflet is equivalent to a doctor's advice.

The spina bifida story

Allowing the food industry's interests to dictate health policy can have tragic consequences. In the early 1980s research was carried out by Professor Richard Smithells in the UK into the role of vitamin deficiencies in spina bifida and other birth defects known as neural tube defects, where the baby's brain and nervous system do not develop properly[3]. This leads to deformity or major disability such as total absence of the skull, defective brain development or absence of the brain and spinal cord, resulting in death. This research showed a clear link between spina bifida and a deficiency of the B vitamin known as folic acid or folate. But when the research was published, no announcement was made by the UK government that all women anticipating pregnancy should ensure an adequate intake of folic acid from green vegetables and orange juice. Doctors were not instructed to give this advice. What did the Government do instead? It stopped setting a Recommended Daily Allowance (RDA) for folic acid. The RDA (now known as an RNI) was normally set for nutrients that the Government wanted to publicize as being at risk of deficiency[270]. This is a clear example of how organized medicine, industry and government work together to marginalize any research which does not suit them. It is only the tip of the iceberg.

Ten years and many more trials later the Government's Chief Medical Officer was finally forced to admit that the British diet causes serious birth defects—he advised that all pregnant women and those planning to conceive should take supplements[4]. Now, these supplements and advice on food sources of folic acid are available to all pregnant women.

In the mid 1970s, before spina bifida was routinely detected during pregnancy and women offered abortions, the rate of spina bifida was one in 100 births in Scotland, Wales and Ireland[270]. Thousands of cases occurred in the ten years between Professor Smithells' research and the change in government policy. Most of these cases could have been prevented if the Government had applied the precautionary principle. The precautionary principle is used to make quick decisions when important public health issues are at stake. For instance, if there was a suspected danger that one in 100 babies might die from a particular additive used in baby food, that additive would be instantly withdrawn as a *precaution*,

The Healthy Plate

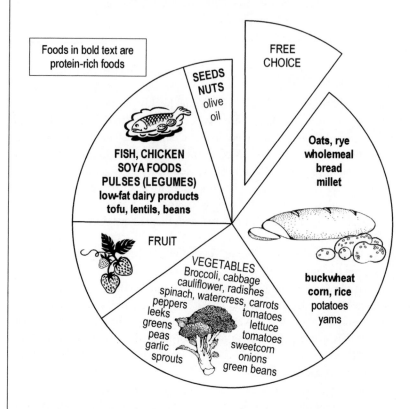

Foods in bold text are
protein-rich foods

FREE
CHOICE

SEEDS
NUTS
olive
oil

Oats, rye
wholemeal
bread
millet

**FISH, CHICKEN
SOYA FOODS
PULSES (LEGUMES)**
low-fat dairy products
tofu, lentils, beans

FRUIT

VEGETABLES
Broccoli, cabbage
cauliflower, radishes
spinach, watercress, carrots
peppers
leeks   tomatoes
greens   lettuce
peas   tomatoes
garlic   sweetcorn
sprouts   onions
        green beans

**buckwheat
corn, rice**
potatoes
yams

Imagine the chart above is a picture of a plate containing the ideal proportions for a day's menu. The nearer you can get to this ideal, the better your body will be able to perform for you. After all, if you don't give a car the right fuel, it will break down eventually. Your body has more anti-breakdown features than your car does, but it can't cope forever with a faulty diet!

Think of these proportions as something to aim for over a period of time. The chart is also a useful yardstick which you can refer to over and over again since a lot of published health advice can be quite confusing. The recipes in this book follow these healthy plate principles, and give ideas for all meals as well as drinks and snacks. They show you how to incorporate items like sunflower and sesame seeds into your cookery with delicious results.

The *Free Choice* segment means that 10 per cent of your food can be anything else that is not on the chart.

If you are a vegetarian, you should ensure a daily consumption of the plant foods shown in bold text rather than relying too much on dairy products for your protein.

The proportions in this chart are based on the advice of the World Health Organization as well as on results of research carried out into the prevention of major diseases.

even if there was as yet no absolute proof. Any medical or governmental system which does not apply the same principle to nutrition is basically corrupt.

You can be absolutely sure that spina bifida is not the only disease caused by the British national diet. It is just a disease which is relatively easy to trace to a nutritional deficiency using current research methods.

The point of all this political information is to show you how widespread nutritional deficiencies are, even in civilized western countries where we are surrounded by plenty. Also to make it clear that there is too much at stake for the authorities even to admit this, let alone do very much about it. It really is time for us all to stop being complacent about what we eat and start protecting our own health in the best way we know how, making use of the knowledge gained from *all* published research, whether it is being ignored by the establishment or not. Of course everyone has a grandfather who smoked and drank himself silly, ate a really bad diet and died happy and healthy at 95. But can you guarantee that you will be like him? Or will you be one of the vast majority whose senior years are ruined by poor health, pain and disability? Don't be daunted—it's never too late to start putting things right.

The foods that protect your health

On the opposite page you will find a picture of a "Healthy Plate". The proportions are based on advice published by the World Health Organization and also on the results of research carried out into the prevention of cancer and heart disease. Hundreds of research studies now show that the more fruit and vegetables, whole grains, fish and fresh nuts and olive oil we consume in preference to other foods, the better our protection against major killer diseases. People who consume the least fruits and vegetables can have more than double the risk of contracting heart disease or cancer in later life. The protection given by a good diet is very significant indeed. Scientists believe that this is because fruits and vegetables are rich in many different types of antioxidants—chemicals which help to neutralize the toxic substances that can start off a cancer. The more brightly-coloured the fruit or vegetable—e.g. bright purple, orange, red or green—the better its protection, since it is the coloured parts which are the most rich in antioxidants.

Plant whole-foods are also rich in B vitamins, especially folic acid. Only in the last few years have scientists discovered it is not just unborn babies who suffer if they lack folic acid. Adults with this particular vitamin deficiency can develop high levels of a toxin known as homocysteine, which accelerates the build-up of cholesterol deposits on your artery walls, causing high blood pressure and heart disease. We also know that the brittle bone disease (osteoporosis) which affects elderly people also seems to be greatly accelerated when homocysteine levels are high.

So don't just eat wholemeal bread and greens to "keep you regular" - eat them to help protect your heart and your bones. Now is the best time to start! In this book you will find more than 100 recipes to help you learn how to make delicious meals and snacks quickly and easily from the healthiest foods.

Improving your digestion and absorption

Nutritional therapists frequently come across people who eat a good diet but still have some of the nutritional deficiency symptoms listed on page 21. This is because they are not digesting and absorbing their food properly. If your digestion is weak, you probably suffer from a lot of intestinal gas, bloating and discomfort. You may even have reported these problems to your doctor and received medicines for an "irritable bowel". Your bowel is indeed being irritated—by undigested food and by the unhealthy internal environment which a poor digestion creates.

Rule No. 1: Relax while eating

Today's "hurry and worry" lifestyle is responsible for much poor health. Because good digestion begins with good relaxation, stress can have a profound effect on your ability to digest and absorb your food. In short, severe stress switches off your production of stomach acid and other digestive juices, and reduces the activity of the nerves and muscles which help with your digestive processes.

Your body's nervous system can operate in either of two modes, known as sympathetic and parasympathetic. (These have nothing to do with sympathy in the usual sense of the word.) Stress switches off your parasympathetic mode—the one which allows your digestive processes to take place—and switches on your sympathetic nervous system, which shifts energy from your digestive organs to your arms, legs and brain, ready for fighting a battle or a threat, or running away from it.

So you can imagine what happens if you never really manage to relax while you are eating. The energy you need to digest your food is not in the right place, your organs of digestion are not being properly stimulated, and your digestive juices do not flow as they should. The result? A weakened digestion. Instead of being properly broken down into individual nutrients and absorbed through the wall of your intestine into your bloodstream, some of your food will pass down your intestines in a partly undigested state. These undigested particles can be seized and fermented by resident bacteria in your lower intestine, producing gas. People who suffer from chronic intestinal flatulence invariably have a poor ability to digest and/or absorb their food.

People who are not relaxed while eating usually also eat too fast and do not chew their food properly. You don't have to chew each mouthful 100 times, but you should make sure that the contents of your mouth are reduced to pulp and thoroughly mixed with saliva before swallowing them. This also reduces the chances of food remaining incompletely digested and absorbed. And don't use water (or other liquids) to "wash down" food. You will digest better if you drink between meals rather than during them.

Drinking tea and coffee within an hour of a meal is especially harmful to mineral absorption. Substances in these beverages combine with iron, zinc and other minerals, resulting in more than 90 per cent passing through without being absorbed[5]. Drink chamomile tea instead. This has a relaxing effect and helps to promote good digestion. It can be mixed with peppermint tea which, as you will see, is very beneficial for your intestines. Herbal teas too can reduce mineral absorption, but this is unavoidable when they are needed for their therapeutic effect.

Stomach acidity

Learning to relax while eating may be all that you need to improve your digestion and absorption. But sometimes a person's digestion seems to be more seriously damaged. In these cases, people report that their food feels as if it "lies like a stone" in their tummy after a meal. These people can physically feel the lack of digestion.

In these cases, the problem is usually one of stomach acid deficiency. Hydrochloric acid (HCl) in your stomach has the unique task of stimulating the rest of your digestive processes. Enzymes from your pancreas, which do most of the work of digestion, are triggered by this acid. So a lack of acid can have quite serious consequences.

Dr Jonathan Wright, an American medical practitioner who specializes in nutritional treatments, says that patients with low stomach acidity (the problem is technically known as hypochlorhydria) usually report the following symptoms:

- "Gassiness", and bloating, belching or burning soon after meals
- A feeling that food just sits in the stomach, not digesting
- Inability to eat more than a small amount of food without feeling full
- Constipation, but sometimes diarrhoea
- Weak, easily broken, peeling fingernails
- Dilated small blood vessels in the cheeks and on the nose (in non-alcoholics).

Dr Wright uses several laboratory tests to confirm his diagnosis. Because stomach acid is important for the absorption of minerals, he first analyzes mineral levels in a hair sample taken from his patient. If six or more minerals (excluding sodium and potassium) are found to be low, then there is likely to be a mineral absorption problem. Stool specimens can also be analyzed. Individuals with low stomach acidity usually have an excess of undigested meat fibres in their stool, as well as abnormally high levels of resident bacteria, yeasts and fungi in their intestines. One of the most important tasks of stomach acid is to act as a disinfectant in the stomach—destroying bacteria and parasites ingested with your food. People who lack stomach acid often belch a great deal because their stomach is no longer sterile and bacteria can ferment its contents, producing gas.

Acne rosacea, where spots form across the cheeks and nose, together with much facial flushing, can also be a sign of low stomach acidity, and can clear up when hydrochloric acid supplements are administered[6,7]. Conventional treatment with antibiotics will of course kill harmful bacteria in the digestive system just as stomach acidity does, and this may be why antibiotics can temporarily clear the condition. The acne may return with a vengeance as soon as the drugs are stopped because the gut bacteria will simply return again. But if low stomach acidity is treated, the body can in time become well-nourished enough to produce its own acid, thus preventing the problem.

In time, people with a stomach acid deficiency can also have difficulty with absorbing vitamin B_{12}. When the cells lining your stomach slow down or stop secreting hydrochloric acid, then the production of intrinsic factor—a substance needed for vitamin B_{12} absorption—can also slow down[8]. We only need tiny amounts of vitamin B_{12}, but if we do not get them, we can develop nerve damage with symptoms such as unsteadiness, burning feet, fatigue and confusion. These symptoms are common in elderly people.

If your symptoms suggest a lack of stomach acid, there are two ways to treat this. The most natural way is to use herbs and spices which stimulate your stomach to produce more acid. Ginger, used in cookery or made into a tea to drink with meals, is an excellent digestive aid and stomach acid stimulant. A few drops of tincture of the bitter herb gentian mixed into a little water and sipped 20 minutes before a meal will also help to stimulate the digestive juices. Many Indian spices aid the digestion and reduce flatulence, including cardamom, cinnamon and cloves. You can also buy commercial preparations of "digestive bitters" from health food shops. To use them, just follow the directions on the label.

If your HCl deficiency symptoms persist in spite of these measures, you can also take supplements known as "HCl plus pepsin". These are pills or capsules of hydrochloric acid and so are potentially corrosive if incorrectly used. You must read and follow the manufacturer's instructions on the product label, and do not exceed the maximum dose. HCl should only be taken with meals. If the HCl gives you any uncomfortable sensations, simply reduce the dose.

You should not need to take HCl supplements for more than about six months, because as your digestion improves you will become generally better nourished, allowing your stomach to recover its ability to produce HCl.

One final word on stomach acidity: some people with arthritis swear that drinking a couple of teaspoons of organic cider vinegar in a small glass of water with meals is a highly effective treatment. This may be because their digestion is improved by consuming a little acid with their meals. But you should note that on the other hand there are also people with arthritis who are sensitive to acidic foods such as fruit juice, and find that these foods aggravate their symptoms.

Arthritis is of course a problem mostly associated with people over 70. But it's not necessarily caused by old age. Medical research shows that up to one third of elderly people do not produce enough stomach acid to absorb all their food and keep their stomach free of bacteria and parasites[9]. Stomach acid production often begins to decline in middle age, but like many problems that we normally associate with ageing, it may be more to do with our diet and lifestyle than with ageing itself.

Pancreatic enzymes and bile

As food leaves your stomach, the acidity triggers the release of juices from your pancreas and liver. Pancreatic juice is alkaline. It neutralizes the acidity of food coming from your stomach. It is rich in enzymes which break down fats, carbohydrates and protein in your food, rendering them into individual components tiny enough to be absorbed through the wall of your intestine into your bloodstream on the other side. These individual components are:

- Amino acids
- Fatty acids and triglycerides
- Simple sugars: glucose, fructose and galactose

At the same time your gall-bladder releases bile. This is an extremely bitter substance produced by your liver. It has three main tasks:

- To emulsify fats into tiny micro-droplets which your pancreatic enzymes can break down more easily
- To destroy harmful bacteria and parasites in your small intestine
- To act as a vehicle for waste matter produced by your liver, carrying it into your intestines so that it can be evacuated in your stools.

If you still suffer from excessive intestinal flatulence after following the advice on stomach acidity in the previous section, you may be overloading your digestive system with too much food—a very common mistake. If you know that you have a weak digestion, you should *never* eat until you are hungry, and you should never feel completely "full" at the end of a meal. Instead, stop eating when you are two-thirds full as this will place much less stress on your pancreas.

If you still suffer from poor digestion even after these measures, you may need to take pancreatic enzyme supplements for a while. These are available from health food shops and by mail order, and you should follow the directions on the product label. I recommend products based on bromelain. This is a plant extract derived from pineapple stems, used as an aid to protein digestion. In clinical trials, bromelain has been found to have many benefits, including anti-inflammatory action and the ability to break down mucus[10].

You can stimulate the release of bile by consuming foods and herbs known as *cholagogues*. These are:

- Dandelion coffee
- Peppermint tea (taken double-strength)
- Radishes and radish juice
- Turmeric
- Artichoke leaf (available as herbal preparations)
- Milk thistle or its extract silymarin

Gentian, taken as described in the previous section on stomach acidity, also stimulates bile flow. If you do not produce enough bile, fat and oil can end up coating all the food in your intestines, making it difficult for digestive enzymes to act on it. So a lack of bile can result not just in poor digestion of fats, but poor digestion generally.

The Hay Diet, also known as "food combining", can be useful for people with weak pancreatic juices. In simple terms, it avoids the consumption of high-protein and high-carbohydrate foods (especially bread) at the same meal. These foods require different sets of enzymes for their digestion, which is thought to increase the pancreas' workload. The Hay Diet is not for everyone, but if you feel any digestive discomfort after eating, or suffer unduly from gas, then you may find it useful to eat protein and carbohydrate foods at separate times. The Hay Diet also advocates consuming fruit on its own, since this is digested more rapidly than other foods and may begin fermenting if delayed in the digestive tract by being mixed with them.

Absorbing nutrients

Poor digestion causes bloating, wind and discomfort because:

- Undigested food in the lower part of the digestive system is fermented by gas-producing bacteria, which thrive on this food and multiply.
- Undigested food and excessive undesirable bacteria in the lower part of the digestive system are very irritating to your gut wall (the wall of your intestine) and can make its tissues inflamed and swollen.

Inflammation in your gut wall can damage delicate structures located there, especially:

- The mechanisms which allow nutrients through your gut wall to your bloodstream on the other side,
- The barrier which normally prevents undigested particles, bacteria and toxins from passing through your gut wall into your blood,
- The cells in your gut wall which produce digestive enzymes.

Starches and complex sugars like sucrose and lactose are not fully broken down by enzymes from your pancreas. For the last stage of their digestion they need additional enzymes (known as disaccharidases) to convert them to simple sugars. These special enzymes are produced by your gut wall. Unfortunately an inflamed gut has difficulty with this task, and these carbohydrates can simply end up as food for irritating bacteria and fungi.

Clearly it is important to reduce inflammation. Improving your digestion helps because it reduces the population of irritating bacteria and fungi. These starve when your digestion is good, because they can only thrive on undigested food.

The next step is to reduce their numbers even more with natural anti-microbials such as:

- Raw garlic and onions
- Extra-virgin olive oil
- Peppermint tea (taken double-strength)
- Spices: cinnamon, cloves, cardamom, cayenne pepper, asafoetida
- Citrus seed extract
- Golden seal (do not take when pregnant)
- Oregano oil
- Artemisia annua

I would recommend consuming all of these every day for about six weeks. The last four items should be bought as commercial products and taken in accordance with the manufacturer's instructions.

Next you will need to replace the beneficial bacteria which normally ensure that the undesirables do not thrive. This is done by taking supplements of probiotics and prebiotics. These are, respectively, Acidophilus and Bifidus bacteria, and special sugars known as fructo-oligosaccharides (FOS) which these friendly bacteria feed and thrive on. You should use only guaranteed probiotics. Some cheaper products do not contain much live Acidophilus. Others do not contain the right strains which can survive the acid environment of the stomach. Even live yoghurt may do little good for this reason.

Now is also the time to consume foods and products which will help your damaged gut to heal. These include:

- Comfrey tea
- Slippery elm tea

- Liquorice tea
- Fresh cabbage juice
- Supplements of butyric acid and n-acetyl glucosamine (NAG).

Symptoms of inflammation in your intestines can also be aggravated by food intolerances. Later on you will learn how to test yourself for food intolerances so that you can stop eating any problem foods. This will also help to heal your intestines.

Assimilation

Once the nutrients in your intestines have been absorbed into your blood, they will be transported all round your body and delivered to the cells which need them. A cell is the smallest living unit in your body. Each cell is like a tiny plant which has a separate life of its own and absorbs water, oxygen and liquid feed. Specialized cells form different types of body tissues such as skin, bone, brain, liver or kidney.

Sometimes the outer wall of your cells, known as the cell membrane, can simply "soak up" the substances it needs. This is known as passive diffusion. But more often it uses tiny mechanisms like special pumps and receptors on its surface. If there is something wrong with these mechanisms, a cell can develop a nutritional deficiency—problems with assimilating a vitamin or mineral even if that nutrient is in plentiful supply in the surrounding blood.

Another potential problem with assimilation is fluid retention. If too much fluid passes out of your blood and stays in the spaces between cells, nutrients can become too diluted and once again the cells will not be properly nourished.

Fluid retention can be treated by looking for and eliminating its causes. Some of these include

- Food intolerances
- Eating too much salt or sugar and too little protein
- A lack of B vitamins and magnesium
- A lack of flavonoids from fresh fruit and vegetables
- Too little exercise

There is a vicious circle involved in assimilation problems. Nutritional deficiencies themselves can actually damage the mechanisms of assimilation.

When assimilation becomes so poor that a cell can only absorb normal amounts of a vitamin if flooded with a concentration hundreds of times higher than normal, an individual is said to have a vitamin resistance or a vitamin dependency.

The *Merck Manual*, which is a standard medical textbook for doctors, describes a vitamin dependency as *a genetic defect in the metabolism of the vitamin... In some instances, vitamin doses as high as 1000 times the recommended dietary allowance (RDA) improve the function of the altered metabolic pathway.*

Vitamin dependency is recognized for most of the B vitamins as well as vitamin D. The diagnosis is confirmed by measuring enzymes which depend on a particular vitamin. These measurements are made both before and after administering a megadose of that vitamin—for instance 200 to 600 mg per day of vitamin B_6. Any individual who needs megadoses to normalize their enzyme levels can be said to have a vitamin (or mineral) dependency.

Doctors who routinely test all their patients for defects in vitamin metabolism are finding that this condition is becoming very common indeed. Let's take a look at some of the research.

Research from the Department of Neurology, University of Southern California, Los Angeles, USA, 1990

Patients suffering from a variety of problems including depression, dementia, neuropathy and seizures, but with normal levels of vitamins in their blood were tested and then given a trial of B_{12} therapy. The improvements in their condition led the researchers to conclude that damage to the nervous system due to an extra high demand for vitamin B_{12} is common[11].

Research reported in the journal Annals of Allergy, 1975

A double-blind study was carried out in which 76 asthmatic children were given 100 mg of vitamin B_6 supplementation per day. This is 50 times the adult RDA. Their asthma symptoms significantly improved and they were able to reduce their use of conventional medications. Supplementing with half this dose of vitamin B_6 (50 mg per day, or 25 times the RDA) was not effective[12].

Research from the University of Southampton Medical School, UK, 1991

Chronic fatigue patients were found to have low levels of magnesium in their red blood cells. After treatment with intramuscular injections of magnesium their red cell magnesium levels became normal and at the same time their energy levels improved[13].

Research from the Department of Medicine, Columbia University College of Physicians and Surgeons, New York, USA, 1984

Vitamin B_6 levels were measured in the blood plasma of 16 people suffering from sickle cell anaemia, an inherited incurable disease in which sufferers have very fragile red blood cells. The levels were found to be very low compared with normal people, so supplements of 100 mg vitamin B_6 per day were administered. This resulted in an increase in both haemoglobin levels and in the number of red blood cells[14].

Research reported in the Journal of Nutritional Medicine, 1991

The bone density of postmenopausal women given both dietary advice and nutritional supplements (with special emphasis on magnesium) was measured.

Supplementation for poor assimilators

Nutrient	RNI*	Deficiency symptoms	Dose per day
Vitamin A (retinol)	700 mcg (2300 iu)	Abnormally poor vision in bad light. Spotty skin (acne). Frequent colds or infections. Dry, scaly skin. Persistent Itching inside ears.	7,500 iu Do not exceed this dose if pregnant.
Vitamin B₁ (thiamine)	1.0 mg	Depression, irritability, fatigue, insomnia, muscle weakness. Burning and tingling in toes and soles.	25-50 mg as part of B complex
Vitamin B₂ (riboflavin)	1.3 mg	Bloodshot, burning, "gritty" eyes. Cracks and sores in corners of mouth. Dry, cracked, peeling lips. Eyes sensitive to light. Sides of nose red, greasy, scaly. Soreness and burning of lips and tongue.	25-50 mg as part of B complex
Vitamin B₃ (niacin)	18 mg	Depression, dermatitis, fatigue, insomnia, irritability, loss of appetite, muscle weakness, red swollen tongue, psychiatric problems.	50-100 mg as part of B complex
Vitamin B₅ (pantothenic acid)	7 mg	Burning on soles of feet. Depression, fatigue, loss of appetite, poor muscle co-ordination, weakness, "wind pains" in intestines.	50-100 mg as part of B complex
Vitamin B₆ (pyridoxine)	1.5 mg	Anaemia, convulsions or fits, inability to remember dreams, insomnia, irritability, kidney stones, morning sickness of pregnancy, nervousness, premenstrual symptoms. Red scaly patches at side of nose and corner of mouth. Skin rashes, especially on forehead.	25-50 mg as part of B complex. Best also taken with magnesium to help assimilation.
Vitamin B₁₂ (cobalamin)	1.5 mcg	Agitation, anaemia, disorientation, confusion, unsteadiness, mental derioration, fatigue, psychiatric problems. Increased risk of heart disease due to homocysteine levels rising. Loss of sensation in feet and legs. Sore, smooth tongue.	50-100 mcg. In severe cases, injections may be needed.
Folic acid	200 mcg	Anaemia, poor appetite, apathy, birth defects, habitual miscarriage, breathlessness, constipation, fatigue, im-paired growth in children, insomnia, memory impairment, mental confusion, paranoid delusions, reduced immunity, sore tongue, weakness. Increased cancer risk. Increased heart disease risk due to homocysteine levels rising.	400-800 mcg as part of B complex
Vitamin C (ascorbic acid)	40 mg	Bleeding gums or loose teeth. Easy bruising and fragile blood vessels. Fatigue, frequent infections.	500-2,000 mg
Vitamin D (calciferol)	5 mcg (200 iu)	Osteoporosis (brittle bones) or osteomalacia (soft bones) in adults. Rickets (knee pain, bowed legs) and poor growth in children. Bone pain and tenderness. Weakness of some muscles (e.g. in climbing stairs). Waddling gait, deafness.	200 iu
Vitamin E (tocopherol)	10 mg (15 iu)	Age spots, cataracts, damage to cell membranes, fragility of red blood cells, infertility, muscle weakness, neuro-muscular damage. Possibly auto-immune diseases. Increased risk of cancers and heart disease.	50-200 iu

Nutrient	RNI	Deficiency symptoms	Supplement
Calcium	700 mg	Loss of bone density. Softening of bones. Loss of muscle tone. Muscle cramps or spasms.	200-500 mg
Chromium	25 mcg	Adult-onset diabetes[18], atherosclerosis, high cholesterol, muscle weakness, hypoglycaemia (symptoms include fatigue, dizziness, mood swings and fainting when meals are missed).	50-100 mcg§
Copper	1.2 mg	Anaemia (see Iron below), broken blood vessels, sensitivity to cold. Low blood pressure. Nerve damage.	1-2 mg
Iodine	140 mcg	Enlarged thyroid, hypothyroidism. Raised oestrogen levels[19], leading to breast problems (lumps or tumours) and fibroids. Sometimes hearing loss[20].	100-200 mcg (from kelp tablets)
Iron	Women 14.8 mg Men 8.7 mg	Anaemia (weakness, anorexia, depression, confusion, dizziness, easily tired, pale, breathless, palpitations, constipation). Impaired growth and school performance in children[21]. Sometimes hearing loss[22].	10-15 mg
Magnesium	300 mg	Poor detoxification, chronic fatigue, muscle pains, swallowing problem, flickering eyelids, facial tics, jerks and spasms, insomnia, irregular heartbeat, adult-onset diabetes, hyperinsulinaemia (hypoglycaemia), kidney stones, loss of bone density, muscle weakness and tremors, high blood pressure, nervousness and anxiety due to increased release of stress hormones[23], sensitivity to noise, PMS, poor circulation.	100-300 mg Vitamin B_6 deficiency can reduce the assimilation of magnesium
Manganese	1.4 mg	Brittle bones, dermatitis, heavy menstrual periods, blood sugar problems, deterioration of cartilage.	2-5 mg
Molybdenum	50-400 mcg	Aggravation of asthma. Dislocation of eye lens. Gouty arthritis. Poor detoxification.	100-200 mcg
Selenium	75 mcg	Pale fingernail beds. Poor digestion due to pancreas insufficiency. Poor detoxification. Reduced male fertility. Reduced kidney function[24]. Cataracts, cancerous changes, heart disease. Increased susceptibility to viruses[25].	100-200 mcg
Zinc	9.5 mg	Abnormal hair loss, acne, poor appetite, poor taste and smell, reduced male fertility[26,27], poor growth in children, white spots on fingernails. Anaemia.	10-15 mg
Essential fatty acids GLA and EPA		Dry skin, rash, thirst, frequent urination, fatigue, PMS, painful menstruation, schizophrenia, chronic inflammation, arthritis, coldness. Children's problems: hyperactivity, learning difficulties, retarded growth[28,29,30]. To supplement: GLA take 500 mg per day oil of evening primrose, blackcurrant seed or starflower (borage); EPA take 500 mg per day of fish oil. Eating oily fish (sardines etc.) yields more EPA than supplements.	

*Reference Nutrient Intake. Equivalent to the former Recommended Daily Allowance. Where no RNI exists, the estimated daily requirement is given instead. Failing this (for example in the case of vitamin D) American figures have been used instead of British.

§Values given for minerals are elemental. This refers to the amount of the mineral itself rather than the compound. For instance 50 mg zinc citrate yields about 17 mg elemental zinc.

Supplements were found to be 16 times more effective at improving their bone density than dietary advice alone[15].

Research from the U.S. Department of Agriculture, Beltsville Human Nutrition Research Center, USA, 1993

15 research studies were examined, in which chromium supplements were administered to people with impaired glucose tolerance—a condition found in type II diabetes and incipient diabetes, where cells have a reduced ability to use insulin. 12 of these studies showed that chromium supplements improved the efficiency of insulin[16].

Research reported in the Journal of Clinical Psychiatry, 1979

Vitamin B_1-dependent enzymes were measured in 42 non-alcoholic psychiatric patients. 16 of them still had a cellular deficiency of vitamin B_1 despite having received supplements containing the vitamin for up to six weeks before testing[17].

There exist thousands more research studies using nutritional supplements to combat illness. Unfortunately most of these test neither blood levels nor nutrient-dependent enzymes before supplementation. This is a faulty procedure. If blood levels are normal but enzyme levels are low, this is a clear indication that any beneficial effects of supplementation are probably due to treating an assimilation problem. This would explain why some people respond so well to supplementation and others do not.

If you have several symptoms of nutritional deficiency despite eating an average or better-than-average diet, it is likely that you are suffering from poor assimilation and may need vitamin or mineral supplements. Take a look at the table on pages 36-37, which highlights some of the symptoms of individual deficiencies and suggests a dosage range for supplements to correct these.

Can't I just eat more of a particular food?

A lot of people ask whether they need to take supplements or whether they could just eat more of a particular food to get extra B vitamins, zinc and so on. Of course you can do this if you are eating a less than ideal diet. Eating more of all the most nutrient-rich foods is an important part of nutritional therapy.

But if your problem is poor assimilation you will temporarily need higher amounts of certain nutrients than nature can provide in food. This is because at present you may only be capable of assimilating five per cent of the total vitamin B_6 (for example) which is in your blood at any one given time. So to get your recommended daily amount of 1.5 mg of vitamin B_6, you would have to consume 30 mg, which is a virtually impossible amount to get from food.

Supplementation need not be permanent. Once your cells are properly nourished they can start to repair themselves. This means also repairing their ability to absorb nutrients from your blood. So in time your assimilation should improve and you can stop taking supplements. As you will see in the next section, you should allow plenty of time for this.

What causes poor assimilation?

Dr Abram Hoffer is a psychiatrist practising in Canada, who began using nutritional medicine to treat mental illness in the 1950s. These were the days when there were few useful drugs to control the ravaging symptoms of schizophrenia, and all doctors were interested in what nutrition could do.

Dr Hoffer has written many books about his work, and one of his cases illustrates very clearly how poor assimilation of nutrients can develop. This was the case of George Porteous—one of the Hong Kong veterans, Canadian soldiers who had sailed to Hong Kong in 1940 during World War II, were captured by the Japanese and survived 44 months in Japanese prisoner-of-war camps. Twenty-five per cent of the Canadian soldiers died in these camps. They suffered from starvation and severe malnutrition as well as brutality from the guards.

Porteous, a fit physical education instructor, survived and returned home having lost one third of his body weight. On the way home in a hospital ship the soldiers were given nourishing food and extra vitamins in the form of rice polishings. George recovered only partially. He suffered from both psychological and physical symptoms. He was anxious, fearful and slightly paranoid. In a room he had to sit facing the door. He had severe arthritis and could not raise his arms above his shoulders. He needed his wife's help in getting out of bed and to get started for the day. He needed barbiturates in the evening to help him sleep and amphetamines in the morning to help him wake up. He was very sensitive to both heat and cold.

In 1960, Porteous was director of a sheltered home for the elderly, and met Dr Hoffer who wanted to conduct research into the effects of vitamin B_3 megadoses on the people in the home. Porteous first took the supplements himself—1,000 mg after each meal. Within two weeks Porteous could lift his arms normally again, and was free of all his symptoms—every single one. Except for one brief episode in 1962 when he went on a holiday and forgot to take his vitamin B_3 with him, Porteous remained well until his death when he was Lieutenant Governor of Saskatchewan. Dr Hoffer has now treated over 20 ex-prisoners from Japanese camps and European concentration camps with equally good results[31].

Can medical history provide a clue?

Dr Hoffer is also famous for stating that there is no difference between the symptoms of schizophrenia and pellagra, the textbook vitamin B_3 deficiency disease. During the height of pellagra in the United States in the early 20th century, one third of all psychiatric hospital inmates were pellagra sufferers. A 1910 textbook of psychiatry offered only four diagnoses of mental illness: dementia praecox (now schizophrenia), tertiary syphilis, pellagra and scurvy. In the southern United States, where pellagra was rife, hospitals had to try to distinguish whether their patients had pellagra or schizophrenia—a difficult task because the patients have the same symptoms: the same hallucinations, the same delusions and the same skin discolouration. The diagnosis was made by administering vitamin B_3. Those who recovered in a few days were diagnosed with pellagra. Those who did not were labelled with schizophrenia.

"This effectively denied pellagra sufferers the right to recover slowly", comments Dr Hoffer. He says that there are two types of pellagra; one corrected by diet alone, and the other requiring 600 mg a day or more due to a B_3 dependency. This is 30 times the amount found in a normal diet, so few doctors ever thought of giving mental patients vitamin B_3 in that amount. "Many people labelled with schizophrenia would recover if their vitamin B_3 needs were recognized" says Dr Hoffer[32].

So what does this teach us? Dr Hoffer says there is no doubt that every human exposed to stress and malnutrition for a long enough period of time can develop a vitamin dependency. While his own cases are extreme, we should not forget that one in every 100 births in England and Wales in the 1970s was a victim of spina bifida, caused by a B vitamin deficiency. Malnutrition is not restricted to World War II prisoners or to 1930's America. Many of today's children eat no fresh vegetables at all, and live on little more than burgers, chips and sweets. Many people have gut inflammation and intestinal absorption problems. If Dr Hoffer is right that vitamin dependencies are caused by malnutrition, then we could be justified in reasoning that when only high-dose supplements seem to reverse deficiency symptoms, the individuals in question may have suffered from malnutrition at some point in their lives—perhaps even before birth[239-241]. Supplements raise the concentration of nutrients around cells and so help them to absorb more.

Food supplements are consumed by over 30 per cent of the British population[271]. We are talking about very large numbers of people who experience benefits from these products. If medical decision-makers do not stop trying to marginalize such issues then they will continue to waste billions of pounds of our money.

How to treat nutritional deficiencies

Step	Assessment	Instructions
1	Compare your diet with the chart on page 26. How well are you doing?	Use the recipes in this book to help you make positive changes. After one month reassess your nutritional deficiency score using the questionnaire on page 21.
2	Is your score now below 3?	Keep up the good work—that's all you need!
3	Score still 3 or more? Any maldigestion symptoms (much gas, bloating, discomfort)? Score still 3 or more but no maldigestion symptoms? Proceed to step 7.	Do not eat unless you are hungry. Do not overload your stomach. Relax while eating. Avoid stress. Eat slowly. Chew properly. Don't drink with or soon after meals except a little chamomile and peppermint tea to aid your digestion. Don't drink tea or coffee near mealtimes. If your food intolerance score was 2 or more, proceed with food intolerance testing as described in the next chapter.
4	Intestinal flatulence and bloating persist?	Your pancreas may be under stress. Bromelain and/or pancreatic enzymes may help. Take as directed on the product label. To stimulate bile flow, drink dandelion coffee and peppermint tea. Use turmeric in cooking. Take artichoke leaf and milk thistle supplements.
5	Food lies like a stone? Can't eat more than a small amount without feeling full? Constant burping? Constipation (sometimes diarrhoea)? Peeling fingernails? Dilated blood vessels on cheeks and nose? Acne rosacea?	Sip a few drops of tincture of gentian or digestive bitters in a little water 20 minutes before meals. Use ginger and cayenne pepper in cooking. Reduce flatulence with tea after meals made from ground cinnamon and cloves. If these symptoms persist, take HCl pepsin supplements as directed on the product label.
6	If gas and bloating persist, especially if there is also fatigue and nagging headaches, you may have intestinal inflammation due to dysbiosis. Here is an extract in summary form from the intestinal healing programme on page 50. If you have nutritional deficiencies combined with maldigestion and food allergy symptoms, then follow that programme in full.	(1) Follow anti-microbial treatment for 6 weeks: raw garlic and onions, extra virgin olive oil, peppermint tea double strength, cardamom, cayenne, cloves, asafoetida (Indian spice). Take supplements of citrus seed extract, golden seal (not if pregnant), oregano oil, Artemisia annua. (2) Follow bacterial replacement programme for two weeks: supplements of acid-resistant Acidophilus and Bifidus, fructo-oligosaccharides (FOS). 3) Gut wall healing programme for two weeks: comfrey tea, slippery elm tea, liquorice tea, fresh cabbage juice. Supplements of butyric acid and N-acetyl glucosamine (NAG).
7	If your nutritional deficiency score remains 3 or more you may have an assimilation problem.	Use the chart on pages 36-37 to assess which vitamin and mineral supplements you may need, and take them for a minimum of three months before re-assessing your symptom score.

See page 294 for suppliers of the products mentioned on this page.

Food Intolerances

Your symptom score suggests that you might suffer from a food intolerance. In this chapter we will look for answers to the following questions:

- What is a food intolerance
- How often is it wrongly diagnosed by doctors?
- What can it do to your health?
- How can it develop?

It will help if you can read all the explanations, since this will help to motivate you. But if you want to skip straight to testing yourself for food intolerances (allergies) then go to page 47 now.

Most people feel wonderful when they have eliminated food intolerances. It is like gaining a new lease of life—a fabulous, rapid and totally unexpected freedom from pain and misery, and a new confidence as you regain control over your health. People too chronically exhausted to walk have become physically active again. Weekly migraines that always lasted 48 hours have vanished forever. Chronic sinus congestion has miraculously cleared. Bowels have begun to work normally again. Chronic eczema has disappeared. Burning rheumatic pains which the doctors cannot explain have melted away. Arthritic joints have stopped hurting. Waterlogged body tissues have given up years of retained fluid resulting in permanent weight loss of up to 10-15 lbs—the list goes on and on. I have personally seen all these results. All these people had been misdiagnosed by their doctor. They did not have any of the illnesses described—they had food intolerance symptoms.

Food intolerances are often referred to as food allergies, but it is better to keep the two terms separate, especially when talking to your doctor. Both food allergies and food intolerances are unpleasant reactions triggered by eating a particular food. An allergy causes an immediate, often severe reaction such as swellings, sudden rashes, or even life-threatening anaphylactic shock, where the blood pressure suddenly drops to dangerously low levels. Peanuts and shellfish are famous for causing this type of problem. It is often diagnosed with a skin prick test, where the offending food quickly causes a rash if an extract is placed on your skin.

On the other hand a food intolerance usually involves foods which people eat all the time, every day. It cannot be diagnosed with a skin test. Rather than life-threatening reactions it is more likely to cause the following symptoms:

- Chronic fatigue or unexplained drowsiness

- Head feels "foggy" all the time
- Sudden bouts of unusual aggression or depression
- Behavioural problems in children, including hyperactive and autistic behaviour
- Chronic skin rashes
- Frequent severe headaches
- Diarrhoea or severe constipation or both (alternating)
- Griping tummy pains with or without mucus discharge
- Painful or swollen joints
- Frequently congested sinuses
- Fluid retention (and resulting weight gain)
- Chronic catarrh
- Wheezing and breathing difficulties
- Dark colour under your eyes
- Rheumatic pains
- Symptoms of poor digestion and absorption: frequently bloated, uncomfortable tummy with much gas. Sometimes undigested food in stools.

If you have a food intolerance, the symptoms are not caused by the food itself, but by your reaction to it. Thus one individual may develop headaches from eating bread; another may get catarrh. The symptoms often come and go at random, or they may be present most of the time. Although the above list of symptoms is long, you will probably only have one or two of them depending on which of your organs is your "weakest link". It is relatively rare to suffer from a large number of different food intolerance symptoms.

Doctors who specialize in nutritional therapy believe that a lot of people with common ailments such as eczema, asthma and migraine, have been misdiagnosed by their doctors. They do not believe that they have these ailments at all, but simple food reactions. In fact they estimate that up to one third of the western population suffers from undiagnosed food intolerance symptoms, and instead of receiving proper treatment are just being prescribed painkillers, cortisone (steroids) and other drugs which temporarily control the symptoms[33].

What causes a food intolerance?

Unlike an allergy, which is usually inherited and with you for life, a food intolerance can develop quite suddenly. Nobody knows exactly what brings it on, but damage to the intestinal walls caused by chronic poor digestion and inflammation is thought to play an important part. This damage makes the intestines "leaky".

When the intestinal wall becomes leaky, bits of partly-digested protein from your meal (known as peptides) leak through the walls of your digestive system into your bloodstream. This leakage of food should never normally occur. When it does, your immune system treats the peptides as if they were bacteria. It attaches IgG antibodies to the peptides to make them easy targets for destruction[34]. When these peptide/antibody complexes come into contact with histamine-producing white blood cells (basophils or mast cells) they stimulate them to release histamine.

Histamine is a chemical responsible for the physical symptoms experienced by allergy sufferers. If you have ever suffered from hay fever or insect bites, you will be familiar with some of its effects. Histamine dilates your blood capillaries, producing symptoms such as skin redness, swelling and irritation, and can also constrict the bronchi of the lungs, causing wheezing (asthma). Inflammation occurs when capillaries affected by histamine become leaky, and more fluid passes into the surrounding tissues in order that more white blood cells can be carried to the sites of the "foreign invader". Because of these effects on the body, histamine can cause any of the symptoms listed on page 43.

Food intolerances and your liver

A leaky intestinal wall can result in much stress for your liver. Not only peptides, but also bacteria and their toxins, and pollutants from your food and drink can escape through a leaky intestinal wall into your bloodstream. Your liver has to deal with these as well as with its regular workload, and it uses up precious resources to do so. Feeling ill when exposed to alcohol, medicines, fumes or chemicals is a sign that your liver is not able to make enough enzymes to cope with its job. This kind of sensitivity can also be experienced as headaches after eating chocolate and matured cheeses.

Testing for food intolerances

As already mentioned, skin prick tests are not suitable for identifying food intolerances. Food intolerances involve complex reactions in the body, sometimes taking a day or more to result in symptoms.

The most reliable test to find out which foods (if any) you may be intolerant to, is known as the Avoidance and Challenge test, and this is what you will learn how to do on page 47.

Most experts do not recommend any other tests for food intolerances. Blood tests are expensive and unreliable because they rely on mixing food with your blood to see how it behaves. Undigested food is not supposed to come into contact with your blood. If it does, as when your gut is inflamed and leaky, we would expect any food to be able to trigger the processes which lead to histamine release and food intolerance symptoms. The accuracy of other methods such as kinesiology (muscle testing) and vega testing (electrical measurements carried out on the skin) depends so much on the practitioner's unique gifts that it is a minefield for most of us.

The Avoidance and Challenge test works by identifying which foods result in unpleasant symptoms for an individual when consumed. A carefully controlled procedure is required because symptoms may take 24 hours or more to appear. By then you probably have no idea which food has set them off. The culprit can only be tracked down by avoiding the main suspects for long enough to allow the symptoms to disappear and to clear the problem foods completely out of the system. The foods are then reintroduced one by one while you watch to see if the symptoms return.

Don't make the mistake of thinking that you can cut corners. For instance, eating a piece of bread and then waiting to see if you get a headache will leave you none the wiser. The four foods which you will test are responsible for over 90 per cent of unidentified food intolerances for one simple reason—we eat them so frequently, often several times every day.

Foods responsible for more than 90 per cent of food intolerance reactions

Wheat (found in bread, flour, biscuits, sauces, puddings etc.)
Dairy products (found in milk, cream, cheese, yoghurt, butter, and anything containing these)
Yeast (found in alcoholic drinks, stock cubes and other savoury flavourings, gravy mix, bread and pizza)
Egg (found in egg dishes, egg pasta, many brands of ice cream, desserts, batter, pancakes etc.)
Soya, corn, gluten, nuts, citrus fruit, tomatoes, pork, beef and chicken can also be problem foods occasionally.

If you have a food intolerance, the chances are that one of the four foods listed above in bold type will be responsible. The instructions for testing these foods are given on page 47. Follow them very carefully, especially the ones which ask you to stick to the Diagnostic Diet on page 46. Many convenience foods do not have all their ingredients listed on the label. If you unknowingly eat a little of the test foods when you are not supposed to, the test will not work.

You will notice that the diagnostic diet also cuts out foods like sweets and chocolate, tea and sugar. This is because they can have stressful effects on your internal chemistry, which may muddy the waters when we are assessing the effects of the diet.

The diagnostic diet

Permitted foods

- All fresh vegetables including raw salads, lightly steamed or stewed vegetables, soups made with fresh vegetables, potatoes (without butter), preservative-free vegetable juices, additive-free frozen vegetables. Do not use canned vegetables except for pulses (beans) in water.
- All fresh fruits and pure fruit juices. Juices must not contain added ingredients such as sugar or colouring. Canned fruit is allowed occasionally if packed in fruit juice without syrup or added sugar.
- All fresh or frozen fish, especially oily fish like mackerel, herrings and sardines. Canned fish is also permitted if packed in pure oil, not brine.
- All fresh or roasted nuts and seeds (unsalted), e.g. almonds, Brazils, walnuts, cashews, hazelnuts, pecans, sesame seeds, linseeds (will pass straight through you unless ground up in a coffee grinder), sunflower seeds, pumpkin seeds, pine kernels. **Important**: ensure nuts are not mouldy. Brazils and cashews in particular usually need washing before you eat them.
- Pure nut butters and tahini (sesame seed paste) are also allowed if sugar-, salt-, and additive-free.
- All pulses (legumes) e.g. lentils, kidney beans, butterbeans, peanuts, haricot beans. They can be home-cooked or canned in plain water.
- All products made from natural soya (soy) e.g. soya milk, miso, tofu, but not textured vegetable protein or soya protein isolate.
- All cold-pressed (unrefined) vegetable oils. These are available from health shops. Extra virgin olive oil from supermarkets is also suitable.
- Grains other than wheat: brown rice, spelt, oats, rye, barley, millet and buckwheat, as well as flours and flakes made from these grains. Since grains are very small, they can absorb more pesticide, so try to get them organically grown if available.
- Use arrowroot or cornflour as thickeners.
- Pure herbal or fruit teas except Maté (high in caffeine).

In Part V you will find many recipes allowing you to make delicious meals using these foods. You can use any of the recipes without restriction.

Foods not allowed

- Cow's milk products: butter, cheese, milk, yoghurt, or anything containing dairy products, lactose or whey, in even the smallest amounts.
- Wheat grains and products: bread or pastry, sauces or gravies, pasta, batter, cakes or biscuits made with wheat flour.
- Stock cubes/powders, or gravy/sauce mixes. These should be avoided as they can contain disguised wheat (in the form of hydrolized vegetable protein) or yeast. Use miso paste (from health food shops) instead, dissolved in hot water.
- Eggs
- Stimulants: sugar, tea, coffee, alcohol, beer, wine, salt. Do not eat sweets or chocolate.
- Artificial additives: colourings, preservatives, "instant" foods etc. Please check all labels carefully to ensure that everything you eat is free of these items.
- Yeast: yeast extracts, fermented foods, sauces or drinks except for miso and tamari.
- It is also advisable to eat meat only once or twice a week, if that. Meat is hard to digest and can contain contaminants unless organically raised. Organic poultry is better.

DON'T CHEAT. EVEN TINY AMOUNTS OF THE WRONG FOODS CAN PERPETUATE YOUR SYMPTOMS!

How to test yourself for food intolerances

	Testing Procedure	Results
Weeks 1 & 2	Follow the Diagnostic Diet: eat *only* from the foods and drinks in the list on the previous page. Avoid all the foods in the Not Allowed list. You can use any of the recipes in this book to prepare food.	
Week 3	In addition to the Diagnostic Diet, also consume egg-free wheat pasta, wheat flour or plain wheat crackers every day for 5 days, then stop. If you get any unpleasant reactions, such as headaches, sinus congestion or severe fatigue, or if your weight rises by several pounds during that time, make a note of them in the Results column and stop eating the wheat before the 5 days is up. There is no point in continuing, because it is extremely likely that you have a wheat intolerance and need to continue avoiding wheat. Whether or not you experience a reaction, stop the wheat after 5 days, and follow the Diagnostic Diet for the next two days.	
Week 4	Repeat what you did in Week 3, consuming cow's milk products daily instead of wheat, particularly fresh milk, cheese and yoghurt. The procedure is exactly the same as for Week 3.	
Week 5	Repeat what you did in Week 3, consuming eggs daily instead of wheat. If you do not want to eat a whole egg every day, make a 2-egg omelette with plain egg and water, cook it very thinly, and eat a small strip each day for the test period.	
Week 6	Repeat what you did in Week 3, consuming yeast daily instead of wheat. Buy a small jar of low-sodium yeast extract from a health food shop, and make it into a hot drink with boiling water. Drink this each day for the test period.	

What to do next?

Any chronic (long-term) symptoms which did not clear within the first two weeks of this test and return when you tested one of the foods, are probably not due to a food intolerance.

If you do find that you react badly to one or more foods, you should avoid those foods for about six months, after which levels of protective secretory IgA will be restored, allowing you to eat the foods from time to time without a return of your symptoms. You may also need to follow the Intestinal Healing Programme on page 50. If, on the other hand, the diagnostic diet seems to *aggravate* some symptoms, this is probably because you are intolerant to one of the permitted foods. Try cutting out soya products and gluten (from spelt, oats, rye and barley as well as wheat). If this fails, keep a diary of foods eaten and symptoms experienced. This will help you track down the culprit(s).

Did you get a positive result?

Well done if you managed to identify any problem foods and eliminate some or all of your symptoms. You are well on your way to recovery, but you have not got there yet. Although you may feel a thousand times better by avoiding wheat, dairy products or some other problem food, this avoidance is not a proper cure. It is a bit like taking an aspirin—the symptoms only go away for as long as the treatment is applied, and in the meantime the underlying illness continues to progress.

In this case, the illness is the digestive weakness and gut inflammation which allowed undigested food to get into your bloodstream and body tissues where it made your body produce histamine. If digestive weakness and gut inflammation are not treated, more food intolerances usually develop.

If you think it is hard enough to avoid wheat, imagine how hard it would be if you also started reacting to milk and cheese. Some people end up consulting nutritional therapists because they have become intolerant to so many foods that they no longer know what to eat.

Take a look at the diagram on page 49. This shows how bad digestion leads to intestinal dysbiosis and food intolerances. Dysbiosis simply means too many of the wrong kind of bacteria or yeast/fungal type microbes. You may have heard of a yeast known as Candida albicans. It is a particularly common type of dysbiosis because it is mainly caused by taking antibiotic medicines. Antibiotics kill the bacteria in your gut, especially the friendly ones which normally keep yeasts under control. It takes a while for the friendly bacteria to re-establish themselves, and in the meantime Candida can become rampant and no longer controllable, like weeds on a lawn. Here is a very useful tip: next time you take antibiotics, take them along with citrus seed extract, which is an anti-fungal supplement and will help to control Candida and other yeasts and fungi. It is not enough just to eat yoghurt, which some people do when they take antibiotics, to keep up the numbers of friendly bacteria. The friendly bacteria in yoghurt may not be acid-resistant and, like some Acidophilus supplements, could be killed by your digestive juices as well as by the antibiotics.

Antibiotics manufacturers should really put a harmless anti-fungal agent into their products since antibiotics have such a well known harmful effect on gut ecology. It is a complete mystery why they do not bother to do this.

The intestinal healing programme on pages 50-51 gives you all the information you need to know in order to restore your intestines to good health. Do work at it, and at the same time continue to avoid any foods which seem to give you symptoms. After six months' complete avoidance you can cautiously try eating them again to see if you can now tolerate them.

The vicious circle of dysbiosis

Aggravated by debilitating illness, immune system weakness, smoking, sugar, steroid drugs (including cortisone, contraceptive pill and HRT)

Bad Digestion

Gut Infections, alcohol, painkillers, toxic drugs

Increased irritation damages intestinal lining and its ability to produce sugar– and starch-digesting enzymes. Digestion and absorption worsen.

Undigested food irritates intestinal lining

Irritation causes histamine release

Bacterial/yeast overgrowth in small intestine forms barrier to food absorption. Aggravates irritation of intestinal lining. Bacterial toxins absorbed into bloodstream cause liver overload and toxicity symptoms such as severe fatigue.

Intestinal lining becomes "leaky"

Inflammation-promoting bacteria and yeasts thrive, and can begin to spread upwards into the small intestine (*dysbiosis*).

Absorption of digested nutrients is impaired. Undigested particles are more easily absorbed into blood.

Undigested food provides nourishment for resident toxin– and acid-producing bacteria and yeasts in the bowels.

Immune system reacts to particles. More histamine is released. Food intolerance symptoms occur.

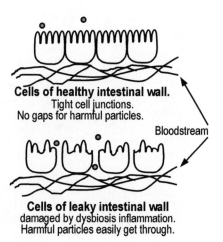

Cells of healthy intestinal wall.
Tight cell junctions.
No gaps for harmful particles.

Bloodstream

Cells of leaky intestinal wall
damaged by dysbiosis inflammation.
Harmful particles easily get through.

Intestinal healing programme

Step	Procedure	Comments
1	**10 to 20 minutes before eating,** slowly drink a small tumbler of water containing a few drops of tincture of gentian or golden seal. Eat only when you are hungry. Relax well when eating. Eat slowly and chew your food thoroughly. Do not overload your stomach.	The bitter taste of these herbs helps to stimulate stomach acid production. (You must allow yourself to taste the liquid.) Golden seal is also a useful liver herb and an anti-microbial for the intestines. Do not take golden seal in pregnancy.
2	**During each meal,** take 1-3 (depending on the size of the meal) capsules of HCl pepsin or betaine hydrochloride. As the meal ends, take supplements of bromelain and/or pancreatic enzymes as directed on the product label. To aid digestion and soothe inflammation, sip peppermint and chamomile tea with meals. Add ground cinnamon and cloves to the tea to help reduce flatulence. Do not consume too much liquid.	HCl is a hydrochloric acid supplement. This stomach acid helps to start off the rest of the digestive process. Reduce the dosage if you experience any discomfort. Do not take HCl if you have a peptic ulcer. Bromelain is a digestive enzyme made from pineapple stems and especially aids protein digestion. Pancreatic enzymes help to complete the digestive process.
4	**Food:** For the first two months restrict sweet and starchy food, also dried fruit and fruit juices. Try to make your diet 90% as follows: • Fish, chicken, soya products • Vegetables (cooked and as salads), beans, lentils, chickpeas, raw onions • Nuts of all types (especially Brazil nuts) and sunflower and sesame seeds. • Extra virgin olive oil in liberal amounts. Make liberal use of radishes, cayenne (chilli) pepper, fresh ginger, cloves, cinnamon, turmeric, cardamom, asafoetida. Stir minced raw garlic into meals just before serving.	Starchy food, sugars and grains cannot be digested completely when your intestine is inflamed, because the walls of your intestine cannot produce the necessary enzymes. By avoiding these foods for two months you reduce the amount of undigested food particles that feed toxin-producing bacteria and yeasts. Raw garlic and onion and the spices mentioned help to control these undesirable micro-organisms while promoting good digestion.
3	**Gut repair (1)** (2 months): To reduce harmful bacteria and parasites in your intestines, take grapefruit (or citrus) seed extract. Whenever you can, take one clove of fresh garlic, chopped and swallowed with water, three times a day. If you have ever taken a lot of antibiotics (especially if recently) also take enteric-coated oregano and clove oil capsules*.	*These help to destroy *Candida albicans* and other harmful fungi. Follow the directions on the product label when taking these products. Always rinse your washing-up. Tiny traces of detergent can damage delicate intestinal cell membranes.
5	**Gut repair (2)** (1 month): After the first two months, your intestines should be getting less inflamed. It is now time to begin replacing your beneficial intestinal bacteria. Take a guaranteed quality combination of Acidophilus/Bifudus bacteria for one month.	Not all products contain live beneficial bacteria. Those in yoghurt are killed by stomach juices. To repopulate your intestine an acid-resistant product is required. For the first seven days, "Replete", although expensive, is ideal.

6	**Gut repair (3)** (1 month): Tissue restoration. Comfrey tea: 1 cup (double-strength) 3 times a day. Once a day combine this with slippery elm. Also drink the juice of fresh cabbage leaves as often as you can with meals. Supplements: Enteroplex: 1 capsule with each meal. Butyric acid, n-acetyl glucosamine (NAG)*.	Enteroplex contains a combination of herbal liquorice and cabbage extract. Cabbage juice with each meal can be used instead. Comfrey is a great healer which has sometimes had a bad press, but does no harm in moderate amounts. *Gut repair nutrients
7	If your gut symptoms have not improved after this four-month programme, you are advised to obtain a special stool analysis (CDSA). This can be arranged through a nutritional therapist. Be patient; successful treatment can take time.	The test will show which types of irritant bacteria are still damaging your intestines, and the best anti-microbials to use against them.

For suppliers of any products mentioned, see page 294. Take all supplements in accordance with the directions on the product label. This three-month Intestinal Healing Programme sets out to reverse the harmful changes shown in the diagram on page 49. This will result in less inflammation in your intestines, due to better digestion and fewer toxin-producing bacteria. You should then suffer less from food intolerances and liver overload problems (see the symptoms listed on page 22).

Eat organic if you can

Wheat, dairy products, eggs and yeast do seem to be such common causes of food intolerance reactions that I usually advise people to consume them only in moderation even if they no longer cause symptoms. Modern wheat strains have been bred to have a very high gluten yield. Modern yeast strains have been bred to a very high degree of virulence. Dairy cows and laying hens are often fed a rather unnatural diet, which may include yellow colouring to make cream and yolks look more appetizing. I would certainly recommend eating organic versions of wheat, dairy products and eggs. I have come across children who become hyperactive after drinking ordinary milk but not after drinking organic milk.

Liver Overload

Your liver has the monumental task of taking unwanted waste products and toxins which have been absorbed into your blood, and transforming them into substances which are easy to excrete. But the efficiency with which a person's liver can do this job can vary as much as 60-fold. This means that in theory, one person who smokes 60 cigarettes a day and whose liver is very efficient at detoxifying the cancer-causing substances in cigarette smoke, may be no more likely to get cancer than another who smokes only one cigarette a day, or one who is even a passive smoker, but has a particularly inefficient liver.

Your liver overload score of two or more suggests that your liver might be struggling a little to cope with its daily load of toxins. This chapter provides the necessary knowledge for you to give your liver a helping hand. As a result you will not only begin to feel better, but you should drastically reduce your chances of getting a major illness in later life. Research at Birmingham University suggests that people with a well-functioning liver are less likely to get Alzheimer's disease, motor neurone disease, Parkinson's disease and multiple sclerosis[1,2]. A well-functioning liver can also help to protect you against cancer. Since the incidence of cancer in the UK is now one in three, this is very good news indeed. Your liver can break down and neutralize many chemicals which are known to set off the cancerous process. Do try to read the explanations in this chapter as these will help to motivate you. But if you want to skip straight to the Liver Rejuvenation Programme, turn to page 61 now.

Toxins

Toxins are harmful substances which can interfere with your body's functioning. They fall into three basic categories:
- *Xenobiotics*, which means substances foreign to your body, such as fumes, mercury, lead, drugs, medicines, pesticides and other chemical pollutants,
- *Metabolic wastes*: harmful substances such as ammonia, aldehydes and unuseable oestradiol (oestrogen) produced in the course of your body's normal metabolism,
- *Endotoxins*: harmful waste matter produced by the bacteria which normally live in your intestines. These toxins can be absorbed from your intestines into your bloodstream.

The removal of these from your body depends on four main organs:

- Your liver, which processes toxins and prepares them for excretion,
- Your intestines, which eliminate fat-soluble toxins in your stools,
- Your kidneys, which extract water-soluble toxins from your blood,
- Your skin, which excretes a variety of toxins in your sweat.

Your body needs to excrete harmful wastes and toxins as quickly as possible to prevent them from interfering with its functioning. But many toxins cannot be directly excreted—either because your kidneys keep sending them back to your blood or because they do not dissolve in water. Your liver's job is step by step to change them until they do dissolve in water and so can be excreted in your urine or bile. We usually describe this job as "detoxification", but this is not strictly accurate because some necessary intermediate stages of the liver's work can make a chemical more toxic than it was originally. The strict term for it is biotransformation—the transforming of one substance into another, more excretable one.

How the liver breaks down toxins

There are two main stages of liver detoxification known as Phase I and Phase II. In Phase I unwanted chemicals are usually combined with oxygen. This can make them very toxic, so antioxidants such as vitamin C, flavonoids and selenium-based enzymes must then act on them to neutralize the oxygen. In Phase II toxins are combined or react with a variety of other detoxification aids, including:
- Indoles from broccoli, brussels sprouts, cauliflower and cabbage
- Sulphate
- Acetyl groups
- Glucuronic acid
- Amino acids (protein).

Step by step, the toxins are turned into "intermediates", and then into acids. Since these acids are water-soluble, they can be extracted from your blood by your kidneys and excreted in your urine.

It may surprise you that one of the most important detoxification aids is certain amino acids found in protein. Protein is made from chains of amino acids joined together in different ways. The most important amino acids which aid detoxification are:
- **Cysteine**: helps to detoxify mercury, lead and arsenic, paracetamol, steroids, contraceptive pill, aniline food dyes, terpenes, phenols and tyramine,
- **Glutathione**: helps to detoxify penicillin, tetracycline, petroleum products (including diesel smoke) toxic metals, bacterial toxins and alcohol,
- **Methionine**: helps to break down excess histamine and hormones and to detoxify phenols, sulphites, hypochlorites, morphine, paraquat, mercury,

lead, arsenic and tin,

- **Glycine**: helps to detoxify phenols, aspirin, toluene, xylene, benzene, benzoate preservative, bile acids,
- **Taurine**: helps to detoxify chlorine compounds (including carbon tetrachloride) and to prevent the formation of toxic aldehydes, such as acetaldehyde.

Ammonia and ketones

The amino acid carnitine reduces levels of lactic acid, a metabolic waste which is formed in muscles (and makes them ache) when they are exercised without enough oxygen. Certain amino acids, namely arginine, ornithine, aspartic acid, glutamic acid and glutamine are also needed to break down ammonia. Ammonia is produced by the natural breakdown of protein in your body, and is toxic to your liver and brain. Alcoholics who have a very severely damaged liver often suffer brain damage because their liver can no longer control levels of ammonia.

Another type of metabolic toxin known as "ketones", is formed when you go on a low-calorie diet and start using your body fat for fuel. High ketone levels make your body acidic, which is harmful. The amino acid alanine, found in nuts, seeds and oats, helps to prevent the formation of ketones, and carnitine helps to control ketone levels.

Fruit and vegetables, which often form the basis of the "detox diets" that you read about in magazines after Christmas every year, supply many antioxidant nutrients which help in Phase I of your liver's work. But due to their lack of protein they contain only small amounts of amino acids. It is not advisable to restrict yourself to eating only fruit and vegetables if you want to help your liver break down and excrete toxins. You should also include nuts and sprouted seeds (see page 130 for advice on sprouting).

Environmental medicine

Some doctors—known as environmental medicine specialists—have much experience in working with people suffering from an overloaded liver. Like other doctors they are consulted for help with illnesses such as:

- Asthma
- Severe chronic fatigue and ME
- Childhood autism
- Multiple allergies
- Gulf War syndrome (a debilitating illness which many troops came down with after the Gulf War in 1991)

- Autoimmune diseases such as rheumatoid arthritis. (In autoimmune diseases the cells of the body's own tissues begin to appear abnormal for unknown reasons, and the immune system then attacks and destroys them).

The difference is that unlike other doctors, one of their first steps is to carry out tests to see which toxins are not being cleared very quickly from the patient's body.

Making detoxification aids

As we know, the liver's ability to clear toxins depends on a good supply of detoxification aids which come from your diet. Others, e.g. sulphate, taurine, glutathione, are made by your body itself. But some people seem to have very low levels—they lack the ability to make them properly. Once again your diet can play a part. The enzymes which help to make these detoxification aids must have a sufficient supply of B vitamins, magnesium, selenium, molybdenum and many other vitamins and minerals. Environmental medicine specialists now know so much about the diet/liver connection that they are able to tell you precisely which nutrients you are lacking by dosing you with common chemicals like aspirin and caffeine and later on testing your urine to see whether your liver has broken these chemicals down within the normal time limit.

I hope you are now beginning to see how intimately nutrition is intertwined with health. Perhaps you started reading this book because you suffer from an illness such as asthma, and did not see nutritional deficiencies as very relevant or important. But look at it this way. If just a slight deficiency of selenium, for example (selenium deficiency is actually very common) can reduce your ability to make one of your liver's most important detoxification enzymes, then how do you think your body is going to cope with pollutants and wastes as they build up over the years? Will any nerve or brain cells be damaged? Will your cell membranes go on allowing the right substances in and out of cells? Will something go wrong with cholesterol control? Will cancer-causing pollutants be rendered harmless? Will higher toxin levels cause any internal inflammation, sending up histamine levels to cause spasms in your airways? What symptoms will you get? What name will your doctor give to your symptoms if and when they begin to appear?

A disease is simply a major breakdown in body function. Which functions will most suffer from a toxic overload just depends on your "weakest link".

Ailing livers

Whatever your illness, environmental medicine specialists prescribe a healthy diet together with supplements to help bypass assimilation problems. They also check whether you have any food intolerances. But most of all they will prescribe "environmental control" - reducing your exposure to pollutants, many of which are probably found in your own home.

This type of approach has resulted many times in a return to health in seemingly hopeless cases. It is not really surprising when you know that, according to Dr Jean Monro of the Breakspear Hospital in Hertfordshire, the livers of up to 58 per cent of her patients have difficulty in processing even mildly toxic substances like caffeine and alcohol[35]. It is not just Dr Monro who says this. ME sufferers have a well-known intolerance to alcohol[36]. They usually feel ill very quickly after drinking it because their liver cannot produce enough enzymes to cope with it.

There are thousands of natural chemicals in food, including man-made pesticides and even natural insecticides known as "secondary plant metabolites". Ammonia is a natural toxin which comes from eating protein. If he or she cannot

---

Common chemical pollutants found in the home

Home care materials

Lavatory cleaners
Oven cleaners
Spray polish
Artificial air fresheners
Carpet cleaners
Detergents
Fabric conditioners
Bleach
Shoe polish
Metal polish

Cosmetics and personal hygiene

Nail varnish
Nail varnish remover
Hair spray
Perfume
Artificially scented soap , talc, shampoo, moisturizer, deodorant, aftershave etc.
Toothpaste

Pest control

Wood preservative
Garden sprays
Fly spray

Heating

Fumes from gas boilers, paraffin, gas, wood or oil stoves. Free standing butane or propane heaters are particularly bad.

Decorating

Paint stripper
Paint
Varnish
Fungicide in wallpaper paste
Turpentine
White spirit

Motor vehicles

Gases from upholstery
Petrol or diesel
Evaporating oil from engines

Fumes from garages built underneath or adjacent to living quarters

Miscellaneous

Dry cleaning fumes (clothes should be aired outdoors after cleaning)
Tobacco smoke
Recreational drugs
Over-the-counter medicines
Mould spores from damp surroundings or damp cloths
Artificial food additives
Dust
Gases released by new carpets and furnishings, foam rubber, mattresses,
Fumes from gas cookers
Newsprint (open newspapers outdoors before bringing in to read)
Creosote
Butane in spray cans
Surgical spirit
Glue

Always keep a window open, even if just a little, to maintain good air circulation in your home

---

process these chemicals, someone whose liver is in a very weakened state can feel ill most of the time. When they try to eat to keep up their strength, they feel worse.

Overworked and undernourished

These livers are not diseased, they are overworked and undernourished, and the resulting toxic overload leads to malfunctions in the individual's body. These malfunctions can turn into diseases. Work carried out at Birmingham University by Dr Guy Steventon and Dr Rosemary Waring has shown that the livers of people with chronic fatigue syndrome, parkinsonism, motor neurone disease and Alzheimer's disease are consistently more sluggish than those of healthy people[1,2]. Similar work has been carried out at King's College, University of London[272]. All this research has been published in several medical journals, including *Nature* and the *Lancet*, but little attention is being paid to it in the medical world.

Unfortunately most of us have no way of knowing how efficient our liver is before we start smoking, drinking too much alcohol and caffeine, or eating too many of the foods which fail to nourish our liver properly. We may have no idea that our liver is letting us down until we are badly overloaded with internal pollution and our health is failing. On the other hand, knowing more about how your liver processes toxins can help you look after it.

A helping hand for your liver

The first priority is to reduce your liver's workload. You can help it considerably by cutting down on your exposure to chemicals in your home. Take a look at page 57 which gives a table of common chemical pollutants found in the home. Try to substitute natural, unscented products for these whenever you can. And most of all, try to keep a window open all the year round even if just a little. Our modern sealed buildings charged with fumes from chemically-treated furnishings may be one reason for the modern epidemic of chronic fatigue syndrome and other mysterious illnesses that never used to plague us. Sealed workplaces can be even worse, especially in buildings where air is simply recycled without taking in any fresh air. To prevent this from spreading fungal and Legionella infections, the water in the humidifier is sometimes laced with dilute pesticide. The occupants of the building—without their knowledge—are then constantly sprayed with this pesticide. Extra-low frequency radiation and positive ions emanating from electrical equipment like VDUs are also recognized problems. Keeping plants on your desk helps to combat the effects of positive ions by generating negative ions.

Eating the right foods can also help your liver. It should be no surprise that foods which are good for the other organs of your body are also good for your liver. But you can also ensure that your diet helps your liver in more ways than one. The right food choices can help to

- Keep to a minimum the amount of unwanted chemicals which your liver has to deal with
- Increase the production of detoxification aids
- Drain wastes from your liver by stimulating the production of bile and stimulating your gallbladder to empty.

Don't forget fibre

Foods high in dietary fibre are especially important for preventing constipation, which is one of the prime causes of internal pollution. Fat-soluble wastes drain from your liver into your gall-bladder, which empties into your intestines. If you do not have regular bowel movements, these wastes will be reabsorbed through your intestinal walls back into your bloodstream.

Your Liver Rejuvenation Programme is on page 61. It should be applied for an initial six-week period, after which you should reassess your symptoms. Depending on how you feel, and the severity of your condition, you can either continue with it on a permanent basis, or have a break and then repeat it every few months or once a year. You may also find some additional guidance in Part III, which looks at specific health problems.

Your liver and oestrogen

You may have been surprised to see in the diagnostic questionnaire on page 22 that premenstrual mood changes, breast cysts and tumours, fibroids and endometriosis are connected with the liver. This connection was reported as long ago as 1943, by Dr Morton Biskind, a physician from Westport, Connecticut. He realized that because the liver needs B vitamins to break down oestrogen and excrete it in the bile, B complex deficiencies could cause an oestrogen overload[38]. We know now that all the health problems listed above are linked with an oestrogen overload, because we know that all can be reversed by artificially reducing oestrogen. For instance breast tumours are often treated with the anti-oestrogen drug tamoxifen, and endometriosis is treated with drugs that inhibit the menstrual cycle or to removal of the ovaries, which produce oestrogen.

Excess oestrogen (including HRT and the contraceptive pill) can also encourage gall-stones by reducing the flow of bile from the gall-bladder.

Apart from B vitamins, indoles in the brassica family of vegetables: broccoli, cabbage, cauliflower and brussels sprouts also help the liver to break down excess oestrogen, and are useful aids to treatment[39,40,187]. Soya products contain isoflavones which can bind to excess oestrogen, thus helping to neutralize its effects[80]. I have come across at least one case where endometriosis was cured after the patient started to consume half a litre a day of soya milk. (Soya milk can be used to make delicious porridge and rice pudding—you do not have to drink it on its own if you do not like the taste).

Foods rich in dietary fibre help you to excrete the oestrogen waste that your liver sends to your gall bladder[41]. So a diet low in fibre encourages higher oestrogen levels. This may be why it also encourages breast cancer. Another cause of high oestrogen levels can be iodine deficiency, which seems to stimulate the sex glands[19].

Although we hear a great deal about "inheriting the breast cancer gene", we should also remember that there really is no such thing. Breast cancer can certainly run in families, but then eating habits also run in families and are inherited. You may inherit a gene which makes your breast cells more sensitive to oestrogen than the average. But this does not absolutely guarantee that you will get breast cancer. You may just need larger than average amounts of antioxidants, iodine, brussels sprouts or dietary fibre to avoid your oestrogen levels getting into the danger zone. If breast cancer runs in your family, you should take the advice in this book very seriously, especially the principles of the Liver Rejuvenation Programme, which can be carried out for a few weeks every year even if you are healthy.

Liver Rejuvenation Programme

Step	Procedure	Comments
1	If necessary, ensure regular daily bowel movements, using a varied programme of: • Enemas • Ground linseeds or psyllium[1] • Epsom salts[1] • Gentle laxatives[2] (*not* liquid paraffin) • Bromelain with meals[3].	Daily exercise such as brisk walking helps to prevent constipation. Eating dates is also helpful. It is essential to drink plenty of water. **Notes** 1. One dessert-spoon in a large glass of water. 2. As per label instructions. Take no more often than once every three days. 3. Poor digestion can contribute to constipation.
2	Try to avoid tea, coffee, alcohol, food additives, saturated fat, refined carbohydrates and other highly processed foods. Consume the following as often as possible, and use this recipe book as regularly as you can, including the Detoxification Soup on page 153. • Beetroot and beetroot juice • Artichokes and watercress • Radishes (including the mooli variety) and radish juice • Dandelion coffee and peppermint tea • Turmeric (yellow Indian spice) • Broccoli, cabbage, cauliflower, brussels sprouts. Can be juiced. • Sunflower seeds, oats, Brazil nuts • Bilberries, blueberries, blackberries.	By encouraging your liver to produce bile and stimulating the drainage of the bile into your gall-bladder, these beneficial foods help wastes dissolved in your bile to reach your intestines as soon as possible, after which a bowel motion will remove them from your body. Broccoli etc. actually help your liver to make detoxifying enzymes. Dandelion coffee can be bought from health food shops. Or make your own by drying and roasting dandelion roots, crushing them and boiling the pieces. If you make your own raw beetroot or radish juice, allow it to stand for 20 minutes before drinking. Avoid drinking grapefruit juice, which can interfere with the action of some of your liver enzymes. Turmeric has numerous beneficial effects on the liver, including helping to protect it from inflammation. Sunflower seeds, oats and Brazil nuts are a good source of cysteine and methionine.
3	Take the following herbs and supplements daily: Magnesium[1] ....100-300 mg N-acetyl cysteine[2]........500 mg Methionine[2] ....1,000 mg Lipoic acid[3] ....100 mg Silymarin[4] .... As per product label [Wild Yam[5]........ As per product label] Vitamin C and flavonoids[6], especially black grape or cherry skin extracts, pycnogenol or Ginkgo biloba Lecithin[7]................... 1 tablespoon Multivit/mineral providing B complex, selenium, manganese, molybdenum.	**Notes** 1. Needed for most liver detoxification processes, but assimilation is often impaired. 2. Strongly liver-protective amino acids which also help make taurine and glutathione. 3. Helps to keep up glutathione levels[37]. 4. Stimulates the gall-bladder, and has a protective and repairing effect on liver cells. 5. As needed to prevent pain of liver spasms when liver is overloaded. Or use chamomile tea instead. 6. Help to prevent toxins from being formed while the liver is working. 7. Helps liver cell membranes to excrete toxins which could damage them.
4	Take regular saunas to help your liver by excreting toxins through your skin.	See page 294 for suppliers of the products mentioned here.

Part III

A-Z of health problems

So far you have learned how to analyze some of your symptoms—to look at what they suggest is wrong with your diet or with your ability to digest and use your food. You have learned how dysbiosis in your intestines can interfere with your nourishment and produce many harmful toxins. You have learned about food intolerance, the workings of your liver, and how to help your liver minimize levels of harmful substances in your body.

Armed with this information, you are already well on the road to self-repair. All that remains is to focus on some common illnesses, with a view to giving you more information on how they start and on the medical research which suggests more specific ways of helping them with nutritional therapy.

Alzheimer's, dementia and senility

These are very similar conditions. Although it is associated with specific changes in the brain, Alzheimer's disease is often just taken to mean premature senility. It can begin in middle age, and starts with a serious decline in short-term memory—a reduction in your ability to recall recent events, telephone numbers, or where you put your car keys.

Certain things can accelerate the ageing of those parts of our body which are responsible for memory. Three types of deterioration have so far been identified:

- Loss of nerve cells
- Damage to nerve cells
- Reduced production and increased breakdown of the important brain chemical acetylcholine.

The adrenal hormones adrenaline, noradrenaline and dopamine are also important for memory and concentration.

The nitric oxide connection

Some research has shown that supplements of vitamin E, which works as an antioxidant and also has anti-clotting properties, can slow down the progression of Alzheimer's disease[42,54]. Other research has shown great benefits from supplementation with the amino acid arginine, found in nuts and sunflower seeds, and needed for the body's production of nitric oxide. Nitric oxide helps to keep blood vessels relaxed, thus improving the circulation to the brain. In one study, elderly people were given 1.6 grams a day of supplementary arginine. Their score for mental ability improved by more than 50 per cent in three months. This improvement was lost when the arginine supplements were stopped[45]. Supplements of the herb Ginkgo biloba also enhance the blood circulation in the brain, and have been tested on Alzheimer's patients with good results[46]. Flavonoids from blue and purple berries help to maintain the integrity of the blood-brain barrier, which normally keeps toxic substances away from sensitive brain cells. They can even do this when the blood pressure is high—normally a time when the blood-brain barrier is particularly at risk[244].

The amino acids methionine and carnitine, have been found to have a positive effect on Alzheimer's disease, probably because they help to enhance production of the memory aid acetylcholine[46,47].

Phosphatidylserine research

Several research studies have shown that supplementation with phosphatidylserine (PS)—a combination of phosphate and the amino acid serine—can help reverse age-related memory problems and the deterioration of mental ability. Several encouraging scientific studies have so far been carried out. Functions measured include:

- Learning names and faces
- Recalling names and faces
- Facial recognition
- Telephone number recall
- Misplaced objects recall
- Ability to concentrate while reading
- Recall of details of events from the previous day or the past week
- Word acquisition and recall.

Individuals treated with PS supplements experienced significant improvements in these functions, in some cases reversing their mental decline by the equivalent of up to 12 years. Those worst affected often showed the most improvement[49,50,62].

PS appears to work through its role in the conduction of the nerve impulse, the accumulation, storage and release of neurotransmitters (which regulate the nerve impulses), and the receptor sites on cell surfaces.

It is a very interesting fact that people with osteoarthritis on long-term treatments with large doses of aspirin and similar anti-inflammatory drugs, seem to have a 50 per cent lower chance of getting Alzheimer's disease[44,51].

Gluten can be bad for your brain

Recent research reported in the journal *Neurology* in 2001 found that early-stage dementia may be linked with sensitivity to gluten—the protein found in wheat, oats, barley and rye. Dementia symptoms improved in nine patients with abnormal brain scans after they were given a gluten-free diet[53].

Low vitamin B_1, B_{12} and folic acid levels, in association with high homocysteine levels are also common in Alzheimer's patients[43,55]. High homocysteine encourages the clogging of arteries and so impairs the circulation. Homocysteine can be reduced with supplements of vitamin B_6, B_{12} and folic acid—in fact high homocysteine levels are now being used as an indicator of deficiency and/or poor assimilation of these three nutrients.

On the other hand levels of toxic metals such as aluminium and mercury are often high[57,58].

Saturated fat can starve your brain of oxygen

A diet high in fat (i.e. chips, crisps, burgers, biscuits, cakes, cheese, cream, ice cream, chocolate, pastry and deep-fried foods) and relatively low in essential polyunsaturated oils results in saturated fat being absorbed into the membrane around your red blood cells. This also has a harmful effect on your circulation; it makes your red blood cells less flexible—less able to pass down the very narrow blood vessels which feed your brain cells and other delicate and sensitive areas such as eyes and ears. As "log-jams" develop, the flow of oxygen and nutrients to brain cells can be impeded, which may seriously affect their functioning and survival. Boosting essential polyunsaturated oil levels has been shown to improve both red cell flexibility and mental functioning in Alzheimer's patients[59].

Arthritis

Osteoarthritis is an inflammatory condition which causes the cartilage gradually to degenerate until the bones are rubbing together. It is said to affect about 90 per cent of people over the age of 70, so don't be put off by reassurances that it is hereditary. It is often curable by nutritional means. Some of the leading causes of osteoarthritis are:

- Food intolerances.
- Too much acidity in the body from consuming too much protein.
- A deficiency of essential polyunsaturated oils.
- An overloaded liver, often made worse by long-term constipation.

Long-term inflammation caused by undue stress on a joint (due to injury, overweight, poor posture etc.) can lead to long-term fluid retention around the joint which encourages degeneration of the cartilage (see also page 71).

Useful treatments for osteoarthritis

- Find out whether you have any food intolerances by carrying out the test on page 47.
- Regularly use the recipes in this book, which are mostly not high in protein, and provide the right oils.

- Follow the Liver Rejuvenation Programme on page 61.
- Regularly massage the affected areas, imagining that you are squeezing out fluid and stroking it towards the centre of your body.
- You may also find great relief from taking supplements of evening primrose oil, especially if alcohol seems to aggravate your arthritis. Alcohol inhibits an enzyme which helps to turn the oils in your diet into GLA. A lack of GLA—which is also the active ingredient in evening primrose oil—encourages inflammation.

Some people with osteoarthritis find that it is made worse by eating acidic foods such as fruit. In some cases citrus fruit in particular seems to be a problem. In other cases, acidity seems to help—some people swear by taking two teaspoons of cider vinegar in a small glass of water before each meal.

A small percentage of osteoarthritis sufferers improve when they stop eating foods belonging to the "deadly nightshade" family: potatoes, tomatoes, peppers and aubergines. Tobacco also belongs to this family of plants.

Another, although rarer, cause of arthritis-like symptoms is "iron overload" caused by a history of consuming too many iron supplements or eating a lot of food which has been in contact with iron[60].

Supplements can help

Medical research has found that certain nutritional supplements have proved very useful in the treatment of osteoarthritis, particularly:

- S-adenosyl methionine (SAM) - helps to reduce inflammation by keeping down levels of histamine[61]
- Glucosamine sulphate—helps rebuild cartilage (you will need to take 1,500 mg per day)[63]
- Green-lipped mussel extract. Some people find that it helps to rehydrate shortened tendons as well as helping arthritis. It contains anti-inflammatory substances, chondroitin sulphate (similar to glucosamine sulphate) and other compounds.
- Shark cartilage and bovine tracheal cartilage—probably help stimulate cartilage production[64]
- Fish oils—anti-inflammatory
- DL-phenylalanine (DLPA) - has painkilling properties[65,66]
- Bromelain—an enzyme extracted from pineapple stems—has been found to reduce pain and swelling after sports injuries by breaking down fibrin[10,273]. Combined with other digestive enzymes, has also helped arthritis[67,274,275].

The Indian spice turmeric has a joint rebuilding effect[68]. Use it in cookery or mix it to a paste with water, form small balls and swallow them with water.

The herb devil's claw is a natural painkiller often used by arthritis sufferers as an alternative to aspirin and similar drugs.

Asthma

Asthma attacks occur when the bronchial tubes of your lungs go into spasm due to histamine, a substance associated with inflammation. (Histamine is also a cause of allergic symptoms such as swellings and itching.) Factors which contribute to asthma include:

- Allergies to inhaled matter such as dust mite droppings,
- Food intolerances,
- Magnesium and B vitamin deficiency,
- Excess salt consumption,
- Liver overload.

So it's worth carrying out the Food Intolerance Test and the Liver Rejuvenation Programme (pages 47 and 61). Use the recipes in this book as regularly as you can: they are rich in vitamins and minerals and very low in salt. Foods with a natural anti-histamine (anti-inflammatory) effect such as onions, purple berries, turmeric and oily fish (mackerel, herrings etc.) should be consumed as often as possible. It is important to drink plenty of water, as dehydration stimulates histamine release.

Gut bacteria can complicate asthma

Asthma varies enormously in its response to nutritional therapy. Some cases clear up quite quickly by mere avoidance of a food to which you are intolerant. On the other hand some of the more resistant cases of asthma do not really clear up until intestinal dysbiosis (see page 49) has been treated for some months.

Large amounts of histamine can be produced when the intestines are in a state of constant irritation due to Candida albicans overgrowth (candidiasis). This can aggravate a tendency to asthma[43]. The problem is that people with severe asthma— especially children—are usually given fairly frequent courses of antibiotics to prevent or treat chest infections. Each time antibiotics are taken, Candida is encouraged to thrive even more.

Some supplements which researchers have found helpful in reducing asthma attacks include:

- Lycopene (an antioxidant found in tomatoes) supplemented at 30 mg day can help to reduce symptoms in people with exercise-induced asthma[71]
- Magnesium and high-dose vitamin B_6[69,70]
- Selenium[72,73]

Autism

Researchers specializing in nutritional medicine are beginning to find clues to the causes of this devastating illness, which is increasing in frequency. Many research studies have been carried out using different avenues of treatment. Each type of nutritional treatment seems to help only a proportion of austistic children, suggesting that it is a disease with many contributing factors. Here are summaries of what researchers have discovered so far.

1. Some cases of autism occur as a result of vaccine damage. In the USA it is thought that responsibility may lie with the toxic metal mercury, used as a preservative in some vaccinations given to children. A major lawsuit is now being brought by families of autistic children affected in this way[127]. In the UK, the MMR (measles, mumps, rubella) vaccine has been especially implicated. In Norfolk, the Austistic Society were told that they should expect only 3-4 sufferers in their area, but there are already 46 and the numbers are growing daily, says Dawbarns, a firm of solicitors working with 150 families whose children became autistic following the MMR vaccine. A concern is that the vaccines are being given too early, before the child's immune system can cope with them[135].

2. Dr Mary Megson, Director of Developmental Pediatrics at the Children's Hospital in Richmond, Virginia has found that a high proportion of autistic children and their families have an abnormally high need for vitamin A due to problems with absorbing this vitamin. Water-soluble forms of vitamin A found in supplements do not help, but vitamin A as cod liver oil has produced many dramatic improvements[128].

3. Laboratory expert Dr William Shaw has found many abnormal substances in the urine of autistic children, suggesting that they have many metabolic abnormalities. One of these substances is tartaric acid—a by-product of certain yeast. Another is arabinose, produced by Candida albicans. Both can profoundly interfere with energy production in the body, and arabinose can also damage the nervous system. Both tartaric acid and arabinose levels come down when the children are given anti-fungal treatments such as nystatin and supplements based on oil of oregano[129,134].

4. Some of the earliest nutritional research into autism found that supplements of magnesium and high doses of vitamin B_6 helped many children. Parents often considered them more effective than prescribed medications[131,136].

5. Another avenue of research uses a gluten-free and/or milk-free diet, since the digestion of some autistic children (and also some sufferers of chronic fatigue syndrome or ME) seems to form antibodies and abnormal substances known as opioids from gluten and milk protein. Opioids act a little like opium or its derivative morphine—causing drowsiness and over-relaxation[132].

6. Other researchers have found that 100 per cent of autistic individuals have a reduced liver detoxification ability and most have a high body burden of toxins known to affect the nervous system—including pesticides—which the liver has failed to eliminate[133].

To address these factors, parents of autistic children should consider carrying out the Food Intolerance Test, the Intestinal Healing Programme and the Liver Rejuvenation Programme in this book plus daily cod liver oil supplements.

Autoimmune illness

Including rheumatoid arthritis, multiple sclerosis, lupus erythematosus

Autoimmune diseases occur when the body's immune system, designed for protection against infections and toxic injuries, for unknown reasons begins to attack and destroy normal tissue.

The very first comment I should make about these illnesses is that they are frequently misdiagnosed. I have personally treated two people who were diagnosed with rheumatoid arthritis but most certainly did not have this disease. They had a simple food intolerance which was giving them symptoms similar to rheumatoid arthritis. Once the offending food was withdrawn from their diet, all symptoms disappeared (to their enormous relief).

The next comment I should make is that perhaps the immune system is being wrongly accused. Perhaps it is not attacking normal tissue, but tissue which has been altered in some way so that it no longer appears normal.

For instance, if any part of your body suffers from damage—perhaps due to high levels of pollutants or other toxins—your immune system will rush to the scene of the damage, aided by histamine, which is produced in the surrounding area. Histamine makes the tiny blood vessels (capillaries) in this area "leaky" so that they can release extra fluid into the tissue spaces—the spaces between your cells—thus allowing white blood cells to get into these spaces and "clean up" the damage. Protein particles also escape with the fluid. This whole process is called inflammation. It causes swelling, and the swelling causes you pain and stiffness, especially if it is around a joint.

How your body deals with inflammation

Next, white blood cells called macrophages produce enzymes which split the protein particles up into much smaller fragments that can then be reabsorbed by the capillaries. The aim is that once the excess protein has been removed in this way, the excess fluid will drain away in the blood or lymph, and the painful inflammation ceases. But things are not always that simple.

What if the damage or toxicity which stimulated the inflammation does not cease? To put matters in very simple terms, white cells could be permanently present, producing enzymes designed to break down proteins in that area. How can these enzymes distinguish between proteins that should and should not be there? In the short term this does not matter, as short-term damage can be repaired. But in the long term could we be looking at the gradual destruction of healthy tissues and calling it "auto-immune attack"?

Eminent Australian lymphology researcher Dr John Casley-Smith—one of the top specialists in this field—says that this could certainly be true. He also points out that chronic inflammation can lead to a hardening of the tissues known as fibrosis. Fibrosis traps fluid and blocks it from getting back to the lymphatic system. This also has the effect of perpetuating the inflammation[74].

Massage and vegetables can help

It is no wonder that in the ancient Ayurvedic medical system of India massage is a standard treatment for arthritis. Massaging the fluid away from inflamed areas can help to reduce inflammation and prevent fibrosis.

It is also no surprise that traditional naturopathic (nature cure) diets are based on fruits and vegetables and their juices. They contain large quantities of flavonoids— nutrients now known to be very important in helping to prevent the abnormal leakage of fluid and protein from blood capillaries. Dr Casley-Smith's writings point out that a diet deficient in B vitamins and flavonoids causes capillaries to become fragile and susceptible to leaking with very little provocation.

Food intolerances can also cause chronic inflammation and so may play a part in the development of autoimmune attack. The "target tissues" - joint cartilage, skin, nerve cells, pancreas, thyroid gland and so on, may vary according to their affinity for the toxin that damages them. For instance phenols—toxins which come from plastics—have a special affinity for blood vessel walls, and tend to accumulate there. Swelling and inflammation of blood vessel walls is known as vasculitis, and is common in people with severe chemical sensitivities[75].

Self-help techniques

So, armed with these possible insights into your condition, how might you proceed to help yourself if you suffer from an autoimmune illness? Conventional medical treatments based on cortisone are not designed to reverse your illness. Although they may help you to feel a lot better, they can lead to problems of their own such as thinning of the skin and suppression of the immune system.

If I was unfortunate enough to be diagnosed with an autoimmune illness, my first step would be to test myself for food intolerances as described on page 47. I would then avoid any problem foods, and concentrate on eating as wide a variety as possible of foods with natural anti-inflammatory properties, particularly fruits and vegetables, and to drink their fresh juices in large quantities. I would also eat nuts, seeds, pulses and whole-grains. Although I am now a vegetarian, I would consider eating oily fish such as herrings and sardines because their oils have anti-inflammatory properties. I would take care to ensure that I digest all these foods properly by following the advice on digestion given earlier in this book. I would take digestive enzyme supplements based on bromelain, which has been shown to find its way into the bloodstream and from there to reach areas of inflammation, help reduce swelling and break down fibrin which causes fibrosis[10,273].

Clover tea and intestinal cleansing

I would drink celery juice and red clover tea, which are good sources of coumarin—a substance which helps fluid to drain out of tissues. And I would follow the Liver Rejuvenation Programme on page 61 and take up to 10 grams a day of supplementary vitamin C with flavonoids plus Ginkgo biloba, to help get rid of toxic substances from my body. I would also follow the Intestinal Healing Programme on pages 50-51 since many yeasts and bacteria which live in the intestines can produce harmful toxins. Research has also shown that elevated levels of antibodies to Candida albicans are found in up to 60 per cent of autoimmune patients, so I would want to follow all the advice given in this book for eradicating Candida from my system[76].

Finally I would have regular lymphatic drainage massage sessions, and also help my lymphatic drainage by walking briskly for at least half an hour a day if I was not yet too disabled to do so.

Try a tropical holiday

Yes, it is all exceptionally hard work, especially without a doctor's encouragement and guidance, and you may not begin to see results for some months. But knowing a little about how your body works can give you so much more inspiration to do that work rather than remaining in the dark feeling that you have no control over your future health.

If you have the means, you may also want to consider taking an extended holiday in a warm climate. It is an extraordinary fact that autoimmune illness—especially multiple sclerosis—is far more prevalent in North America and Europe[77]. Exposure to sunshine of course helps us to make our own vitamin D, and researchers have found that autoimmune sufferers do tend to have low vitamin D levels compared with healthy people. Very few foods contain natural vitamin D.

Cancers

Medical science is now 100 per cent behind the strategy of preventing cancer by eating more fruit and vegetables, which contain the antioxidant vitamins and minerals, the carotenes and flavonoids which help to prevent normal cells from becoming damaged and cancerous as a result of exposure to the thousands of cancer-causing substances (carcinogens) found in our modern world.

Cancers are also said to be a problem of the immune system, since it is normally responsible for destroying abnormal cells. Many factors, including emotional ones, faulty nutrition and an overloaded liver can weaken the immune system.

Using the recipes in this book will give you the best possible nutritional protection. Some nutrients are also highly protective against specific cancers, so you should eat soya foods plus broccoli and other members of the cabbage family to prevent breast cancer[78,79,80], tomato sauce to prevent prostate cancer[79] and whole-grains (rich in dietary fibre) to prevent colon cancer[81,82]. It goes without saying that if you smoke, you should give up as soon as possible. Even the best diet cannot really protect a smoker from lung cancer.

Don't confuse supplements with vegetables

The research into food and cancer is sometimes badly interpreted. When researchers found how protective vegetables can be, they surmised that individual vitamins such as vitamin C and beta carotene contained in the vegetables could be responsible for the anti-cancer effect. But the statement "beta carotene may help to prevent cancer" was interpreted by the average person as "beta carotene supplements may help to prevent cancer" - not the same thing at all! There are a lot of other protective ingredients in vegetables.

Anti-cancer diets

Many people want to know what they can do to help themselves if they have been unfortunate enough to develop cancer. A number of anti-cancer diets are available—the best-known one probably being the Gerson diet, designed by Dr Max Gerson in the 1930s. The Moerman diet, popular in Holland, is based on similar principles. These are complex diets, beyond the scope of this book, but the Resources section on page 294 suggests sources of further information. Most anti-cancer diets are based on healthy eating principles similar to those in this book, plus the consumption of copious quantities of fresh fruit and vegetable juices made at home with a juice extractor. Carrot, lemon (with pith), cabbage, beetroot, broccoli and celery juice are all good.

By all means try out any other systems you have heard about, but only if they are recommended by other cancer sufferers. Internet newsgroups are a good place to look for such recommendations. Always remember that if there really was a quick, easy and reliable natural cure for *everybody's* cancer, we would all know about it. Vitamin C therapy probably comes the closest to this, and has the added advantage that it has been scientifically tested. Two people personally known to me have cured themselves of cancer by taking 10 grams a day of powdered vitamin C dissolved in water and drinking it in divided doses between meals. Nobel Prize Laureate Dr Linus Pauling and his colleage Dr Ewan Cameron were the original researchers in this field, and successfully restored several terminal cancer patients to health when their doctors had given up on them[83,84].

Special help for breast cancer

For breast cancer, there is some very encouraging research into the use of high-dose antioxidant supplements together with large doses of coenzyme Q10. 32 women whose cancer had spread to their lymph nodes (this is normally a very bad sign) were treated with this combination in a study carried out by Danish doctors in the early 1990s. Of these, six experienced a complete halt to the disease. None experienced any progression of their cancer, and none died over the 18-month period of observation although 12 per cent of the women would normally have been expected to die during this time[215].

High levels of oestrogen can encourage the development of breast cancer. Women with breast cancer often have a defective ability to break down excessive oestrogen in their liver[197]. For these women it is essential to take the advice given on pages 59-60 and to follow the Liver Rejuvenation Programme on page 61. Breast cancer is often found together with hypothyroidism, indicating a possible iodine deficiency. Iodine deficiency can cause raised oestrogen levels[19].

Help for side effects of conventional treatments

Several research studies show that antioxidant supplements can be helpful when used together with chemotherapy[52]. Consuming 2-3 teaspoons a day of the yellow spice turmeric while on chemotherapy can help to prevent your liver from becoming inflamed and may also inhibit tumours by reducing their blood supply. Your liver needs to stay as healthy as possible to help you cope with the chemotherapy, which is just a little less toxic to your own cells than to cancer cells.

After you have finished chemotherapy, take large doses of N-acetyl cysteine, and lipoic acid, and follow the Liver Rejuvenation Programme on page 61 to help your liver cells recover and clear the drug residues from your tissues.

Consuming flavonoids, as found in orange peel, blue and purple berries, onions and apple skins, help to lessen burning and redness of the skin due to radiotherapy.

This is because of the role they play in the strength of your capillary walls[276].

Magnetic therapy—the application of the north pole of a magnet to the skin—also has powerful anti-tumour effects[85]. See page 294 for where to get therapeutic magnets. The north pole is usually coloured blue on these magnets.

Psychological therapy may also be important in cancer. Depression and lack of fulfilment has a depressant effect on the immune system, and many people develop this illness within a few years of losing a loved one, for example.

Candidiasis

This is a type of dysbiosis—a condition where the intestines become overgrown with the wrong type of bacteria or yeasts and fungi (in this case the yeast Candida albicans). These micro-organisms produce toxic substances which irritate the intestines and are absorbed into the bloodstream. In large amounts they can be particularly stressful to the liver.

The diagram on page 49 shows how dysbiosis occurs, often starting with bad digestion, irritation and inflammation of the intestine. Yeasts such as Candida albicans are especially encouraged by antibiotics and by sugar consumption.

For candidiasis you need the Intestinal Healing Programme on pages 50-51.

Chronic fatigue syndrome and fibromyalgia

When leading a normal life leaves you feeling exhausted, you are said to suffer from chronic, or persistent fatigue. Often, sleep does not refresh you. If they are able to get out of the house at all, chronic fatigue sufferers may go to bed straight after getting home from work. Many people with this problem are bed-bound. Symptoms that can accompany it include muscle pain (known as fibromyalgia) and "brain fag" - a frightening loss of the ability to concentrate on anything and to get your head round any but the simplest thoughts.

Some known causes of chronic fatigue

- The lingering effects of viruses such as the Epstein-Barr virus which causes glandular fever,
- Sensitivity to chemicals (often as a result of a liver overload),
- Nutritional deficiencies, especially magnesium, where there often seems to be a profound assimilation problem,
- Food intolerances. One of these is known as "opioid excess syndrome" and occurs when gluten in your diet seems to encourage the production of chemicals in your brain which act a little like sleeping pills,

- Dysbiosis: a toxic condition of the intestines which overloads the liver and is often brought on by taking antibiotics (see diagram on page 49),
- Research shows that some people develop chronic fatigue syndrome soon after taking a course of antibiotics, or after receiving vaccinations[296].

The first step in treating this problem is to follow the Food Intolerance Test instructions on page 47. This will show you which of your symptoms are caused by a food intolerance and which are not. Symptoms like headaches and digestive discomfort often disappear when problem foods have been removed from the diet.

Most people with chronic fatigue would benefit from the Liver Rejuvenation Programme on page 61, which helps to treat chemical sensitivity, and from the Intestinal Healing Programme on pages 50-51, which treats dysbiosis.

I have also treated a case of chronic fatigue syndrome which seemed to be mainly caused by environmental factors. This lady's bedroom seemed to be a problem: she felt worst of all after a night's sleep and was free of all symptoms if she was able to get out of her house for 12 hours or more. We managed to get rid of all her muscle pains by switching to anti house dust mite bedding and ensuring that her mattress and bedroom were thoroughly vacuumed. Some houses have a lot of mould spores, which can result in chronic fatigue as an allergic symptom. Outgassing from wood preservative and other chemicals impregnated in timbers etc. can also be a problem.

Muscle pain in chronic fatigue can also be caused by toxins (especially tartaric acid) produced by harmful bacteria and yeasts in your gut, and by abnormally high levels of lactic acid produced by your muscle cells (see below).

Watch out for chemicals

Chemicals can damage the processes which take place in your mitochondria—the part of your cells where energy is produced. When the mitochondria are over-stressed, or when your cells cannot get enough oxygen, your body relies on a process called glycolysis to make energy. Glycolysis is very inefficient, and not capable of producing very much energy. It forces your muscles to produce a lot of lactic acid. This is the substance which makes everybody's muscles hurt when they have been over-exerted. Chronic fatigue patients' muscles feel like this all the time.

If you live or work in a sealed building, chemicals in the atmosphere can linger for much longer and at much higher levels than in a building with a good air flow. Take especial note of any premises where you seem to feel worse. Your fatigue may be partly caused by something in them. Try to avoid as many as you can of the items listed in the table on page 57.

If you live or work near a farm, you may be affected by organophosphorus pesticides, either sprayed on crops or used in sheep dip. These can produce identical symptoms to all those associated with chronic fatigue syndrome. One of their effects is on the circulation, and chronic fatigue sufferers are known to have a slower than normal circulation, with a reduced blood flow to the brain[86]. One of the treatments which some chronic fatigue sufferers have found helpful is lying in cold water. This may be because the cold helps to stimulate your mitochondria as well as reflexes which boost your circulation. Magnesium injections are also an effective treatment for some chronic fatigue sufferers[13]. Magnesium helps with detoxification, and helps your muscles to decontract, which improves your circulation. Many chronic fatigue sufferers cannot absorb enough magnesium from their food or even from supplements. Vitamin B_6 aids magnesium assimilation.

Another source of chemical toxicity is mercury in "silver" tooth fillings. Mercury is a highly toxic substance and it is a mystery why it is allowed in the mouth. Claims that it does not escape from the teeth have been many times disproved[87,277]. Research suggests that one of the earliest targets in the body for damage caused by mercury is the mitochondria—the part of your cell which produces energy[294]. Consuming coriander leaf can help you eliminate mercury[252].

Toxic chemicals can also affect your adrenal glands, and low adrenal function is also common in chronic fatigue syndrome[98].

"Stealth" bacteria and viruses

If all these suggestions do not bring about a considerable improvement in six months or less, then it is possible that you have an active virus which has evaded detection by your doctors. Some bacteria, such as mycoplasmas, lack cell walls which would normally allow them to be spotted in medical tests and by your immune system. They are sometimes known as "stealth pathogens". The Epstein-Barr virus can also behave like a stealth pathogen[278,279].

The Liver Rejuvenation Programme includes measures for boosting the amino acid glutathione in your liver. This is absolutely essential to combat viruses. International chronic fatigue expert Dr Paul Cheney has stated that a glutathione deficiency is very common in chronic fatigue syndrome. It allows viruses to proliferate whereas high glutathione levels will stop virtually any virus from replicating. He points out that one of the most common causes of glutathione deficiency is a dietary selenium deficiency[90]. In the UK, our average selenium intake since our entry into the EU led to importing EU wheat instead of Canadian wheat, has dropped to about 30 micrograms a day—less than half of the recommended daily intake[91]. Viruses are more easily able to mutate, perhaps into unrecognizable forms, in the presence of a selenium deficiency[25].

Anti herpesvirus techniques can help

If the virus is of the "lipid-coated" type it may be possible to combat it by using coconut oil in your cooking. Such viruses are sensitive to a substance known as lauric acid found in coconut oil[92]. Lauric acid can also be purchased as a supplement. On the other hand the amino acid arginine found in nuts, seeds and grains helps to encourage the growth of the herpesvirus family to which the Epstein-Barr virus belongs. You can control the effects of arginine by avoiding these foods and taking lysine (another amino acid) supplements—about 2 grams a day[93]. The flavonoid quercetin, found in onions, cabbage and apple skins, also has pronounced anti-viral properties[145,250].

Another useful asset in the treatment of chronic fatigue is the medicinal mushroom Coriolus versicolor (see page 294 for sources). And why not look for Shiitake mushrooms in the supermarket? These oriental mushrooms have anti-viral properties[264].

Above all, never give up. "Diet and supplements" are reported by the British support group Action for M.E. to be the most helpful therapy for chronic fatigue sufferers according to surveys of its members.

Graded activity programmes

Research has clearly shown that even the worst-affected chronic fatigue sufferers can benefit from a properly designed programme dividing rest and activity into small, manageable portions spread throughout the day (for example, three 5-minute walks daily rather than a 45-minute walk once a week)[94]. The patients work with a specialist therapist to plan their own programme. The patient is asked to keep a diary of their normal activities and their symptoms. This diary is then used to set short-term goals, particularly the following:

- Stabilize activity and rest,
- Increase activity (within the patient's abilities),
- Establish a sleep routine,
- Address unhelpful thoughts,
- Identify what the patient needs to do to achieve goals,
- How to deal with problems when they arise.

Once a structured schedule is established, the activity level is gradually increased. Using this method, research has found that in 15 sessions over six months, a 70 per cent improvement can be achieved. The therapist aims to:

- Shift the focus from discussing symptoms to managing them,
- Ensure the patient feels he/she has been listened to and believed,
- Challenge any belief that "nothing can be done",
- Help the patient understand how "graded activity" helps him/her.

The most severely affected chronic fatigue patients believe that they are not capable of any activities at all and that they could not follow such a programme.

Nothing could be further from the truth. Even brushing your hair, reading a newspaper, listening to the radio and talking to other people are activities. By properly programming these activities the chronic fatigue sufferer can conserve energy and use it as constructively as possible. The great sense of achievement which can be gained in this way reduces depression and hopelessness, which in themselves are great drains on energy. The energy saved can be put towards more constructive uses.

Common Cold

Drinking orange juice won't cure a cold, since it doesn't contain enough vitamin C. But research into the effects of large doses of vitamin C on the immune system has generally shown benefits. The number, size and mobility of white blood cells can be improved[95]. Vitamin C also seems to work directly against viruses, perhaps by helping you to make more interferon. Many people are now taking vitamin C at the first sign of a cold and finding it a highly effective treatment.

Vitamin A is used in large amounts by the body when an infection occurs. Cod liver oil is a rich source of vitamin A. The traditional wisdom about cod liver oil preventing colds now has scientific evidence to back it up. In a recent study in New Zealand, researchers gave children small daily supplements of vitamin A. The result was a 22% reduction in the number of cases of colds and flu. The children's vitamin A intake had previously been considered adequate.[96]

Zinc is needed in adequate amounts for stored vitamin A to be released. Zinc itself (as do most nutrients) plays an important part in the immune system—our body's natural defences against infection.

Some herbs—particularly Echinacea—are also thought to be able to "boost" immune function. Radishes and radish juice have decongestant properties and so can help to eliminate cold symptoms.

Homoeopathic aconite and belladonna (taken together) can be extraordinarily and rapidly effective in treating colds and flu which have a very sudden and violent onset (e.g. raging sore throat, violent sneezing). Homoeopathic gelsemium is a specific for flu which begins more slowly and is associated with hot and cold sensations and shivering.

How to treat a cold

Vitamin C therapy started just as a cold is beginning can get rid of it in hours. Once the cold has started, vitamin C therapy can no longer get rid of it quickly, but it can help decongest your nose, give you more energy and speed up recovery. Here are the instructions for how to use it.

1. *At the first sign* of a cold or the flu, take 1 level teaspoon of pure vitamin C

powder dissolved in a glass of cold or lukewarm water or juice. The first signs of a cold are: beginning to sneeze, with a slight loss of energy and probably a slightly raw feeling in the throat, as if all is not quite right.

N.B.: It is important to develop awareness of your body. Early symptoms are often ignored but if left too late the cold may have to run its course.

2. Repeat this dose every 2 hours until symptoms disappear. They usually will if caught at this very early stage. I usually find that one or two doses of vitamin C are enough.

3. If your symptoms are appropriate (see above) you could also take the relevant homoeopathic remedies. Use a potency of 6c, and take every 2-3 waking hours for two days.

4. **If the symptoms disappear rapidly**, take 1 quarter teaspoon vitamin C powder or 1 gram (1,000 mg) tablet every 8 hours for the next 24 hours, then every 12 hours the day after. You may wish to continue with this as a maintenance dose.

5. **If the symptoms take longer to disappear** (2 days or more), tail the vitamin C off more slowly, gradually reducing the dose and increasing the interval over about 4 days. If you do not do this, the cold or flu may return with a vengeance. Vitamin C seems to work first by suppressing the symptoms and second by fighting the infection. If you stop taking it too soon the infection-fighting action may not yet be complete.

6. I also recommend taking 1 tablespoon cod liver oil and 15 mg zinc per day for one week. If you wish to add the herb Echinacea, take this for one week in accordance with the manufacturer's directions. Eat several radishes a day. If you have a juicer you could juice the long white mooli radishes. Leave the juice to stand for 20 minutes before drinking, to reduce the peppery taste.

Important

As long as vitamin C is being absorbed from the intestines it is well-tolerated and causes no discomfort. Once it is no longer being absorbed, it causes loose bowel motions, rather like a laxative. This happens at a daily intake of 1-10 grams (1,000-10,000 mg) in most healthy individuals.

Vitamin C users agree that the worse the infection, the more vitamin C can be absorbed. Someone with severe flu may have no loose bowel motions even at an intake of 20 grams a day. If you do experience bowel discomfort or a laxative effect, you should reduce the dosage to a comfortable level.

Vitamin C powder is recommended because it must be dissolved in liquid before swallowing. This prevents stomach irritation, which can be caused by swallowing the equivalent in tablets or capsules. It is also a more economical form of vitamin C. Large doses of vitamin C should be taken away from mealtimes, as they could interfere with the absorption of minerals from food.

More advice

The cheapest form of vitamin C powder is ascorbic acid, and this is easy to find in the shops. But if you dislike the taste or the acidity, you may prefer a buffered (non-acidic) form of vitamin C powder. I recommend magnesium ascorbate, which can be obtained from mail order sources. Magnesium ascorbate also has the advantage of providing extra magnesium, which is frequently in short supply in the average diet.

Constipation

Although the treatment for constipation seems obvious—a high-fibre diet—I am including it here because I ate a high-fibre diet for years yet still suffered from constipation. I did manage a small bowel motion most days, but the motions were very hard, and very difficult to expel. Here is a list of all the things which I have found can encourage constipation:

- A lack of fibre-rich foods: vegetables, pulses, porridge, wholemeal bread, brown rice, dates, prunes, linseeds. As fibre absorbs liquid it swells and provides bulk for your intestines to act on.
- Lack of exercise. A daily brisk walk will help your bowels. Cycling and tummy exercises are especially good. Poor muscle tone in your lower abdomen is a major cause of constipation.
- Magnesium deficiency. Your abdominal muscles can become too contracted if your diet is low in magnesium, and the rippling motion (peristalsis) which helps to push your bowel contents along is inhibited.
- A lack of water. Tea, coffee and alcohol are diuretics—they can dry you out so that there is not enough water to help bulk out the contents of your bowels.
- Poor digestion due to a lack of stomach acid or pancreatic enzymes. This was the problem in my case. I had done everything else right for years, but I was still constipated until I started to take bromelain with each meal.

No-one is sure exactly why badly digested food is more difficult to expel, but this cause of constipation first came to my attention in the writings of US nutritional medicine expert Dr Jonathan Wright[6] and sure enough, in my case he was spot on.

Cystitis

Inflammation of the bladder. Although often treated with antibiotics, it is not always due to an infection. Other common causes are food intolerance, candidiasis and the use of artificial bath or personal hygiene products and harsh laundry detergents. A very severe chronic form of cystitis known as interstitial cystitis can be an autoimmune condition. Helpful treatments for cystitis include:

- Drinking a glass of water or cucumber juice (for soothing) every waking hour.
- Eat nuts. Their arginine content helps to reduce symptoms by increasing nitric oxide production[288]. Avoid fatty, sugary, salty foods and excess protein. Eat according to the Basic Healthy Plate on page 26.
- Research has shown a 78 per cent reduction in cystitis episodes for women who use an Acidophilus pessary once a week as a preventive measure[293].
- Cranberry juice or capsules of cranberry extract help to prevent bacteria from adhering to your bladder wall[287].
- Carry out the Food Intolerance Test.
- If you also suffer from thrush and/or candidiasis symptoms, follow the Intestinal Healing Programme.
- Take the herbs Uva ursi, echinacea and Saw palmetto. Uva ursi works best when you avoid acidic foods and drinks.

Deafness

Consuming too many chips, crisps, sweets, burgers, biscuits, cakes and sugary drinks, and too much cream, ice cream, white bread, chocolate, pastry and deep-fried food can take its toll in more ways than one. These foods encourage all the health problems associated with nutritional deficiencies because they provide a lot of calories in the form of saturated fat and sugar but very few vitamins and minerals. Several nutritional deficiencies seem to encourage deafness, in particular vitamins A, B_{12}, D and folic acid, and the minerals iron, iodine, magnesium and zinc. In a research study carried out at the University of Georgia in 1998, elderly people with impaired hearing were found to have B_{12} levels 38% lower and folic acid levels 31% lower than people with normal hearing. Much of the hearing loss is believed to occur in the cochlea of the ear, which is nourished by many small blood vessels. Vitamin B_{12} and folic acid deficiencies inevitably lead to high homocysteine levels, which encourage cholesterol deposits on blood vessel walls and so can reduce the blood flow to the cochlea. B vitamin deficiencies also damage the auditory nerves (those related to hearing)[97].

A diet high in saturated fat and relatively low in essential polyunsaturated oils (i.e. one which contains a lot of the foods listed above) means that saturated fat will become incorporated into the membrane around your red blood cells. This also has a harmful effect on your hearing; it makes your red blood cells less flexible—less able to pass down the very narrow blood vessels which feed your nerve cells, eyes, ears and other delicate and sensitive areas. As "log-jams" occur, these cells can become deprived of nourishment and oxygen. In a research study carried out in 1988 on children with hearing difficulties, fluctuations in their hearing were found to vary according to their fat intake. Dietary changes led to a drop in cholesterol levels and a return to near-normal hearing[98].

Not only deafness but also tinnitus—a continuous ringing in the ears—seems to be linked with circulatory problems in the small vessels (the microcirculation)[245].

Your microcirculation can be considerably helped by what you eat:

- Oily fish (herrings, salmon, mackerel, sardines) help to prevent "log jams" in your capillaries[59].
- Blue and purple berries and ginkgo biloba supplements, rich in flavonoids, have long been known to help the micro-circulation[46,247]. Copper also plays an important role[246], and is considered in Rudolph Steiner's anthroposophical medicine system to be a warming element.
- Warming foods such as ginger and chillies act as circulatory stimulants.
- Nuts are very rich in arginine, needed to make nitric oxide which helps to keep blood vessels dilated.

Depression

The adrenal hormones dopamine, adrenaline and noradrenaline are thought to play a part in abnormal mood disturbances. Individuals with depression excrete reduced amounts of these hormones and other similar compounds in their urine. Individuals with mania, on the other hand, excrete increased amounts. Drugs used to treat depression work by inhibiting an enzyme which breaks down adrenal hormones, thus keeping larger amounts of them circulating in your body.

The amino acid tyrosine is the raw material from which your body makes adrenal and thyroid hormones. Because of this connection, researchers have tried giving tyrosine supplements to people with clinical depression. These trials have produced encouraging results[99].

Amino acid therapy

Your body synthesizes tyrosine from the amino acid phenylalanine, and some trials have shown that this too can be an effective treatment for depression. In fact, in some double-blind trials, where neither the patients nor the researchers knew who was getting phenylalanine and who was getting the antidepressant drug imipramine, both products were found to be equally effective. The form used was DL-phenylalanine (DLPA) in a dose of 75-200 mg per day and was administered to depressed patients for 20 days. 12 patients were discharged with a complete or good response and only 4 patients did not respond[100].

Doctors sometimes prescribe the amino acid L-tryptophan for depression, because it forms serotonin in your brain. Serotonin helps to keep you happy.

Another amino acid which has had good results in research on depression is methionine, in the form s-adenosyl methionine (SAM)[101]. SAM donates methyl groups needed for making carnitine, nucleic acids and adrenal hormones.

Vitamin and mineral deficiencies

According to the medical literature, vitamin and mineral deficiencies should be investigated in people suffering from clinical depression. Of particular concern are the vitamin folic acid, which can reach dangerously low levels in people who rarely eat fresh vegetables, and the trace element selenium, the average consumption of which has fallen below the official deficiency level in the UK[91]. In one 1989 research study, folic acid (folate) levels were estimated in depressed patients and found to be significantly lower than in normal controls. The lower the folate the more severe the depression[102,104]. This effect of folic acid deficiency is probably because this vitamin is needed to convert tyrosine and tryptophan respectively to adrenal hormones and serotonin, which both govern mood[47].

In another study, 11 healthy men were given a selenium-rich or selenium-poor experimental diet for 99 days. Those who were initially low in selenium experienced depressed moods[103].

Other useful treatments

In contraceptive pill users with depression, anxiety and other symptoms, vitamin B_6 supplements can help by restoring normal metabolism of the amino acid tryptophan[105].

Inositol is a member of the B complex family of vitamins but is not strictly a vitamin. In a 1995 study, after receiving 12 grams of inositol per day, 13 patients with clinical depression felt significantly better[106]. Lecithin is an easily available nutritional supplement which is extremely rich in inositol.

In 1996 the *British Medical Journal* reviewed all the studies which have tested the herb St John's Wort against mild to moderately severe depression. They found that extracts of this herb are just as effective as standard antidepressant drugs and produce less than half the side effects[107].

The insulin connection

Chronic low blood sugar (see page 86) can lead to profound depression. If blood sugar swings are too severe, this can be reflected in extreme mood swings—mania when blood sugar is high, followed by depression as insulin surges and makes it drop. You know if you have this kind of depression because it turns you into a sugar junkie. A tendency to low blood sugar makes you crave sugary foods and drinks to avoid the depression. Sometimes these mood swings are misdiagnosed as manic depression or bipolar disorder.

Two of the most important nutritional deficiencies involved in developing blood sugar problems are chromium and magnesium. The late Dr Carl Pfeiffer of the Brain Bio Center in New Jersey also used to treat manic depression (bipolar disorder) by addressing vitamin B_6 and zinc deficiencies.

Severe depression can also be associated with high levels of histamine in the body, which is another reason why methionine supplements may help. Methionine and calcium can help to reduce histamine[117]. Vitamin C, quercetin and magnesium also reduce excessive histamine[119,146,147].

Post-natal depression is thought to be due to the temporarily high copper levels which linger after pregnancy. High copper levels are encouraged by a zinc deficiency[110]. Zinc is especially depleted by pregnancy and breastfeeding.

Diabetes and hypoglycaemia

Both diabetes and hypoglycaemia are disorders involving insulin. Insulin is a hormone needed to carry glucose from your blood into your cells, which can then use the glucose to make energy.

There are two types of diabetes, known as type I and type II. Type I usually begins in childhood. It is thought to be possibly an "autoimmune" condition, i.e. your own immune system destroys the cells of your pancreas—your insulin-producing organ. The result is a lack of insulin. Type I diabetes can also be inherited. Scientists do not know whether this is due to a faulty gene, or to the mother's diet in pregnancy. A diet high in fat and sugar may impair the development of the baby's pancreas, and when the baby is born, he or she may not be able to produce enough insulin.

Insulin resistance

Type II diabetes, which begins in adulthood, is when your muscle and fat cells become "resistant" to insulin, so sugar remains in your blood and these cells cannot use it to make energy. Your body may then produce more insulin in an attempt to overcome this, resulting in hyperinsulinaemia—chronically high insulin levels. But some of your organs cannot cope with this extra insulin. Too much insulin makes your kidneys retain sodium, causing fluid retention, high blood pressure and high levels of uric acid[111]. When insulin over-stimulates your liver, your blood fat levels can rise. A woman's ovaries can begin making more testosterone when there is too much insulin around, leading to symptoms of polycystic ovary syndrome (PCOS) [112]. Another effect of hyperinsulinaemia is a change in body shape. Body fat begins to collect mainly in your abdomen and around your waist.

Diabetic complications

Left untreated, both type I and type II diabetes cause fatigue, weakness and great thirst—and in severe cases blindness, kidney disease, coma and death. Raised blood fats increase the likelihood of heart disease, and nerve damage combined with circulatory problems can lead to foot ulcers and gangrene.

At present the only effective treatment for type I diabetes is insulin replacement. But type II diabetes is entirely a different matter. Here are some natural treatments which according to research can improve insulin resistance and so reverse type II diabetes:

- Losing weight
- Taking exercise—even just walking for half an hour a day—can reduce insulin resistance by up to 40 per cent[113].
- Taking supplements of vitamin E, magnesium, zinc, chromium, vitamin B$_3$, maitake mushroom, carnitine, taurine, coenzyme Q10, lipoic acid, silymarin, fish oil and conjugated linoleic acid (CLA)[115].

Which supplements are best?

Of all these supplements, magnesium, chromium, vitamin B$_3$, maitake and lipoic acid probably have the most significant benefits against insulin resistance, while other supplements may be useful in combating diabetic complications[16,115,216]. At the 57th Annual Scientific Session of the American Diabetes Association meeting in Boston, June 1997, the results of an important study using a chromium supplement were announced. Obese adults with insulin resistance were supplemented with 1,000 mcg chromium per day. After 4 months, insulin resistance was reduced by a highly significant 40 per cent and this dramatic improvement was maintained for 4 months after the supplement was discontinued[18].

Fenugreek seeds, a flavouring used in Indian cookery, can help to reduce blood sugar in diabetics. Take 15 grams of powdered seeds mixed with water after a meal, or add the powder to a curry[116].

A compound found in cinnamon may also help to combat insulin resistance. The US Agricultural Research Service has filed a patent on methylhydroxy chalcone polymer (MHCP), which has been shown to increase glucose metabolism by about 20-fold in a test tube assay[248].

The fact that vitamin and mineral supplements can have such a beneficial effect speaks volumes about the causes of type II diabetes. Supplements have no inherent medicinal effects. They can only cure conditions caused by a failure to consume, absorb or assimilate enough of the nutrients in question. The modern low-vitamin, high-fat, high-sugar diet not only makes us fat but deprives us of the nutrients which our bodies need in order to make and utilize insulin. By improving your diet and following the general nutritional treatment procedures outlined in this book, you have a good chance of improving your type II diabetes and of reducing or coming off your medication—with your doctor's permission of course.

Hypoglycaemia

Hypoglycaemia literally means low blood sugar and is caused by your pancreas "over-shooting the mark" and producing inappropriately large amounts of insulin after a meal. These remove sugar from your blood far too rapidly, causing havoc with your blood sugar control hormones and making you feel faint, nauseous and shaky if you miss a meal. You can also suffer from headaches and depression. Hypoglycaemia turns people into "sugar junkies" - they feel better almost immediately if they consume something sweet because this temporarily reduces their high insulin levels. The problem is that sugar stimulates insulin production, and within a short time their insulin will be high again. I have known people who had such violent mood swings due to the sugar junkie syndrome that they were diagnosed with manic depression.

No-one knows exactly why chronic hypoglycaemia occurs, but nutritional therapists believe that since researchers have found it responds well to supplements of chromium, vitamin B_3, zinc and magnesium in particular, it may be a condition where the body's feedback mechanisms are in some way defective due to nutritional deficiencies, and cannot quickly detect that enough insulin has been produced[217,218].

Of course nutritional therapists do not use these supplements on their own. They recommend a regime of small frequent meals and snacks so that your blood sugar is not allowed to fall too low. It is also very important to avoid consuming sugary food and drinks as well as stimulants such as tea, coffee and alcohol, which make extra demands on insulin as well as on other hormones involved in blood sugar control.

Gall-stones

By storing bile needed for your digestion, your gall bladder helps you to break down your food properly and so to avoid developing nutritional deficiencies. But by middle age, many people (usually women) are admitted into hospital to have their gall bladder removed owing to gall-stones. Now known to be mostly due to a faulty diet containing too much sugar and fat, and too few whole-grain foods, gall-stones are usually an entirely preventable condition. Because they are fibre-rich, the recipes in this book are ideal to help keep your gall bladder healthy.

Beware of complaining too much to your doctor if he/she has diagnosed you with gall bladder disease. If you persist in complaining he will offer you an operation to remove your gall bladder.

Bile needs to be stored so that it can be released at the right time—when you eat fatty food. If you lose your gall bladder, bile drips into your intestines without proper control and at mealtimes there may not be enough present to help you digest fats and oils. These can then coat other foods, hindering their digestion too.

Once you have received your diagnosis, you can go home and try out some nutritional therapy.

A radical new approach

Dr Jonathan Wright—one of the icons of nutritional medicine in the USA—has found that very few instances of gall bladder pain are actually due to gall-stones. In fact he says that the pain is virtually always caused by a food intolerance[6]. What happens is this. If you are intolerant to wheat, for example, or dairy products, or some other food, inflammation will develop in your body when you eat it. If the inflammation tends to be in the blood vessels of your head you may develop migraines. If in your skin, eczema. But if the inflammation is in your bile duct, which is the exit from your gall bladder, the result can be spasmodic pain whenever your gall bladder contracts to allow bile through the duct[6]. It's as simple as that. So please do make sure you carry out the Food Intolerance Test on page 47 and see if the diagnostic diet takes away your gall bladder pain.

Chamomile tea taken double strength is a natural anti-spasmodic (prevents spasms), and is very useful for gall bladder pain, as is the herb wild yam.

A fat-free diet is not the solution. It may appear to help because your gall bladder usually contracts when there is fat or oil in your diet. But it is unhealthy for your gall bladder not to contract. This can cause stagnation of its contents and subsequent inflammation.

Dissolving gall-stones

If an X-ray shows that you do in fact have gall-stones, it may not be necessary to have them removed. Gall-stones can be slowly dissolved over the course of time by daily consumption of fresh lemon juice and dandelion coffee. Supplements of lecithin, the amino acid taurine (1 gram per day) and the herbs silymarin (extract of milk thistle) and barberry also help dissolve gall-stones[219,220]. Silymarin can stimulate your gall bladder to contract, which can cause spasms, so make sure you take it with luke-warm chamomile tea, plus (if necessary) wild yam capsules.

If you are a woman, then eating broccoli and its relatives cabbage, cauliflower and brussels sprouts may also be helpful, since these help the liver to break down oestrogen. Excess oestrogen (especially HRT and the contraceptive pill) is known to encourage gall-stones by reducing the flow of bile from the gall-bladder. This may be why women seem to suffer from this problem so much more than men.

No-one has so far managed to convince me that the old-fashioned olive oil and lemon juice "liver flush" really flushes out gall-stones rather than just creating globules of bile-coloured wax. This involves drinking half a pint of olive oil mixed with the juice of a lemon, followed by a dose of epsom salts. In any case it can be dangerous if a gall-stone becomes dislodged and lodges in your bile duct. The pain is very severe and you could end up needing emergency surgery. Some people have very narrow bile ducts and even small stones could cause this problem.

Hay fever

People with hay fever may believe that nutrition is not relevant to their problem. The sneezing and watery eyes of hay fever sufferers are caused by histamine and inflammation, produced in response to pollens such as ragweed, to which they are sensitive.

In fact, nutrition is very relevant. If you can reduce the amount of histamine produced, you can reduce or eliminate the inflammation. So it's important to cut out any foods in your diet that might also be stimulating your cells to produce too much histamine. How to find out whether any foods are doing this? Test yourself for food intolerances as described on page 47.

Other useful tips for reducing histamine include consuming lots of magnesium– and methionine-rich foods, especially nuts and sunflower seeds, plus oats and leafy greens. Cabbage, onions and apple peel also contain quercetin, a flavonoid with antihistamine effects, so you should do your best to eat these as often as you can. Purple berries, rich in other types of flavonoids, are also anti-inflammatory.

Additional nutrients in the form of supplements can also help reduce histamine, especially calcium, magnesium[118], methionine[117], quercetin[159], high-dose vitamin C[119]. Some people also find supplements of bee pollen very helpful. Bee pollen should be taken starting in early spring.

Heart attacks, strokes, angina, high blood pressure high cholesterol

These have been grouped together because they all form part of the same problem—high cholesterol levels and arteries narrowed by cholesterol deposits. If you are using this book because either you or someone in your family is at risk of, or suffers from, any of these problems, you can feel reassured that medical science fully supports the effectiveness of nutritional therapy in combating them.

Causes of all these problems include:

- Eating a diet lacking in vitamins and minerals, especially B vitamins, magnesium and selenium. This happens when your normal diet is high in convenience foods, fried, fatty or sugary foods, red meat and alcohol.
- Eating too much saturated fat (as in burgers, pastry, cakes and biscuits), which makes your blood sticky, and so prone to forming tiny clots in small blood vessels.
- Not eating enough fresh vegetables, especially leafy greens rich in folic acid, magnesium and carotenes.
- Not eating enough fresh fruit, which is rich in flavonoids that help keep arteries strong and prevent fluid retention (which raises blood pressure).
- Not eating enough fresh nuts and seeds (e.g. sunflower and sesame seeds) which provide essential polyunsaturated oils as well as the amino acid arginine, needed to make nitric oxide. (Nitric oxide helps to keep your blood vessels dilated).
- Smoking and lack of exercise.
- Consuming too much salt, which makes you retain fluid[120]. Fluid retention raises your blood pressure[121,122].
- Eating a lot of sugary food which raises your insulin levels too quickly. The extra insulin raises blood fats, makes you retain sodium and encourages fluid retention and cholesterol deposits on artery walls.
- Diabetics also have an increased risk of developing heart disease.

Heart disease—a collagen problem?

According to the late Linus Pauling, twice a Nobel Prizewinner, heart disease begins as a weakness of the collagen which forms the walls of arteries. The strength of collagen depends on adequate amounts of vitamin C and flavonoids, which of course come from the fruit and vegetables in your diet. Weak collagen in arteries can be damaged by the mechanical stresses of blood flow. Your body tries to repair that damage by incorporating fatty particles of lipoprotein (a) into your artery walls. This attracts cholesterol deposits, which form on the inside of your artery walls, leading to narrowed arteries and a restricted blood flow to your heart muscle[123]. A lack of blood means a lack of oxygen, and although you may not notice a problem while you are resting, over-exertion may start to cause pains in your chest as your heart struggles to get more oxygen. These pains are called angina. Angina is a progressive problem, and medicines from your doctor cannot cure it although they can temporarily slow down your heart and dilate your arteries to relieve some of the distress. There is a price to pay for this—the beta-blocker drugs normally used have side effects such as impotence, memory loss and depression. They can also cause fluid retention, which brings weight gain.

Heart attack or stroke

Unless you do something about your diet, your arteries will usually become progressively more blocked, and if a tiny clot becomes lodged in a part of the artery which is very blocked, this could cut off the blood supply completely. If this occurs in an artery in your brain, you may experience a stroke—part of your brain dies due to the lack of oxygen. If it occurs in the coronary artery of your heart you may experience a heart attack. If the blood flow to your heart resumes, your heart can start beating again, but it is usually damaged and in time can become enlarged and develop congestive failure. Although you can still continue to live for some years, this is a progressively disabling condition which makes you weak and exhausted. Excess fluid can build up, especially in your lungs, causing a chronic cough. This must be treated with diuretics.

Angina sufferers are often offered a bypass operation so that the blood vessels which supply their heart can bypass the most clogged arteries, but do not assume that it will make you feel 100 per cent well again. And unless you do something about your diet, the new arteries will just clog up in a few years. If you have angina, high cholesterol or high blood pressure, the time to do something about it is now. Believe me, you don't want to wait until some real damage occurs.

Your doctor is not likely to tell you all this because it is pretty scary stuff and most people do not want to hear it. But I have never believed in keeping people ignorant of the limitations of conventional medicine.

Some heart attacks are caused by spasms

Not all heart attacks are caused by clogged arteries. Some years ago, there was a story in the press about a young man of 25 who had a heart attack and died. It turned out that he loved milk and drank at least five pints every day, having been told that it was good for him. I also personally know two people—one man aged 22 and another in his fifties, who were rushed to hospital with all the symptoms of a heart attack, but were later told that their arteries were fine and they had probably just had a "panic attack" due to stress. But the people in question had not been under any stress.

If you know where to look in the medical literature, you will find reference to "cardiac spasms" which can be fatal. They are like getting a stitching pain in your chest so severe that you cannot move or breathe. These spasms shut off the blood supply to your heart just like a heart attack, but are brought on by an imbalance between calcium and magnesium. Most people eat a very magnesium-poor diet. If at the same time you consume dairy products, which are very rich in calcium but poor in magnesium, you can aggravate the effects of your magnesium deficiency. The result? Spasms or twitches, irritable nerves and an irregular heartbeat. I have had mild heart spasms myself, in the days before I studied nutrition, when I used to suffer from a magnesium deficiency. They seem to be common. You can avoid getting them by eating magnesium-rich foods every day: fresh vegetables (especially leafy greens), nuts, sunflower seeds, porridge oats, wholemeal bread.

An oil-free diet is not healthy

If you have high blood cholesterol levels or high blood pressure, these foods will also help to bring them down. They work not just by helping you to lose weight, but by nourishing you better. But do not make the mistake of going on an oil-free diet. The oils in nuts and seeds as well as oily fish (salmon, sardines, herrings, mackerel) are very beneficial. Arginine in nuts makes nitric oxide, which helps keep blood vessels dilated and so can in turn help male impotence and other problems linked with artery blockage. Fish oil supplements contain less fish oil than a meal of the fish themselves.

Olive oil is also healthy, and plenty of recipes in this book use it.

Don't underestimate the power of healthy eating to prevent and treat all these health problems. The day is not far away now when your medical insurance will penalize you if you do not eat a heart-protective diet. Hospitals are full of middle-aged men having completely avoidable bypass operations, and some day the Government will get fed up with funding this. Smokers already pay for the costs of their cancer treatments through the high tax on cigarettes, but there is as yet no tax on sugar, crisps, chips, cakes, doughnuts, sweets, cream, chocolate, pastry, sausages, burgers, white bread and biscuits.

Food supplements which can help your heart and arteries

- Conjugated linoleic acid (CLA). Research shows it is an effective inhibitor of the artery-clogging process (atherogenesis) and can help to clear arteries which have already become clogged[124].
- The amino acid lysine, taken at a dose of two grams a day, increases the "slipperiness" of artery walls, thus preventing cholesterol from clinging to them[4].
- Vitamin C taken at a dose of two grams a day helps to strengthen collagen and prevent artery walls from developing structural weaknesses which can attract cholesterol deposits[4].
- According to research, coenzyme Q10 and the amino acids carnitine and taurine can help to reduce the symptoms and extend the life expectancy of people with congestive heart failure.[126,158,221,222,223]
- Vitamin E supplements at extremely high doses (400-800 mg per day) have been used by researchers to help prevent heart attacks. Like fish oil they act

as anticoagulants, so helping to prevent blood clots. I would recommend trying the other supplements in this list first and only adding such a large amount of vitamin E if for some reason your arteries remain blocked. Take it under a doctor's supervision as large doses of vitamin E can raise the blood pressure.

Hepatitis

Hepatitis means "inflammation of the liver". The inflammation is mostly due to a virus infection, but can also be caused by over-exposure to drugs and toxic chemicals.

Viral hepatitis known as the A, B and C types are the most common, but other forms can exist. Hepatitis can also be caused by autoimmunity.

- Hepatitis A is transmitted by contamination of food with faeces.
- Hepatitis B is transmitted through infected blood or blood products, or by sexual contact.
- Hepatitis C is mainly spread by shared needles in intravenous drug use. It has a higher mortality rate than the other types.

Acute viral hepatitis is very debilitating. Most patients recover completely within 16 weeks. But some will go on to suffer from chronic viral hepatitis. Typical signs and symptoms are fatigue, lack of appetite, nausea, fever, weakness and headache, with discomfort or pain in the liver area. Clearly any natural approach to the treatment of chronic hepatitis or to restore health to the liver after hepatitis, should be twofold, and should aim to:

- Combat viruses
- Reduce inflammation.

The most effective anti-viral treatments in nutritional therapy are

- Vitamin C, taken at the rate of 10 grams a day in divided doses[224]
- Selenium supplements, 200 mcg per day[25]
- Boosting glutathione with

  Lipoic acid supplements (100 mg daily)

  Silymarin supplements (140-210mg 3 times daily)

  A cysteine-rich diet including oatmeal and sunflower seeds, soaked overnight to make them more digestible.

In one research study on naturally-occurring flavonoids, published in the journal *Antiviral Research*, quercetin was found to have the most pronounced anti-viral effect[145,250]. Quercetin is also a powerful anti-histamine, and so helps to reduce inflammation[146,147,159]. The best food sources of quercetin are onions, cabbage and apple peel. It may be that French onion soup should replace chicken soup as the cure-all for the 21st century!

Silymarin also helps prevent toxins from entering liver cells and can reverse damage to the liver. Other anti-inflammatory treatments include:

- Powdered liquorice root 1-2g three times daily
- Turmeric 1 teaspoon three times daily
- The juice of purple fruits and berries.

Chamomile tea taken triple strength helps to controls the pain of liver inflammation by relaxing the area and preventing spasm.

Research has also shown benefits from supplements of the maitake and shiitake mushrooms[137,138,264], vitamin B_1 (thiamine)[143], and particularly vitamin E[140,141,148] against hepatitis. Hepatitis B infections are more prevalent in selenium-deprived parts of China[139], and selenium deficiency is thought to encourage the spread of viruses[25,90].

One published report describes three case studies where chronic hepatitis was treated with high-dose lipoic acid, silymarin, coenzyme Q10, selenium, vitamin C, vitamin E and B complex. All these patients had complications such as cirrhosis, portal hypertension, splenomegaly and thrombocytopenia. All recovered sufficiently to return to their jobs or college education[142].

Eat according to the principles of the Basic Healthy Plate on page 26, and particularly avoid "bad" fats. Also see the information on coconut oil on pages 77-78, as the herpes viruses can also cause hepatitis.

Hyperactivity and attention deficit disorder

Hyperactivity—now becoming known as "attention deficit disorder" (ADD) or "attention deficit hyperactivity disorder" (ADHD)—describes children with certain behavioural problems. The recognized symptoms, which may be added up into a "score" for diagnostic purposes, are:

- Restless or overactive
- Excitable, impulsive
- Disturbs other children
- Fails to finish things. Short attention span.
- Constantly fidgeting.
- Inattentive. Easily distracted.
- Demands must be met immediately. Easily frustrated.
- Cries often and easily.
- Mood changes quickly and drastically.
- Temper outbursts. Explosive and unpredictable behaviour.

Hyperactive children sometimes don't sleep at all at night. They may physically attack their parents or others without provocation, or violently destroy other people's property without a second thought. Many are repeatedly in trouble with the police.

Research has found that in hyperactivity, glucose (sugar) metabolism is reduced in the frontal lobe of the brain, which then doesn't work properly[149].

Will your child "grow out of it"?

Statistics show that 40 per cent of hyperactive children eventually "grow out of it", although without psychological counselling to deal with the effects that the illness has left on their lives, problems may still remain. The remaining 60 per cent may grow up disturbed, psychopathic and delinquent.

Not so long ago, doctors used to deny that hyperactivity existed, and simply blamed parents for not bringing their children up in a properly disciplined way. Others blame social factors on disturbed behaviour. But when a drug (Ritalin) was developed to control the symptoms of hyperactivity, diagnosing the disease rapidly become much more popular, and in the UK prescriptions have doubled every year from 4,000 in 1994 up to a record high of nearly 158,000 in 1999. In the USA more than 4 million children are on Ritalin, including some as young as one year old. In some classrooms up to 40 per cent of children are on the drug, which is a type of amphetamine. It is not a cure for the disease.

Despite Ritalin's side effects and the potential long-term damage which all drugs are capable of causing, very few doctors are prepared to use treatments based on nutritional research. Yet some of the research studies show clearly that hyperactivity statistics could be dramatically reduced with nutritional therapy.

1985 research study—Institute of Child Health, London

In 1985, Egger and colleagues at the Institute of Child Health, London, gave 72 hyperactive children a hypoallergenic diet (low in foods likely to cause allergic reactions). 62 improved and 21 of these achieved normal behaviour. 28 of the children were then given foods previously excluded. Hyperactivity symptoms returned much more frequently in these children than in others given a placebo (inert substance). Artificial colourings and preservatives provoked reactions most frequently, but no child was sensitive to these alone[150].

1989 research study—Kaplan and colleagues

In 1989, Kaplan and colleagues gave 24 preschool-age hyperactive boys a baseline diet and then randomly assigned them to either a placebo (control) diet for three weeks or an experimental diet for four weeks. This experimental diet was free from added sugar, artificial colouring and flavouring, chocolate, MSG, preservatives and caffeine, as well as any food which the family said affected their child. Parents recorded a 58 per cent improvement among the children on the experimental diet but little improvement in the placebo group[151].

1992 research study—National Society for Research into Allergy

In 1992, the National Society for Research into Allergy (UK), working with Superintendent Peter Bennett of the West Yorkshire Police, carried out a study on ten random habitual young offenders with an average age of 11 years. Most were destined for institutional care. On psychological testing, every child was found to be hyperactive. On nutritional testing, all the children were found to be very low in zinc. Some also had manganese and chromium deficiencies.

The children were given a diagnostic diet, low in all the foods which allergic people most commonly react to. Foods were then reintroduced one by one into the diet to see if a relapse would occur. If it did, that food was then excluded permanently.

All the eight children who finished the programme responded to the diet with a dramatic reduction in their behavioural problems. Six months later, five of the children still remained free of problems. At the same time, the rates of shoplifting, car theft and criminal damage in Shipley dropped by up to 50 per cent. These five children (who lived in Shipley) had in fact been responsible for a large proportion of the local crime statistics[152].

1994 research study—Annals of Allergy

In 1994, the journal *Annals of Allergy* reported that the hyperactivity ratings of 19 out of 26 hyperactive children given a diet excluding wheat, corn, yeast, soy, citrus, egg, chocolate, peanuts, and artificial colours and flavours, dropped from an average of 25 to an average of eight[153].

Nutritional deficiencies

Hyperactive children have also been found to have nutritional deficiencies, especially zinc, chromium, manganese, essential fatty acids and B vitamins[28,154,155,156,157]. Their bodies may also contain excessive levels of copper and elevated levels of the toxic metals lead and cadmium. A lack of stomach acid and digestive enzymes is common, and so is a Candida albicans overgrowth in their intestines.

The Feingold diet, which is sometimes prescribed for hyperactive children, is based on avoiding caffeine, food colourings and other additives as well as salicylates—found in aspirin and as naturally occurring in quite a wide variety of fruits and other foods. Salicylates can block the production of prostaglandins, which are made from the essential polyunsaturated oils in our diet. Avoiding all salicylates leads to a very restrictive diet. Now that we can give children evening primrose oil and other supplements to help with the production of prostaglandins, it is probably no longer necessary. Along with chromium, zinc and B vitamins, evening primrose oil can be very useful for the treatment of hyperactive children[28].

Side effects of Ritalin

The *British National Formulary* (the standard doctor's drug handbook) warns doctors to: *Monitor height and weight as growth retardation may occur during prolonged therapy.* Other side effects include *insomnia, restlessness, irritability and excitability, nervousness, night terrors, euphoria, tremor, dizziness, headache, convulsions, addiction, sometimes psychosis, anorexia, tummy and digestive problems, dry mouth, sweating, heart pains, heart damage, abnormal heartbeat, palpitations, increased blood pressure, visual disturbances, skin rash, fever, joint pains, hair loss, abnormal liver function. Also tics and Tourette syndrome in susceptible children.*

Infertility

Before you opt for expensive fertility clinics, why not consider some of the research which shows how faulty nutrition can affect sperm counts and cause miscarriages? No-one has told you about it? That's because nutritional measures come under "self-help". You're assumed to have already done everything to ensure that you are in the best of health.

Some factors known to cause a low sperm count or weak sperm which cannot swim well:

- Selenium, zinc or vitamin C deficiency from eating a faulty diet[163,164].
- Excess alcohol and caffeine consumption[165,166,167].
- Smoking.
- Environmental oestrogens (toxins in the environment which can mimic female hormones)[168,190,191,192].
- Up to 50 per cent of miscarriages are due to the male partner—i.e. to sperm defects which prevent the embryo from developing normally, as demonstrated by Swedish research[160].

Similar nutritional and lifestyle imbalances can affect women's fertility. For instance women who miscarry are often found to have significantly lower than normal selenium levels. Women can also be infertile if they are very overweight or underweight.

Anorexia, PCOS, endometriosis

I have treated several women who had stopped ovulating due to anorexia nervosa. Once they began eating normal amounts of protein again, their menstrual periods only took a few months to come back. To help them along I also prescribed zinc and vitamin A supplements, since both these nutrients are needed to help make hormones.

Another cause of infertility is polycystic ovary syndrome (PCOS). About 50 per cent of women with this condition suffer from excessively high insulin levels—an imbalance which can be linked to a faulty diet (see page 85). The extra insulin stimulates the PCOS sufferer's ovaries to make testosterone, which suppresses ovulation[112]. Insulin levels can be reduced by correcting the diet and nutrient levels in accordance with the general principles in this book. As testosterone drops, periods can return to normal.

Endometriosis can also cause infertility and can be treated with nutritional therapy. See pages 112 for more information.

Inflammatory bowel diseases

Crohn's disease and ulcerative colitis

Inflammatory bowel diseases—serious chronic diarrhoea conditions associated with intestinal inflammation and damage—are well-named. In orthodox medicine they are treated with anti-inflammatory drugs. But what causes the inflammation? We should not overlook the obvious. The bowel contains the remains of food, and also contains a very large number of bacteria and other micro-organisms—in fact several hundred species.

Now it is a known fact that Crohn's disease often goes temporarily into remission if the patient takes antibiotics which kill these bacteria. It is also known that a diet high in sugar and refined carbohydrates can exacerbate the disease[170]. In a 1981 clinical trial carried out by German researchers, 20 patients with Crohn's disease were given either a diet excluding refined sugar, or a sugar-rich diet. In the most severe cases, the sugar-free diet reduced the severity of the disease whereas the sugar-rich diet increased it[169].

Poor eating habits encourage Crohn's

In 1979 the *British Medical Journal* reported a study of the diets of 30 patients with Crohn's disease compared with 30 controls (people who did not have the disease). The Crohn's patients consumed more than twice as much sugar and only a quarter as much raw fruit and vegetables a day as the controls[170].

As you know, dysbiosis—an excess of inflammation-promoting bacteria and other micro-organisms in your intestines—is an important cause of gut problems. Sugar consumption helps to stimulate the growth of these micro-organisms, but sadly, most doctors are not advising low-sugar diets. Yet they certainly know that dysbiosis contributes to Crohn's, since many of them prescribe antibiotics to treat it. Antibiotics temporarily destroy most of your gut bacteria, good and bad, therefore they can give temporary relief from inflammation caused by bacterial-type dysbiosis although in time they will encourage fungal-type dysbiosis from Candida albicans and other harmful yeasts.

As we saw in Part II, dysbiosis is a resistant problem and requires a vigorous approach, especially cutting carbohydrate consumption. Inflamed intestines cannot produce the enzymes required to complete the digestion of sugars and carbohydrates. The resulting undigested particles are simply seized and consumed by the inflammatory bacteria and yeasts, helping them to thrive uncontrolled. To combat this, the Intestinal Healing Programme on pages 50-51 is recommended for all sufferers of inflammatory bowel disease.

Food intolerances are also a cause of intestinal inflammation. Cutting out the worst problem foods can make a big difference to inflammatory bowel disease.

Parasitic infections can mimic Crohn's and ulcerative colitis

Some parasitic infections such as Blastocystis hominis, Cryptosporidium, and Giardia lamblia can mimic Crohn's disease and ulcerative colitis, and are easily missed by doctors. If you believe that your problems may perhaps have started after a holiday abroad, do press your doctor for tests. Some herbal medicines—especially Artemisia annua, quassia and golden seal—can combat these parasites, so if you are not satisfied with the test results, you could add them to your Intestinal Healing Programme. Do not take golden seal during pregnancy.

The medical literature describes an interesting case where an ulcerative colitis sufferer treated herself with two capsules of the pineapple enzyme bromelain at each meal. Her disease went completely into remission and her colon appeared to be completely healed[249].

Irritable bowel syndrome

This is a term used by doctors for any combination of
- Bloating
- Flatulence
- Pain or discomfort
- Diarrhoea and/or constipation (alternating)

when no serious disease is present. The treatment consists of helping you to cope with these symptoms.

Causes of IBS

- Stress
- Food intolerances
- Dysbiosis

- Undiagnosed parasitic infections, especially if you developed symptoms after a trip abroad.

If you believe that stress is not the main cause in your case, carry out the Food Intolerance Test on page 47 to see if any foods are responsible. If not, you may benefit from the Intestinal Healing Programme on pages 50-51.

Kidney problems

Kidney stones usually occur when abnormal calcium deposits form in the kidneys. Research shows that over-consumption of sugar[290] and deficiencies of magnesium and vitamin B6 can considerably increase your risk of getting them. In one research study, 16 kidney stone sufferers were given supplements of magnesium and vitamin B6. Their excretion of oxalate fell, indicating a significant decrease in kidney stone risk[289].

Another common type of kidney disease is nephrotic syndrome—an inflammation of the kidneys. One French researcher finds that in many cases the inflammation is caused by nothing other than food intolerances[291].

Due to their arginine content, nuts are a beneficial food for the kidneys[292]. Too much sugary, fatty food encourages kidney problems[295].

Migraine and headaches

In my experience, the main cause of these is food intolerances, often aggravated by a spinal alignment problem. If your doctor can identify no other cause, a course of chiropractic adjustments, together with carrying out the Food Intolerance Test on page 47 and avoiding problem foods, may turn out to be a permanent answer to this distressing problem. Coffee is often a big culprit. I get a bad headache as a withdrawal symptom about 24 hours after cutting coffee out of my diet. Other people get headaches when they have had too much coffee to drink.

Try both types of chiropractic: conventional first, followed by McTimoney, since they work in different ways.

If you have other symptoms apart from migraine or headaches, this simple approach may not be enough to help you. In that case you should complete the questionnaire on pages 21-22 and turn to the relevant sections depending on your scores.

Osteoporosis

This is the brittle bone disease which women are prone to develop after the menopause. Causes include:

- Not getting enough magnesium and other minerals in your diet. Calcium alone is not enough to prevent osteoporosis—research shows that magnesium, zinc and other minerals are needed too. Magnesium helps your bones to retain calcium[15,171].
- A lack of exercise.
- A lack of vitamin D, found in oily fish and cod liver oil and formed by the action of sunlight on your skin.
- A lack of vitamin K, which is found in fresh vegetables such as broccoli, brussels sprouts, cauliflower and cabbage[172].
- High levels of homocysteine, caused by a lack of vitamins B_6, B_{12} and folic acid in the diet.
- Too much salt, sugar, protein, and phosphorus-containing food additives, especially those in soft drinks[15].

Don't take HRT—go to a gym!

Beware of hormone replacement therapy. It only protects you while you take it, while at the same time increasing your risk of getting certain cancers. It is also highly addictive. Once you start taking it, it is very difficult to stop because of withdrawal symptoms in the form of severe hot flushes. If you want to come off HRT, do so by very slowly reducing the dose over a period of about one year.

In 1994 the *Journal of the American Medical Association* reported the results of a study on postmenopausal women who underwent a strength training programme. Strength training is usually carried out in a gym. It is similar to body-building except that it does not aim to create a muscular physique but simply to increase physical strength. In this study, osteoporosis was actually reversed, as the women's bone density was increased by the strength training exercises[173]. Exercise really is the best way to halt osteoporosis and to begin restoring density to bones. At the same time a mineral-rich diet is also important. Mineral assimilation problems may be present. In a study reported in the *Journal of Nutritional Medicine* in 1991, vitamin and mineral supplements which particularly emphasized magnesium were found to be 16 times more effective in the treatment of osteoporosis than dietary advice alone[15].

Barbara: a case of
high blood pressure in pregnancy

Barbara consulted me in 1992 when she was seven months pregnant. She was aged 23 and a vegetarian, and it was her first baby.

She came somewhat reluctantly, at the instigation of her mother-in-law, because food was frankly a problem. Her appetite was so poor that she only ate foods for their taste, not from hunger. While the rest of the family had a complete meal, she might pick only at a piece of cheesecake.

Barbara was badly anaemic. Her haemoglobin levels had been progressively dropping since the early stages of pregnancy, despite increasing doses of iron prescribed by her GP and then by the hospital she attended. By the time she consulted me, her skin was extremely pale, and the anaemia was giving her severe fluid retention, especially in her legs. The extra fluid was in turn pushing Barbara's blood pressure sky high—a condition known as pre-eclampsia—and both Barbara and the baby were at risk. Barbara agreed to see me because her doctor wanted to keep her in hospital in order to give her iron injections. She had refused this, and was desperately seeking alternatives.

Barbara's diet history was problematic, with a lot of fat, white bread, chocolate, crisps and biscuits. She had received counselling about iron-rich foods recently from a hospital dietician, but told me that she couldn't follow the advice because she had no appetite.

In taking Barbara's history, I found that she also suffered from permanent sores inside her nose, and that during the first three months of her pregnancy she had felt nauseous 24 hours a day. In my opinion, these symptoms plus the anaemia and fluid retention pointed to quite a severe zinc deficiency. Her diet excluded meat and fish, from which most people get their zinc, and was also lacking in whole-grains, which are a vegetarian source of zinc.

To make matters worse, both iron and folic acid supplements can interfere with the absorption of zinc from food[161,162], yet Barbara's GP was prescribing very large amounts of both.

I believed that Barbara was anaemic because she was zinc deficient, so I asked her to obtain permission from her doctor to stop the supplements. I gave her multivitamins and minerals plus zinc, and also gave her some nutritional counselling.

To her doctor's amazement, Barbara's haemoglobin levels started to rise within days. She went on to produce a healthy baby.

Pregnancy-related problems

Including morning sickness, pre-eclampsia and birth defects

No-one seems to be very clear about what causes "morning sickness" in pregnancy. This can be quite severe; some pregnant women feel nauseous all day and lose a great deal of weight.

Most nutritional medicine experts seem to agree that vitamin B_6 supplements can help this condition. Based on research, there is also broad agreement that taking capsules of powdered ginger is also helpful. (Making tea with boiling water and fresh grated ginger is probably just as good.) But sometimes these two treatments are not enough.

Until the early 1990s, nutritional therapists used to prescribe vitamin B_6 plus folic acid, iron and zinc, because all these nutrients are needed for growth, and all can be depleted by pregnancy. But no-one really knows whether the same degree of morning sickness relief could have been achieved with vitamin B_6 on its own. Nowadays most doctors prescribe quite large amounts of folic acid, and may also prescribe iron to prevent anaemia in pregnancy. This happened in one case which I treated in 1992 (see page 102). This lady turned out to be extremely zinc-deficient, and I suspect that if she had been given zinc supplements in early pregnancy, together with vitamin B_6 supplements, her nausea would have been much less severe. French research reported in 1990 has found that on the basis of low zinc levels found in serum, hair and white blood cells, women need at least 5 mg more zinc per day than normal. The researchers believe that the risk of deficiency is real and is associated with miscarriage, toxaemia of pregnancy, treatment-resistant anaemia, abnormally prolonged pregnancy and difficult delivery. In babies it is leads to decreased immunity, learning or memory problems or birth defects.[175]

Broccoli juice for morning sickness

Dr Jonathan Wright, who is a very well-known nutritional doctor in the USA, says that if all else fails to help morning sickness, try a combination of vitamin C and vitamin K supplements. In one study carried out in the 1950s by Dr Richard Merkel it helped 64 out of 70 cases, with complete relief of symptoms in three days[225]. If you don't want to take (or can't find) vitamin K supplements, try making raw broccoli and cabbage juice with a juice extractor and drink that every day. Green vegetables are very rich in vitamin K.

The case of Barbara on page 102 is about high blood pressure in pregnancy, a dangerous condition known as pre-eclampsia. In Barbara's case it was caused by zinc-deficiency anaemia, made worse by her doctor's high-dose folic acid and iron supplements[161,162]. Severe anaemia can result in fluid retention, which in turn raises the blood pressure. But other cases respond to large doses of magnesium supplements, and since 1995 this has been one of the standard medical treatments for this condition.

Multivitamins prevent facial deformities

Birth defects sadly affect thousands of babies every year, and range from the terrible spina bifida, where the baby's brain and spinal cord are not properly developed, to mental retardation and facial deformities such as cleft lip.

What is even more sad is the appalling lack of research examining the association between birth defects and the mother's eating habits before and during pregnancy. Research is extremely scanty, which means that people who try to make this connection are told that there is "no evidence" to support it.

In 1995, however, the *Lancet* medical journal did publish a study comparing the use of multivitamins between 731 mothers of babies born with a facial cleft or cleft lip or palate, and 734 mothers with non-malformed babies. It was found that the mothers who took multivitamins before and during pregnancy reduced the risk of their babies being born with this type of deformity by 25 to 30 per cent[176].

One thing is now very clear, and that is the connection between folic acid deficiency and spina bifida. GPs now routinely prescribe folic acid supplements or multivitamins to pregnant women. But other nutrients are also needed for growth and development, and neither zinc nor selenium, for example, are routinely supplemented although they are at risk of being deficient in many women's diets[91,174,175].

Prostate enlargement

This is a problem which can affect men from middle age onwards. It can respond very well to natural treatments and many men see results within six months.

The enlargement of the prostate gland causes difficulty with bladder emptying. Sufferers often have to get up several times every night to urinate. The problem seems to be associated with:

- Not getting enough zinc from food.
- Eating too much saturated fat from red meat, sausages, pastry, cakes, biscuits etc., and not enough essential polyunsaturated oils from nuts and seeds.
- Pumpkin seeds are rich in zinc and oils, and have a very good reputation for reducing prostate problems. Sunflower seeds and Brazil nuts also contain many beneficial nutrients. Daily consumption of flax seed oil is also helpful[6].
- Also recommended are 15 mg zinc per day in supplemental form[226], plus the

herbs Saw Palmetto, Pygeum africanum and horsetail, and the rye pollen extract Cernilton, which has been prescribed in Sweden for many years[178,179].

German doctors prefer herbs to drugs

If you thought that natural products weren't powerful enough to help medical conditions, think again. In Germany up to 90% of all patients with this condition are treated with herbal products by their doctor. 50% of German urology specialists prefer to prescribe herbal treatments rather than pharmaceutical drugs. In Italy, herbal extracts represent 49% of all medicines prescribed for enlarged prostate[178].

Occasionally an enlarged prostate can turn into prostate cancer. Research shows that the following foods in particular can help to prevent this:

- Soya products: soya milk, tofu, soya flour, soy sauce and miso[227]
- Tomatoes and foods flavoured with tomato purée[79]
- Selenium supplements[180].

The toxic metal cadmium, which may be high in the prostate of smokers, is a risk factor for prostate cancer. One reason why it is important to maintain adequate zinc and selenium levels in your blood is that both help to displace cadmium[177,180].

Schizophrenia

We have already looked at some of the physical causes of this devastating mental illness on pages 39-40. Dr Abram Hoffer believes that schizophrenia is a disease involving extremely poor assimilation of vitamin B_3 and treats it with 3 grams of a vitamin B_3 supplement per day plus several grams of vitamin C. Others physical causes suggested by nutritional research include deficiencies of vitamins C, B_1, and/or B_6, folic acid and zinc, food allergy, gut dysfunction (e.g. schizophrenia associated with coeliac disease), histamine imbalances, heavy metal poisoning, abnormal essential fatty acid metabolism, and starvation[231-238]. While research shows that these factors should be tested for in those suffering from schizophrenia, they rarely are. Starvation or malnutrition leading to schizophrenia may even occur before birth[239-241].

Dr Abram Hoffer

This world-renowned Canadian psychiatrist who specializes in the treatment of schizophrenia with megadoses of vitamin B_3, first discovered that individuals with the most lengthy and most severe deficiencies of this nutrient tend to need much larger amounts of it than normal in order to recover from the mental effects of the deficiency. Some schizophrenia sufferers need fifty times or more the RDA of vitamin B_3 in order to become well and to stay symptom-free. Dr Hoffer's work with ex-prisoners of war from Japanese World War II prison camps who had suffered near-death from starvation led him to make this discovery. He believes that schizophrenia is mostly a form of pellagra—the vitamin B_3 deficiency disease which was believed to have died out in the 1930s in the western world.

Heavy Metal Toxicity

Mental function may be disturbed by heavy metal toxicity, which was well known as a cause of mental illness in times when mercury, for instance, was used to treat syphilis[242].

Dr Carl Pfeiffer (see below) has found that many cases of schizophrenia are associated with a heavy metal overload, including not just mercury but also lead, copper and cadmium[110]. Lead toxicity is known to be linked with excessive levels of aggression[243]. Coriander leaf can help remove heavy metals from the body[252].

Dr Carl Pfeiffer

No discussion of schizophrenia would be complete without mention of the late Dr Carl Pfeiffer, founder of the Brain Bio Center in New Jersey, USA. Dr Pfeiffer identified the following major types of schizophrenia.

Low histamine

Mental symptoms due to a lack of the neurotransmitter histamine in the body, often in association with a copper overload. The low histamine type is not prone to allergies, there is a high pain threshold and the sex drive tends to be on the low side. Treatment requires folic acid and vitamin B_{12} supplementation, and the clearance of excessive copper levels using copper-antagonists such as zinc[108].

High histamine

Mental symptoms due to an excess of the neurotransmitter histamine in the body. The high histamine type is active and often obsessive, prone to allergies, the sex drive is high, the pain threshold is low, a form of agitated depression is common and the patient has a fast metabolism and usually feels warm. Treatment requires large doses of calcium and methionine. Avoid supplements containing folic acid[109]. Quercetin (found in onions and cabbage), magnesium and high doses of vitamin C can also help to reduce histamine.

Food allergy

Mental symptoms due to the consumption of a food to which the individual is sensitive. For instance, gluten sensitivity is well known to be associated with mental symptoms. Treatment requires the initial avoidance of problem foods, followed by attention to the gut, liver and digestive dysfunctions which led to the development of the food sensitivities[109].

Pyroluria

Mental symptoms due to an excessive need for vitamin B_6 and zinc to a degree which cannot be met by the diet. Treatment requires large amounts of both nutrients in supplement form. Porphyria (the mental illness from which King George III suffered) is also associated with a severe zinc deficiency[109].

Mangangese deficiency can also promote schizophrenia[110]. And some very interesting recent research into schizophrenia is getting good results using fish oils[234-239].

Of course someone who has suffered mental symptoms for a long time will have developed behaviour patterns that are very difficult to eradicate. And as Dr Hoffer points out, stress also plays a large part in the development of mental illness. Nutritional therapy for mental illness is always best carried out under the supervision of a sympathetic psychiatrist. Other therapies that have a calming nature—particularly homoeopathy, flower remedies, healing, aromatherapy massage, meditation and certain types of psychological therapy aimed at reducing negative thoughts may also be beneficial.

Skin problems

Including acne (spots), eczema, psoriasis

It should come as no surprise that if you need plenty of vitamin A, zinc, B vitamins, vitamin C and other vitamins and minerals to keep your skin healthy, then if you don't get enough of these you are likely to have a problem skin!

Nutritional deficiencies—especially zinc and vitamin A—are a big cause of acne and spotty skin, even in teenagers—it's not a purely hormonal problem. Although spots are often blamed on fatty food, and it is true that fats can clog up your pores, don't forget that fatty foods (like sugary ones) tend to be high in calories and low in vitamins and minerals, and thus cause nutritional deficiencies.

Eczema can also be caused by nutritional deficiencies, but is more often linked to food intolerances, so do carry out the test on page 47 if you suffer from it.

Although there seems to be a lack of research in this respect, I would attribute psoriasis mostly to nutritional deficiencies such as a lack of essential fatty acids[182], and an overloaded liver. Alcohol almost always aggravates psoriasis because it stresses the liver. The Liver Rejuvenation Programme on page 61 will probably help you.

Sallow skin is also linked with an overloaded liver, combined with lack of oxygen due to smoking or lack of exercise, and dehydration due to drinking too much tea, coffee and alcohol and too little water.

Thyroid disorders

Your thyroid gland is responsible for governing your metabolism; low thyroid function (hypothyroidism) causes fatigue, weight gain, coldness and sometimes hair loss. Your thyroid gland needs a variety of nutrients, including vitamin A, zinc, the amino acid tyrosine and the mineral iodine to help it make the main thyroid hormones (known as T3 and T4) plus selenium, copper and iron to help convert T4 to the more active T3. Iron deficiency is extremely common, especially in women with heavy menstrual periods. In a study carried out at Pennsylvania State University in 1990, ten women with iron deficiency anaemia were compared to 12 women with normal iron levels. They were found to have lower body temperatures and lower levels of thyroid hormones. After receiving iron supplements for 12 weeks, the women's body temperatures increased and their thyroid hormone levels returned to near normal[181].

The presence of one mineral deficiency often suggests that other mineral deficiencies are also present, so supplements of zinc, copper and selenium as well as iron might have worked even better in this study. Vitamin B_1 deficiency also affects the thyroid gland and can cause irreversible damage.

When trying to boost levels of specific minerals, do not take them together, as they often compete with each other for absorption and can cancel each other out.

Fluoride is a thyroid toxin

Beware of giving fluoride supplements to children, or allowing them to swallow toothpaste containing fluoride. Fluoride inactivates iodine and so can cause hypothyroidism. Some have even linked it with thyroid cancer and many action groups are calling for the banning of artificial water fluoridation.

Some foods have pronounced anti-thyroid effects, especially the meat substitutes textured vegetable (soya) protein and soya protein isolate. Other soya products such as soya milk and tofu can be occasionally consumed in smallish amounts. The same goes for raw cabbage and peanuts.

Occasionally the functioning of the thyroid gland is impaired by a food intolerance. You may benefit from carrying out the food intolerance test on page 47.

Your thyroid and insulin

If you continue to suffer from coldness and fatigue despite at least six months of eating a good diet and getting enough vitamins and minerals, plus taking tyrosine supplements (1,000-2,000 mg per day) your thyroid may not be the main problem. Low blood sugar and chronically high insulin levels due to insulin resistance may be affecting your thyroid and also your mitochondria—the part of your cells which generates heat. Once your blood sugar is properly balanced, your body temperature may normalize. Nutritional deficiencies such as chromium, essential fatty acids and magnesium encourage insulin resistance[18,115,216]. See pages 85-87 for further information.

Hypothyroid people may lack the ability to convert beta carotene to vitamin A, so if you suffer from hypothyroidism you should eat some liver occasionally or take vitamin A supplements to prevent a deficiency.

Oestrogen and iodine

Hypothyroidism seems to be common in breast cancer sufferers. There are two likely reasons for this. First, breast cancer is often caused by excessively high oestrogen levels, which are due to sluggish liver function[38]. High oestrogen makes your body produce abnormally large amounts of a protein known as thyroxine-binding globulin (TBG). Its job is to reduce the effects of thyroxine—your main thyroid hormone. Unless your thyroid can produce more thyroxine to overcome the increased amounts of TBG, you can become deficient in thyroxine—i.e. hypothyroid[280].

Second, iodine deficiency seems to have both a depressive effect on thyroxine and a stimulatory effect on oestrogen[19], which leads to the same problem. You can raise your iodine intake by eating fish several times a week or by taking kelp tablets or adding a little seaweed (available in health food shops) to soup. Many Japanese foods, such as powdered miso soup, contain some seaweed.

In the UK table salt no longer contains iodine, although there is a small amount in sea salt. Don't go overboard with the iodine—some people believe they can't have too much of a good thing and have taken dozens of kelp tablets a day thinking they are helping their thyroid gland. They are not. Consuming this much iodine can actually damage it.

Hypothyroidism is sometimes caused by autoimmunity. This is when damage to your thyroid's cells—in some cases due to chemical pollutants—makes these cells look so abnormal that your immune system starts to see them as alien and attacks and destroys them. The Liver Rejuvenation Programme on page 61 will help to detoxify your body and reduce any autoimmune problems caused by pollution.

Eat more radishes

John Heinerman is a medical anthropologist who has researched the medicinal use of foods and herbs around the world. In his *Encyclopedia of Healing Juices* he reports what he learned during a 1979 visit with medical experts at the Soviet Academy of Sciences. Raphanin, the main sulphur component in radishes, is good at helping to keep the hormones thyroxine and calcitonin in normal balance. With enough raphanin circulating in the blood through the daily consumption of radishes or a small amount of radish juice, the thyroid is helped not to under- or over-produce these two hormones.

Hyperthyroidism is a much less common condition. There is little specific information on nutrition with reference to hyperthyroidism, so you should follow the general principles of nutritional therapy as outlined in Parts I and II of this book, not forgetting radish juice. You may also want to consider trying some other therapies which can have a calming effect, such as meditation, acupuncture and homoeopathy. Orthodox medical treatment consists of reducing secretions from your thyroid gland by destroying part of the gland with radioactive iodine.

Women's hormonal problems

Including period pains, heavy menstruation, premenstrual syndrome, menopausal hot flushes, breast lumps

These are mainly due to dietary imbalances: a lack of fruit, vegetables, whole-grains and other vitamin– and mineral-rich food. Medical research has found that these problems often respond to supplements of B vitamins, zinc, magnesium, and fatty acids from evening primrose oil or fish oil[183,184185,186], which suggests that hormonal problems are linked to nutritional deficiencies.

Period pains are a type of cramp or spasm, which suggests a lack of magnesium. I used to suffer from them very badly until I began to study nutrition and to eat porridge and wholemeal bread (rich in magnesium and B vitamins) instead of white bread. That and plenty of exercise (walking) was all I needed to be completely free of them, and it just took a few months.

Eat orange peel for heavy periods

Heavy menstruation can be a sign of high oestrogen levels. It can also be caused by fibroids or other problems which can be diagnosed by your doctor. But if you also bruise easily, your heavy periods may partly be due to have weak blood vessels which bleed easily. Weak blood vessels mean you are not getting enough flavonoids and vitamin C-rich food in your diet, and need to eat far more fruit and vegetables[228,229].

A lot of flavonoids are found in the pith and peel of citrus fruit. One of my patients was quite happy to eat whole oranges, including pith and peel, in order to cure her heavy periods. She was indeed cured within a few months. It is not necessary to go to extremes—just leave plenty of white pith on an orange when you eat it, and you can get similar results. There is also citrus peel in marmalade and in "mixed peel" products used to make cakes. The flavonoids in the skins of dark-coloured berries such as bilberries, blueberries, blackberries and black grapes can also help to keep your blood vessels strong. Supplements of the herb ginkgo biloba have a similar effect.

Millions of women have experienced the discomfort of swollen, painful breasts and bloated tummies around the time of their period. These symptoms are due to fluid retention. If you suffer from them, you will very likely notice that your body weight goes down soon after your period starts.

Writing in the *Journal of Reproductive Medicine*, nutrition specialist Dr Guy Abraham is sure that premenstrual fluid retention is linked with temporary deficiencies of vitamin B_6 and the mineral magnesium, brought on by the extra nutritional demands on a woman's body as her hormone levels change during the menstrual cycle[183]. Oestrogen levels keep rising until ovulation, after which the woman must make more progesterone while her liver breaks down the oestrogen. All these processes make heavy use of many nutrients. Since vitamin B_6 plays a vital role it risks getting quite depleted at certain times, especially if your diet is low in whole-grain foods. You need both B_6 and magnesium to help you produce dopamine and prostaglandins, substances closely involved in controlling your fluid balance. Evening primrose oil (GLA) supplements can also be useful because they help to produce these prostaglandins.

Leaky blood vessels and PMS

Leaky blood vessels due to a B vitamin deficiency and a flavonoid deficiency (a lack of whole-grains, fruit and vegetables) can aggravate premenstrual fluid retention[228]. Protein leaks into your tissues, attracting water from your blood. As your blood volume is reduced, your body tries to replenish it by making you thirsty. It does this by producing the hormone aldosterone which stops you excreting sodium. The higher your sodium levels rise, the more you want to drink.

Medical journals have published various research studies reporting that giving vitamin B_6 supplements to women with premenstrual syndrome can prevent their symptoms: the *Journal of International Medical Research* and the *Lancet* in 1985[184,189], the *Journal of Reproductive Medicine* in 1987[185], and the *Journal of the Royal College of General Practitioners* in 1989[186], among others[188]. But success using this approach has been variable, which is not surprising, and prevents doctors from taking much notice of the nutrition connection. I hope that by now you are beginning to realize that researchers who assume all women with PMS have only one nutritional deficiency are using a hit or miss approach. If the results of all the research studies are merged together they could show roughly how many cases are due *mainly* to vitamin B_6 deficiency and how many are not.

Oestrogen overload

An imbalance in the ideal ratio of oestrogen to progesterone during the premenstrual phase can cause mood changes: anxiety, emotional instability, irritability or even aggression. Again this is linked with nutrition.

As already mentioned, premenstrual mood changes, breast lumps, cysts and tumours, fibroids and endometriosis are problems due to an oestrogen overload—all are medically treated by artificially reducing oestrogen. For instance breast tumours are often treated with the anti-oestrogen drug tamoxifen, and endometriosis symptoms are treated with drugs that inhibit the menstrual cycle, or by removal of the ovaries (which of course produce oestrogen). Another cause of breast lumps is sensitivity to natural chemicals (called methylxanthines) in chocolate and coffee. Researchers have found that breast lumps often disappear when women stop consuming these items.

How to combat high oestrogen

B vitamins (found in whole-grain foods) and indoles found in the brassica family of vegetables (broccoli, cabbage, cauliflower and brussels sprouts) help your liver to break down excess oestrogen, and these foods are useful aids to the treatment of all these conditions[38,39,40,187]. Soya foods contain isoflavones which can bind to excess oestrogen, helping to neutralize its effects[80]. I have come across at least one case where endometriosis was cured and the patient conceived and went on to produce a healthy baby after she started to consume half a litre a day of soya milk. Soya milk can be used to make delicious porridge and rice pudding—you do not have to drink it on its own if you do not like the taste.

Another cause of high oestrogen levels can be iodine deficiency, since this stimulates the sex glands[19].

A deficiency of dietary fibre allows oestrogens found in bile to be reabsorbed from a woman's intestines instead of being excreted in her stools. High levels of fat in your diet (from deep-fried food, pastry, cakes, biscuits, chocolate etc.) also tend to alter hormone balance, and so the general effect of the western diet as a whole is to raise levels of circulating oestrogens. Not all oestrogen is made in your own body. Some major environmental pollutants such as organochlorine pesticides are "oestrogen mimics", with oestrogenic effects thousands of times greater than the real hormone[168,190,191,192]. Dioxins can also affect the hormone system.

Hot flushes may not be a low oestrogen problem

Finally, the menopause. Because oestrogen can be used to treat menopausal symptoms, it is widely believed that the hot flushes of menopause are caused by reduced oestrogen levels due to ovulation having ceased. But as some American scientists are beginning to point out, this does not make sense. Some of the most notorious health problems suffered by post-menopausal women—breast cancer and fibroids—are due not to a lack of oestrogen but to an oestrogen excess. In fact they can be treated by anti-oestrogen drugs. Hot flushes can of course coexist with fibroids in the same menopausal woman, so how can they be caused by a lack of oestrogen?

If you have suffered from hot flushes, you know that they can be brought on by any slightly stressful thought. Your adrenal glands are responsible for producing stress-related hormones such as cortisol. The new scientific theory is that hormonal fluctuations involving several glands set off hot flushes rather than a lack of oestrogen alone[193,196].

Eat rice for hot flushes

You have probably read about many different herbal and nutritional treatments for menopausal symptoms, including Vitex agnus castus, dong quai, ginseng, Ginkgo biloba, vitamin E, soya products and ground linseeds. All these are excellent. But if you have read that oriental women rarely suffer from hot flushes because they eat soya products, think again. The average consumption of soya foods in the Far East is not really all that high. But what is high is the consumption of rice. If you have a mild case of hot flushes, you may find, like I did, that general healthy eating plus a portion of rice—preferably brown rice—and drinking rice milk every day for a year or so is all you need to banish them forever. If for some reason I went without rice for a few days and began to feel hot flushes beginning, a cup of good quality Korean ginseng tea would quickly make me feel fine again.

On the other hand taking HRT could raise your risk of various cancers and get you addicted. Many women find it impossible to come off HRT because of withdrawal symptoms in the form of severe hot flushes. And some find that they have to keep raising the dose in order to maintain a feeling of well-being[230].

High-fat diets increase oestrogen levels in the bloodstream. This is probably why women who eat too much red meat, cheese, pastry, biscuits, ice cream and so on have higher rates of breast, uterine and other cancers. On the other hand research seems to suggest that a low-fat diet may help to reduce menopausal symptoms[281].

If hormonal fluctuations encourage hot flushes, it is also important to curb your intake of sugar and stimulants in order to prevent sudden surges in your blood sugar levels. These surges will set off a whole battery of hormones that could play a part in encouraging hot flushes.

A-Z self-help summary

BHP = "Basic Healthy Plate" - see the chart on page 26. IHP = Intestinal Healing Programme (page 50) LRP = Liver Rejuvenation Programme (page 61)

Condition	Diet	Supplements (For doses see product label)
Alzheimer's, dementia senility	BHP, daily nuts and sunflower seeds, blue and purple berries, oily fish. Ginger and chillies. Avoid wheat due to high gluten content. Avoid foods containing saturated fat.	Arginine, ginkgo biloba, methionine, carnitine, phosphatidyl-serine, B complex, vitamin E, copper, evening primrose oil (GLA)
Arthritis (osteoarthritis)	BHP, food intolerance test, LRP,turmeric, massage, try avoiding acidic food or deadly nightshade food family. Try cider vinegar.	Evening primrose oil (GLA), SAM, glucosamine sulphate, green-lipped mussel extract, shark or bovine tracheal cartilage, fish oils (EPA), DLPA, devil's claw. Bromelain with meals.
Asthma	Food intolerance test, IHP, LRP, anti house dust mite measures, avoid salt	Lycopene, vitamin B_6, magnesium, selenium
Autism	Food intolerance test, IHP, LRP. Eat liver occasionally. May need to avoid gluten.	B_6, magnesium, cod liver oil
Autoimmune illness	BHP, food intolerance test, IHP, LRP, red clover tea, fruit and vegetable juices, celery juice, oily fish, massage, sunshine	For inflammation: bromelain with meals, vitamin C, flavonoids, ginkgo biloba
Cancers	BHP, LRP plus specific protective foods (see text), vegetable juices. Magnetic therapy, psychological therapy. Breast cancer: seaweed.	Vitamin C powder 10 grams/day dissolved in large glass of water. Breast cancer: CoQ10.
Candidiasis	IHP	As per IHP
Chronic fatigue	Food intolerance test, IHP, LRP, coconut oil, coriander leaf, shiitake mushrooms, cold baths, graded activity. Avoid arginine-rich foods, chemicals, mould, places where you feel worse.	As per IHP, LRP. Magnesium (+B_6 to help assimilation) lauric acid, lipoic acid, quercetin, lysine.
Common cold	Radishes and radish juice.	Vitamin C powder, cod liver oil, zinc, echinacea.
Constipation	IHP. Fibre-rich foods, exercise, linseeds. Drink more water.	As IHP. Magnesium. Bromelain with meals.
Cystitis	BHP. Cranberry juice, cucumber juice, nuts, plenty of water. Avoid artificial bath and personal hygiene products and harsh laundry detergents. Food intolerance test. IHP. Acidophilus pessaries for women.	Cranberry extract. Herbs: Uva ursi, Saw palmetto.

Deafness and tinnitus	BHP, oily fish, blue and purple berries, ginger and chillies, nuts, seaweed. Avoid foods containing "bad" fats.	Vitamins A, B complex, D, iron, magnesium, zinc, copper, Ginkgo, kelp, evening primrose oil (GLA).
Depression	BHP. If sugar helps symptoms, treat as for hypoglycaemia (see Diabetes below)	B complex, selenium, tyrosine, tryptophan, phenylalanine, SAM, lecithin, St John's Wort. Post-natal depression: zinc. If B complex aggravates depression use a brand without folic acid.
Diabetes, hypoglycaemia	BHP. Avoid sugary foods and stimulants. Diabetes: lose weight, take exercise. Eat fenugreek seeds, cinnamon. Hypoglycaemia: take small frequent meals.	Chromium, magnesium, taurine, B complex, maitake, lipoic acid.
Gall-stones	Food intolerance test. Chamomile tea, dandelion coffee, lemon juice. Women: brassica vegetables	Wild yam (for pain), silymarin (milk thistle), lecithin, barberry, taurine
Hay fever	Food intolerance test. Nuts, sunflower seeds, cabbage, onions, apples, purple berries	Calcium, magnesium, methionine, quercetin, vitamin C, bee pollen
Heart attacks, strokes, angina, HBP, high cholesterol	BHP, fresh nuts and sunflower seeds, porridge, fruit and vegetable juices, blue & purple berries, exercise. Avoid sugar, salt,	Magnesium, selenium, fish oil, CLA, lysine, vitamins C, E. Congestive heart failure: CoQ10, taurine, carnitine
Hepatitis	BHP. Cysteine-rich diet: oatmeal and sunflower seeds soaked overnight. Juices of blue and purple berries. Turmeric, onions, chamomile tea. Avoid "bad" fats.	Selenium, lipoic acid, silymarin, vitamin C, quercetin, liquorice root, maitake mushroom, B vitamins, vitamin E
Hyperactivity, ADD	BHP, oily fish. Food intolerance test. Avoid colourings and other artificial additives, sugary food and drink, stimulants.	Chromium, magnesium, zinc, vitamin B complex, evening primrose oil (GLA)
Infertility	BHP, avoid alcohol, coffee, smoking. Ensure aequate protein. LRP to combat endometriosis or environmental toxins. Endometriosis may also respond to increasing soya consumption. PCOS: treat as for hypoglycaemia (see Diabetes above).	As per LRP. Also vitamin C, selenium, zinc.
Inflammatory bowel diseases	BHP. Avoid sugary food and drink. Food intolerance test. IHP.	Bromelain with meals. For parasites: Artemisia annua, quassia, golden seal, raw garlic. Avoid golden seal if pregnant.
Irritable bowel syndrome	Ensure adequate fibre-rich foods. Food intolerance test. IHP.	As per IHP
Kidney problems	BHP, nuts. Avoid sugary, fatty food. Nephrotic syndrome: food intolerance test.	Vitamin B6, magnesium.
Migraine, headaches	Avoid coffee. Food intolerance test. Chiropractic adjustments.	As identified by your Nutritional Therapy Questionnaire

Osteoporosis	BHP, leafy greens, broccoli. Avoid phosphorus-containing food additives, salt, sugar, excessive protein. Exercise, especially strength-training.	Magnesium, calcium, zinc, multiminerals, vitamin D, vitamin B complex
Pregnancy problems	BHP. Cabbage, greens, broccoli and their juices. Fresh ginger tea.	Multivitamins and minerals, iron, zinc, vitamin K.
Prostate enlargement	BHP. Pumpkin seeds, sunflower seeds, Brazil nuts, flax seed oil. To prevent prostate cancer, add soya products and tomato purée.	Zinc, selenium, Saw palmetto, pygeum africanum, horsetail, Cernilton
Schizophrenia	BHP, food intolerance test. If diarrhoea, IHP.	These must depend on the results of vitamin and mineral tests, since the wrong supplements can aggravate symptoms.
Skin problems	BHP, LRP, food intolerance test. Avoid alcohol & fatty, sugary food. Bad psoriasis may need IHP.	Vitamin A, zinc, evening primrose oil (GLA) vitamin B complex
Thyroid disorders	Hypothyroid: BHP, food intol. test, radishes, sea food, seaweed, broccoli. Avoid soya protein concentrate,fluoride. If no success, treat as for hypoglycaemia (see Diabetes). Hyperthyroid: BHP, radishes, meditation, acupuncture, homoeopathy.	Vitamin A, B complex, zinc, tyrosine, kelp, selenium, copper, iron
Women's hormonal problems	BHP plus (depending on the problem) LRP, brassica vegetables, soya milk, iodine-rich foods (especially seaweed), rice. Avoid chocolate and coffee, curb sugary foods and alcohol.	As per LRP plus B complex, magnesium, evening primrose oil (GLA), ginkgo biloba, kelp, agnus castus, dong quai, ginseng, vit E

Part IV

Preparing Food

What foods are not included in our recipes, and why?

- Wheat flour, wheat pasta, wheat cereals and all foods containing wheat
- Cow's milk and products made with it: butter, yoghurt, cheese and cream, casein (milk protein) and whey
- Yeast, as found in yeast extract, spreads, stock cubes, gravy and sauce flavourings and mixes, alcoholic drinks and most types of bread and pizza.
- Hen's eggs in any form
- Artificial food additives
- Sugar, syrup and honey
- Red meat/animal fat*
- Hydrogenated fat
- Salt* and sodium-based baking powder

You can see why people on nutritional therapy need a good recipe book. They often exclaim in horror "But what is there left to eat?" if their therapist asks them to avoid these foods. Some people become quite angry, almost as if echoes of childhood are haunting them: their mother's voice forbidding sweets until they have eaten their greens. "It's impossible for me to eat porridge," one told me. "I just can't stand it." Sadly, our desire to eat convenience and fun foods all the time is at the root of most chronic ill health. We don't want to hear the stark reality—we want to hear that it's ok to go on doing exactly what we're doing and that somehow, somewhere, there must be a pill that will make it all right.

If you feel a little daunted by now, here is some comforting advice.

1. THIS BOOK IS TO HELP YOU GET WELL, IT IS NOT FOR LIFE. When your body has been repaired and you are well, you can relax your eating habits. Just keep focused on how wonderful it would be to be well.
2. There are many, many delicious substitutes for the foods you are used to. You will be truly surprised at how tasty some of these recipes are, and what fun it is to try out new things.
3. If you have come to rely on convenience food, don't worry. You can save a lot of money by preparing your own convenience food. Some of the recipes take about as much time as heating up a meal in the microwave.

---

*There is one recipe for liver, and a few call for sheep's yoghurt or goat's cheese, which contain some animal fat. Several recipes call for miso or tamari sauce, which do contain some salt but are otherwise beneficial. Those on a salt-free diet should omit them.

4. If the thought of eating good food makes you feel angry, resentful, hostile, dismissive and so on, it is very important to think about whether your objections are really appropriate. A 50-year old man who won't eat his porridge or greens is behaving like a little boy. The difference is that a grown man can just tell himself that he likes these foods, and eat them anyway, without making a fuss. He no longer has to prove to himself that he can disobey his mother if he wants to.

Let's take a look now at the reasons why nutritional therapy begins with avoidance of the foods listed above, and suggest some alternatives.

Alcohol

Alcohol stresses your liver and harmful toxins are created while it is being broken down. Alcohol also reduces the effectiveness of anti-diuretic hormone (ADH). When your body's fluid levels are getting low, you need this hormone to slows down your excretion of fluid. If it is not working properly you can go on rapidly excreting water even when you are already dehydrated.

ALTERNATIVES: Many people drink alcohol because it helps them relax. Chamomile tea is a good alternative relaxant. If the social element of drinking alcohol is a problem, you may also have to widen your scope of social activities so that you can find other ways to enjoy your spare time.

Artificial food additives

It is hard to avoid these if we eat commercially manufactured foods. Almost everything contains a cocktail of additives: preservatives, colourings, artificial sweeteners, flavourings and flavour enhancers to name just a few. Sometimes the law does not even require additives to be listed on a packet. For instance a chilled meal purchased from a supermarket may appear to contain no additives at all, but this is because items like "stock" do not have to declare small amounts of sub-ingredients they contain.

The problem with additives is that we only know if they harm the health of well-nourished laboratory animals given them singly in large quantities. We have no idea how they affect the health of humans when consumed over a lifetime in dozens of different combinations.

Large numbers of people are sensitive to these chemicals. For instance, sulphur-based preservatives may trigger asthma and digestive inflammation, and colourings can cause rashes or disturbed behaviour in some children. Certain colourings can react with bacteria in the intestines to form cancer-causing compounds[202,204].

Additives originally thought safe to eat have later been banned. The sweetener aspartame, used as tablets and in countless "diet" products such as yoghurt, cola and ice-cream and by diabetics is now causing worries since it has been linked with headaches, memory loss, eye problems and seizures[206].

One thing we do know is that your liver must try to break down these foreign chemicals and uses up its precious resources in doing so. What we do not know is how successful *your* liver is in coping, and whether it forms any toxic intermediate products which linger in your system.

One of the greatest concerns about additives is the unknown effect of mixing them together as we eat different foods containing them.

ALTERNATIVES: There are now many additive-free products on the market. Health food shops often specialize in them. Or make your own additive-free food.

Bad fats

Fat is not a poison, and does not need to be avoided completely, although some people mistakenly treat it that way. In fact it is essential to have some fat (in the form of essential polyunsaturated oils) in your diet. But most of us eat far more bad fats than we realize since the fat in most high-fat foods is invisible. The fats which especially need to be controlled are animal fat and hydrogenated fat.

Animal fat

Animal fat is sold as butter and lard and found in full-fat milk, minced beef and burgers, sausages, pork pies, chocolate, ice cream, fried food, cream, cheese, eggs, biscuits, cakes, desserts and pastry. Too much of these foods can encourage excess cholesterol in your blood, especially if you also consume a lot of sugar-rich food. Animal fat is mostly saturated fat—also known as hard fat because it is solid at room temperature.

While animal fat tends to consist of little more than calories, some hard fats derived from plants do also contain useful ingredients, for instance

- Sterols, found in a variety of plant fats and oils, block the absorption of cholesterol from your diet,
- Tocotrienols, found in palm oil/fat, have cholesterol-lowering properties[282],
- Isoflavones, found in many plant fats and oils, are good balancers of the female hormone oestrogen and can also help to prevent prostate cancer[80,227],
- Lauric acid, found in coconut oil/fat, can inactivate many viruses and bacteria, including the "stealth" microbes which are now thought to be responsible for some types of severe chronic fatigue[92]. Stealth microbes can evade detection by the immune system or by normal medical tests.

One of the dangers of consuming too much saturated fat is that the delicate outer membranes which cover our cells could become too rigid. This affects the ability of oxygen-carrying red blood cells to squeeze through narrow blood vessels (capillaries) in your brain, eyes etc. Inflexible red cells can block your capillaries, leading to a poorer blood (and oxygen) supply to these sensitive areas, especially if you are an elderly person[59].

Most types of margarine are artificially hardened fats and rarely contain the above-mentioned beneficial ingredients.

Hydrogenated fats

These are artificially hardened fats. You may find these listed as an ingredient on packets of biscuits, cookies, ice-cream and many processed or convenience foods. In some catering establishments, fish-and-chip shops and so on, foods are deep-fried in hydrogenated fats. Hydrogenated fats are oils which have been treated with hydrogen to make them hard at room temperature. Many brands of margarine and "vegetable fat" are made in this way. Sometimes they are only partially hydrogenated, which reduces the hardness to a "soft margarine" consistency. Some recent research has linked a high consumption of partially hydrogenated fats with a higher risk of heart disease[283].

Which fats should I eat?

Olive oil

Can be used in salads, dips, mayonnaises and for frying up to medium heat. Use the very beneficial "extra-virgin" variety, which is the very special first pressing of the olives, and is made without heating the oil, if the olive oil will form part of the dish. Use ordinary olive oil (which is cheaper) if it is only needed for frying.

Groundnut oil

Can also be used for frying, especially when the strong taste of olive oil is not wanted. Like olive oil, it is not rapidly damaged by heat.

Polyunsaturated oils

Sunflower, safflower, soya oil, flax seed oil, hemp oil, walnut oil—use only cold, for salad dressings, mayonnaise, dips etc.

Coconut Oil

Is hard at room temperature and so technically is a saturated fat. But studies have shown that it does not raise cholesterol like butter does[207,268]. Use it for pastry- and cake-making. Coconut oil is also a traditional ingredient of many oriental dishes and curries. You can find it in shops that specialize in Asian cookery.

"Trans" fats

Commercial processing of oils and fats frequently creates an unnatural type of fat molecule known as the "trans" form. Once in your body, these trans fats can grab enzymes needed by essential fatty acids—EFAs. EFAs are similar to vitamins. They are substances derived from oily foods like nuts and sunflower seeds. These EFAs must be derived from your food—your body cannot manufacture them.

Essential fatty acids are especially needed by your cell membranes. They keep them supple and able to do their important job of aiding the entry of oxygen and nutrients into your cells and the exit of various waste products. So don't think that all fats are bad. The oily fats found in nuts and seeds are very beneficial indeed, although of course like any fatty or oily food you do have to watch out for the calorie content. Fortunately these naturally oily foods keep you feeling full for longer than carbohydrates, so they may help you to eat less.

If consuming too much trans fat prevents your body from using EFAs, it effectively means that a diet with too much highly processed fat or oil can in time produce the effects of an EFA deficiency even if you are consuming enough EFAs.

Red meat

And non-organically farmed white meat

Red meat (even if apparently lean) and saturated fat contain arachidonic acid, which can encourage inflammation in your skin, joints or other parts of your body. White meat (poultry) is much less fatty and so less likely to be a problem, but it is far better if it has been organically raised. Even free-range chickens may be fed standard commercial feed which contains antibiotics, dung from other chickens, and other unsavoury items. We do not know how well a chicken's liver can cope with these challenges and what kind of residues remain in the bird's meat and fat.

Non-organic chickens are routinely fed antibiotics. The bacteria in the chicken's intestines can become resistant to them and the bacteria in humans who consume the birds can acquire this resistance. This has led to life-threatening cases where salmonella poisoning, for instance, becomes virtually untreatable because no antibiotic is effective.

ALTERNATIVES: Fish, nuts, beans, tofu and other soya products. Nuts are an excellent protein source and very underrated. Rice can also contribute significant amounts of protein to your diet.

Salt

And sodium-rich foods, including:

1. Highly salted or smoked foods such as salami, ham and bacon, sausages, smoked fish, canned foods, salty cheeses, salted nuts, crisps and other packet snacks, bread, stock cubes, yeast extract, soy sauce and ready prepared pies, quiches, sauces, or commercially manufactured "oven-ready" dishes.
2. Sodium-rich drinks, medicines and food additives. Baking powder. Most commercial soft drinks are very high in sodium. Some medicines, such as antacids based on bicarbonate of soda or effervescent tablets of any kind can also contain large amounts of sodium. One of the most common food additives is a flavour-enhancer known as mono*sodium* glutamate or "E621". Other sodium-rich food additives are E211, E223, E250, E251, E262(ii), E281, E339, E350, E401, E452, E466, E500, E514, E524, R541, E576.

These foods, plus adding salt at the table can easily lead to a salt intake of 12-17 grams a day. The World Health Organization recommends no more than 5 grams.

A high salt intake has been linked with

- Fluid retention
- High blood pressure and weight gain (as a result of fluid retention)[120,121]
- Osteoporosis (brittle bone disease)[171]
- A worsening of asthma[209].

In her book *A Matter of Life*, medical doctor and biochemist Dr Nadya Coates points out that when it comes into contact with water in our bodies, salt breaks down to hydrochloric acid and caustic soda—a highly irritating substance which can damage our cells and can occasionally cause odd burning sensations for which no medical cause can be found.

The best way to control salt is to eat food which you have prepared yourself, so you know exactly how much salt you have put in it. Low-sodium salt products are now available in supermarkets, and can help to cut your salt intake by 50 per cent or more. The recipes in this book will also help you to cut your salt intake drastically, but some use a little tamari sauce or miso, oriental flavourings which do contain salt but are also very rich in other nutrients. If you have been placed on a totally salt-free diet you could omit these or use potassium salt instead.

Baking powder contains bicarbonate of soda, which has effects similar to those of salt. See page 294 for suppliers of alternatives to sodium salt and baking powder.

Sugar, honey and syrup

Read the labels, since sugar is also known as *sucrose, glucose, dextrose and fructose*.

Sugar, a form of carbohydrate, is a natural component of fruit and vegetables, where it is not in concentrated form. Concentrated sugar is found in products such as honey, syrup and treacle, which are mainly sugar and water. The most concentrated form of sugar is the brown or white crystals we buy in packets, which are added to drinks or found in soda pops, ice cream, milk shakes, cakes, biscuits, cookies, jam, desserts, sweets and chocolate. In this form, the average person in the UK consumes about two pounds of sugar a week.

Most of us know that eating too much sugar is bad for our teeth and probably not good for our health. The big question is, how much is too much?

Let's look at it this way. We can only eat a certain number of calories a day without putting on excess weight. If one third of those calories come from sugar, you are eating only two thirds of the vitamin-rich food which a person on a low-sugar diet eats, since sugar consists of calories and no other nutrients. If you don't believe that one third or more of your diet consists of sugar, read on.

If you are consuming the national average of two pounds of sugar per week, that comes to about 150 grams a day. Each gram of sugar yields four Calories, making 600 Calories a day from sugar—or about one third of a normal calorie intake for a woman and one quarter of a normal calorie intake for a man.

Add to this the 30-40 per cent of our diet that comes from fat, and you can see how dangerously high your diet could be in "empty" calories—that is to say foods which provide only calories and virtually no other nutrients at all.

Of course, a national average sugar consumption of two pounds a week means that most people will be consuming either more or less than this amount. If you know that you consume a lot of sugary foods and drinks, your total intake of empty calories could be as much as 80 per cent of your diet.

Your body is not going to react right away to being treated like this. It is very good at coping silently. But in time you could develop vitamin and mineral deficiency symptoms, such as

- Skin problems
- Lacking energy and stamina
- Frequent colds or thrush
- Period pains or PMS
- Diabetes
- Enlarged prostate.

If your liver does not get enough vitamins and minerals to make essential enzymes, it could start to have difficulty processing wastes and pollutants, which in turn can

---

Did You Know?

When advertisements for sugar claim that sugar "gives you energy", they are not using the term "energy" in the usual sense of the word— helping you to *feel* more energetic. All our energy needs can be met by consuming a normal diet containing no added sugar at all.
In fact, energy is a scientific term for calories, so the ads are really just telling you that sugar will provide you with calories!

---

lead to inflammation in your skin or joints, fluid retention, headaches, lethargy and accelerated ageing. A weakening of your immune system reduces your body's ability to protect itself against cancer.

Taking vitamin pills to compensate for the empty calories is not the solution— hundreds of medical studies are showing that the people with the highest *fruit and vegetable* consumption are those least likely to get cancer and heart disease. These foods contain a lot of important nutrients besides vitamins and minerals.

Added sugar—and this includes honey and syrup, which are also concentrated sugar—is absorbed very fast, making your insulin rise too quickly and too high. Scientific trials show that high insulin levels encourage high fat levels in your blood, and cholesterol deposits on your artery walls[200]. As reported in *Pure White and Deadly,* a book about sugar written by the late professor of nutrition John Yudkin, your blood also becomes more "sticky", and so prone to tiny clots that could lead to a heart attack as you get older. High insulin levels make you gain weight: you retain sodium, which encourages fluid retention[111], and you form body fat more easily, especially around your middle.

It really is worth curbing your sweet tooth. Wouldn't you like to approach old age feeling fit and well rather than on a cocktail of medications for high cholesterol, high blood pressure and diabetes? Avoiding sugar does not have to mean going without sweet things. This book provides lots of recipes for delicious desserts—even chocolate mousse!

ALTERNATIVES: Use naturally sweet foods like bananas, raisins, dates and cashew nuts. These contain dietary fibre which helps slow down the absorption of the sugar they contain.

Tea and coffee

(including decaffeinated versions)

These have a diuretic effect. They make you urinate more, which encourages dehydration, increased losses of magnesium and other minerals, and also makes your kidneys retain sodium. Taken with meals, tea and coffee substantially reduce the absorption of iron and zinc from your food[5]. This may account for why some researchers believe these drinks can encourage infertility[165,166,208].

Coffee is a nervous system stimulant which may provoke anxiety and panic attacks in susceptible people[210]. It increases your liver's workload. Children who consume it regularly have an increased risk of diabetes[211].

ALTERNATIVES: Chamomile, peppermint, fennel tea, chicory, dandelion coffee.

Wheat, dairy, eggs and yeast

In order to be able to help as many people as possible, this book assumes that you may be one of the estimated 30 per cent of the population with a food intolerance. (The symptoms of food intolerance are listed on page 22.) If you do have a food intolerance, your problem foods will probably be one or two of these four. The recipes omit all of them to keep things simple, not because everyone needs to avoid them. If you have no food intolerance symptoms you will probably be able to eat these foods in moderation without problems. If you do have food intolerance symptoms, you will be able to use the recipes in this book while you are preparing to test yourself as described on page 47. Once you know what your problem foods are, you can just avoid those and reintroduce your safe foods back into your diet.

The Japanese foods miso and tamari sauce, which can be used as substitutes for beef stock cubes and gravy browning, are not fermented with commercial yeasts and are usually safe for yeast-free diets.

ALTERNATIVES TO WHEAT: Spelt, rice, barley, rye, millet flour etc.
ALTERNATIVES TO MILK: Soya milk, nut milk, rice milk
ALTERNATIVES TO EGGS: In cakes, a mixture of soya flour and soya milk can often replace eggs due to the high protein content.
ALTERNATIVES TO BREAD MADE WITH YEAST: Yeast- and wheat-free pumpernickel (black rye bread). Or make your own spelt flour griddle bread, or oat pancakes (see the recipes in Part V)
ALTERNATIVES TO STOCK CUBES & GRAVY MIXES CONTAINING YEAST: Miso and tamari sauce.

What should I drink?

Scientists estimate that most of us need to drink at least 3-4 litres (5-6 pints) of liquid a day—more if you are breast-feeding, or if you suffer from heavy periods, diarrhoea or tend to sweat heavily. You should drink this amount even if you don't feel thirsty. Thirst only begins once dehydration has started. Symptoms of dehydration include lethargy, nausea (including morning sickness of pregnancy), stomach discomfort, gastritis, heartburn, indigestion, constipation and inflammation. Chiropractors sometimes cure back pain and painful joints by asking people to drink water instead of tea and coffee.

Drinking more than 2.5 litres (4½ pints) of liquid a day halves your risk of getting bladder cancer.

The best drink of all is plain water. Drink it on its own, or use it to dilute fruit juice. A mixture of sparkling water and fresh fruit juice is delicious, and much better for you than canned fizzy drinks, which are often high in sodium and sugar or artificial chemicals. Weak fruit or herb teas such as rosehip, blackcurrant, fennel or chamomile—preferably without sugar—are also good choices, and can be drunk hot or cold (with ice). Certain fruit or vegetable juices and herbal teas can help combat health problems. Drinking a glass of cold water is an instant remedy any time your stomach feels unsettled.

The worst drinks for your health are tea, coffee and alcohol, because of their diuretic effect. A diuretic stimulates your body to excrete fluid more rapidly, even when its fluid levels are already low.

Alcohol can particularly dehydrate you as it reduces the effectiveness of anti-diuretic hormone (ADH), a hormone which is meant to slow down your excretion of fluid when you are beginning to get dehydrated. Drinking a pint of water before going to bed after you have consumed a lot of alcohol can help to reduce the dehydration—and the resulting hangover!

Therapeutic juices

If you get a juice extractor, you can make your own delicious fruit and vegetable juices. Many of these have valuable therapeutic uses, for instance

Celery juice

Helps to alkalinize your body. Very helpful against arthritis.

Lemon juice

(Include some of the pith and peel). Contains limonene, which can help to dissolve gall-stones.

Broccoli juice

Helps to break down excess oestrogen and so to combat women's hormonal problems such as fibroids, breast cysts, endometriosis, breast cancer, PMS. Also contains lutein, which protects the eyes.

Radish juice

Rich in a sulphur compound which helps to regulate your thyroid gland. Stimulates bile production, combats harmful intestinal bacteria. Dries up congestion and helps eliminate cold symptoms.

Time-saving tips

Shopping for meals in minutes

If you are using this cookbook to try to overcome any kind of health problem, you'll need to be well-organized from the start. Most people fail at a special diet because they arrive home tired and hungry, open the fridge and find nothing compatible with the diet. "Oh blow it!" they say, "I'll eat this packet of biscuits and go back on the diet tomorrow." Needless to say, tomorrow may never come.

Most of us want to spend the absolute minimum of time shopping and in the kitchen. As I heard someone say recently "I thought cooking was making toast and reading the instructions on the microwave packet". I love good food, but I too find it hard to spend hours making intricate meals. All the recipes in this book reflect that because I use them myself.

Before you get cooking, let's look at some of the ingredients you should always have in your fridge or store-cupboard (see panel on next page). If you make sure you don't run out, you will always be able to whip up a delicious meal in minutes. And it's guaranteed to be a lot cheaper than a shop-bought ready meal.

Most of these foods can now be bought in the larger supermarkets as well as in health food shops. Fresh vegetables are cheaper from a greengrocer, and fresh fish from a fishmonger.

If you would like to take advantage of the recipes which use ingredients that you prepare in advance and then freeze to make quick meals later on, a freezer would be a great advantage. And, since one of the best-value sources of protein is the humble dried bean or pea, I am also recommending that you obtain a pressure-cooker. I gave up years ago trying to cook beans, split peas and so on in a normal saucepan. Two hours after starting to boil them they can still be like bullets! In a pressure cooker, even the toughest bean will yield to pressure in 5-10 minutes.

I also like to use a wok or stir-fry pan (preferably with a see-through lid) for a lot of recipes, but if you cook with electricity, you should substitute a deep frying pan or sauté pan. Another useful piece of equipment is a food processor. If you get one with a vegetable juicing attachment, you will be able to make some of the therapeutic juices mentioned in this book.

Preparing brown rice and beans for the freezer

Frozen rice and beans are a great standby. You can make a lot of really delicious fast recipes by combining these in different ways. You could also use canned beans but they are more expensive and may be loaded with salt and sugar.

Brown rice is nuttier than white rice, with a different texture. It contains all the B vitamins which are lost when rice is "polished". You can buy brown rice from supermarkets and health food shops.

Wash well, then pre-soak overnight in 1½ times its volume of filtered water. Use the same water for cooking. Bring to the boil then cover tightly and simmer on the lowest possible heat until tender (20-25 minutes).

By now the water should all have been absorbed. Leave the rice in the covered saucepan away from the heat for five minutes, after which it is ready to serve.

Once cold, brown rice can be spread out on an oiled baking tray, frozen, then crumbled into grains and bagged for the freezer.

Dried Beans

These should be soaked in water before use. Cover with four times their volume in boiling filtered water and leave overnight.

Throw away the soaking water, place the beans, well covered with fresh water, in a pressure cooker, bring to full steam, and leave on a low-medium heat for 3-10 minutes, depending on size and age. Remove from the heat and place the pressure cooker in a sink of cold water. You cannot open the pressure cooker until it has cooled down enough to reduce the steam pressure inside.

Pressure-cooking breaks down the poisonous lectins found in raw beans. If you do not have a pressure cooker, boil them fast for at least 10 minutes before simmering or slow-cooking.

To freeze, allow to cool and follow the same method as for frozen brown rice. Spoonfuls of split peas which are a little mushy can be frozen in the wells of tart or muffin baking tins before bagging.

Meals in Minutes Shopping List

Alfalfa seeds
Apples
Beans, dried or canned in plain water
Blueberry or black cherry all-fruit jam
Brown rice
Canned plum tomatoes
Carrots
Dried fruit
Filleted fish for freezing
Frozen chopped mixed vegetables
Garlic
Green cabbage
Herbs and spices
Lemons or limes
Lentils
Miso
Nuts (almonds, cashews, walnuts, brazils, unsalted peanuts)
Oatflakes
Olive oil (extra-virgin)
Onions
Potassium salt
Potatoes, especially Desirée or other waxy varieties
Prawns
Pumpernickel bread (long-life, yeast– and wheat-free)
Rice noodles
Soya cream
Soya, buckwheat, brown rice and polenta flours
Sunflower seeds
Sweet peppers
Tamari sauce
Tofu
Tomato purée

See pages 130-134 for where to get and how to use the more unusual items

Using unfamiliar ingredients

Ingredient	Where To Get It	What It's Good For	How To Use It
Alfalfa Sprouts and Seeds	Sprouts: Health food shops Seeds: Health food shops and garden centres	Rich in coumarin, a type of flavonoid or antioxidant which helps the lymphatic system	Alfalfa sprouts can be bought in packets, but it is cheaper to make your own. Place a level tablespoon of seeds in a large jar, then cover the jar with a piece of nylon fabric from an old pair of tights and secure the fabric with an elastic band around the neck of the jar. Run some water into the jar, shake to thoroughly wet the seeds, then leave overnight. In the morning, pour the water away, straining it through the nylon cover. Rinse the seeds by pouring in water and immediately straining it out again morning and night, and in a few days you will have a luscious growth of curly green sprouts which can be added to soups or eaten as salad. Eat them when they are about one inch long. You can also follow the same procedure to sprout lentils, mung beans, aduki beans, black buckwheat grains, barley grains, almonds and clover seeds.
Bilberries (a small cousin of the blueberry)	These grow wild in many areas. May be available in frozen food departments of some larger supermarkets	Rich in flavonoids, vitamin C and minerals	Consume them as they are, or place in an oven-proof casserole dish in a medium oven for 25 minutes or until the fruits split and the juices run. Serve hot or cold, with soya cream, or use in any of the recipes in this book which call for blueberries. Bilberries are not quite as sweet as blueberries. If sweetening is required use a small amount of puréed dates.
Blueberries	Fresh: supermarkets. Frozen: Ardovries Shearway Ltd (see page 294) Dried: Larger branches of Sainsburys	Rich in flavonoids, vitamin C and minerals	Serve fresh with soya yoghurt, or cook as for bilberries. Should need no sweetening as blueberries are sweeter than bilberries.

Ingredient	Where To Get It	What It's Good For	How To Use It
Brown Rice	Supermarkets and health food shops	Rich in B vitamins. A good source of protein	Brown rice is nuttier than white rice and has a different texture. Wash thoroughly, then pre-soak overnight in 1½ times its volume of filtered water. Use the same water for cooking. Bring to the boil then cover tightly and simmer on the lowest possible heat until tender (20-25 minutes). By now the water should all have been absorbed. Leave the rice in the covered saucepan away from the heat for 5 minutes, after which it is ready to serve. Once cold, brown rice can be spread out on an oiled baking tray, frozen, then crumbled into grains and bagged for the freezer.
Buckwheat	Health food shops	Rich in magnesium and in the flavonoid rutin, which helps to build capillary strength	Buckwheat is a grain unrelated to wheat and is a good alternative for wheat allergy sufferers. Buckwheat flour contains no gluten and is the main ingredient of small Russian pancakes known as blinis. To use as an alternative to rice, toast buckwheat grains in a dry frying pan for 10 minutes over a medium heat. Put in a saucepan with twice their volume of water. Bring to the boil and simmer very gently with the lid on for 15-20 minutes, or until the grains are tender.
Chestnut Flour	Health food shops. Infinity Foods and Windmill Organics (see page 294)	Its sweet taste makes it great for cakes and pastries	See the recipes in Part V.
Coconut Oil	Oriental grocers. KTC (Edibles) Ltd (see page 294)	Does not raise cholesterol levels like butter and other animal fats. Contains lauric acid, which combats the Epstein-Barr virus	Use as a replacement for butter in pastry-making and whenever a hard fat is required. Coconut oil is a solid product but is sold in bottles and jars. If the neck of the bottle is too narrow for you to insert a spoon, melt the oil by placing it in a bowl of hot water, then pour it into an old margarine container before refrigerating it, whereupon it will solidify again.

Ingredient	Where To Get It	What It's Good For	How To Use It
Dried Beans, Split Peas, Chickpeas, Marrowfat Peas, Lentils. (Also known as pulses or legumes)	Supermarkets, grocers and health food shops	A very cheap source of protein, rich in dietary fibre, B vitamins and minerals	All pulses except lentils should be soaked in water before use. Cover with four times their volume in boiling filtered water and leave overnight. Throw away the soaking water, place the pulses, well covered with fresh water, in a pressure cooker, bring to full steam, and cook for 3-10 minutes, depending on age and hardness. Pressure-cooking breaks down the poisonous lectins found in raw beans. If you do not have a pressure cooker, boil them fast for at least 10 minutes before simmering or slow-cooking. Conventional boiling can take up to two hours to soften them, depending on age and size. To freeze, allow to cool and follow the same procedure as for frozen brown rice. Lentils need no presoaking. Boil for 20-30 minutes in two and a quarter times their volume in water.
Miso	Darker varieties: Health food shops. Pale varieties: Clearspring or Source Foods (see page 294)	A delicious stock paste made from fermented soya. Lower in sodium than most stock paste, and very rich in vitamins and minerals. Also contains protein	Mix with boiling water and use to make gravy and to flavour soups and stews. One variety of miso is made with wheat, and should be avoided while following the principles of this book. Other types, such as barley miso, are ok. Don't overdo the miso—it does contain salt. Use just enough to get some colour and/or flavour into a dish.
Potassium Baking Powder and Potassium Salt (CardiaSalt)	At the present time in the UK you can only get these by mail order from Biocare Ltd (see page 294)	For baking and seasoning without the added sodium from the usual products. Also increases valuable potassium	Use in accordance with the manufacturer's directions on the container. Potassium salt is also an ingredient in "Low Salt" products, which typically consist of half to two thirds potassium salt and the rest ordinary sodium salt. These are OK to use in recipes specifying "potassium salt" unless you are on a salt-free diet.
Pumpernickel bread	Supermarkets, health food shops	Wholegrain rye bread with a sweetish, nutty flavour. Buy a brand which contains no yeast or wheat	Eat with soups and salads, or make into an open sandwich (see the recipes in Part V). Pumpernickel does contain a very small amount of salt, but this should not be a problem.

Ingredient	Where To Get It	What It's Good For	How To Use It
Rice Vermicelli and Noodles	Vermicelli: Oriental grocers and supermarkets. Noodles: Oriental grocers and some large supermarkets	A good alternative to noodles made from wheat	Thin rice noodles are about twice the thickness of vermicelli. Pour boiling water over them and soak for 2-3 minutes depending on the product. Rinse immediately in cold water. Larger noodles, which are flat and ribbon-like, are also available and can be used as alternatives.
Sheep's Milk Yoghurt	Supermarkets	A nice creamy alternative to cow's milk yoghurt	Use as normal yoghurt.
Soya Cream	Supermarkets and health food shops	A blend of soya protein and oil which can be used as an alternative to dairy single cream	Soya cream is used as a topping for desserts, or can be stirred into soup or gravy to achieve the same effect as single cream. *Look for it under brand names such as Provamel's "Soya Dream" since in the UK, EU officials have told manufacturers to remove the description "soya cream" from the packaging on the grounds that the product contains no dairy produce.*
Soya Flour	Health food shops	High in protein. Provides all the benefits of soy foods, including protection against prostate cancer and menopausal problems	A few tablespoons of soya flour can often be used as an alternative to eggs in baking because of its high protein content.
Soya Milk	Widely available. You may have to try different brands before you find one you like	Provides all the benefits of soy foods	Use in the same way as cow's milk. Contains less protein, calcium and fat, but a good balance of vitamins and minerals. Some brands are enriched with calcium. Add natural vanilla extract to make it taste more like cow's milk.
Soya Yoghurt	Health food shops. Or make your own, using soya milk and some Sojasun as a starter culture	An alternative to cow's milk yoghurt. Provides all the benefits of soy foods, plus the friendly bacteria found in normal yoghurt	Use as normal yoghurt. *N.B. In the UK it has to be sold under descriptions such as "soya speciality with live ferments" (Sojasun, which is a good thick brand), or Yofu, since EU officials have told manufacturers to remove the description "soya yoghurt" from the packaging on the grounds that the product contains no dairy produce.*

Ingredient	Where To Get It	What It's Good For	How To Use It
Spelt Flour	Health food shops. Some large supermarkets	An alternative to wholewheat flour, also known as "ancient wheat". Most people who are allergic to wheat are not allergic to spelt	Use exactly as wholewheat flour. You can also buy pasta made from spelt.
Sugar-Free (all-fruit) Jam and Marmalade	Health food shops. Some larger supermarkets and superstores also sell the excellent St Dalfour brand	All-fruit jams are made using fruit juice as a sweetener. They contain nothing except fruit and juice	Use as normal jam or to sweeten desserts.
Tamari Sauce	Health food shops	A type of soy sauce, made without using wheat	Use tamari sauce sparingly (since it is salty), to flavour stir-fried dishes. For soups and sauces use wheat-free miso (see above).
Tofu	Supermarkets and health food shops	A good source of protein made from soy—as good as eating meat but with added health benefits	Many of the recipes in this book use tofu. For best results, use the right type. Get to know a particular brand and stick to it if it works. "Silken" tofu has the consistency of blancmange. It is sold as soft, medium or firm varieties, although the package does not always tell you (a) that the product is silken tofu, or (b) whether it is soft or firm. Silken tofu is best for liquidizing and making into mayonnaise and other creamy products. The firmer it is, the less water it contains, and the more water you may have to add to get the finished consistency you want. Standard tofu can also be soft or firm. It has a "chewier" consistency and is best for cutting into cubes, dusting with brown rice flour and frying in oil. Can be marinated beforehand. It can also be liquidized with a little soya milk or water, poured into moulds, and baked with flavourings. The finished result has a consistency like quiche or omelette.

Cooking techniques

Maximizing nutrients

I can't help cringing when I visit someone's kitchen and watch a few handfuls of chopped vegetables rapidly boiling in a huge panful of water.

One of the first rules of cookery is that most of the vitamins from vegetables end up in the cooking water. So the second rule is to use only a small amount of cooking water and keep it to make soup, sauce or gravy; or use a cooking method which doesn't need any water. Here are some alternatives to boiling.

Steaming

This is a good method for potatoes, since only an inch of water is needed in the bottom of the pan. You don't need to buy a special steamer. Cheap metal steaming baskets are available which open up to fit inside any saucepan. You may need to allow the potatoes a few extra minutes' cooking time, and do ensure that the water is kept boiling quite briskly.

Potato water contains vitamin C and can be saved (or frozen) for adding to soup. In continental Europe some doctors recommend drinking potato water to help soothe bowel spasms in irritable bowel syndrome. This is because potatoes are related to Belladonna and contain small amounts of atropine-like compounds.

Braising and sautées

Braising is a wonderful way to cook vegetables. You just stir vegetable pieces (add chopped onion for extra succulence) into a little oil over a medium heat, and then add just a few tablespoons of water. After bringing the liquid to the boil, cover the pan very tightly and turn the heat down to the lowest possible setting. The vegetables cook very slowly in their own juices. The result? Delicious!

Sautées are similar but you add more liquid. Once the food is cooked you remove it, reduce the sauce by boiling, and then pour the sauce back over the food.

Stir-frying

This method is also similar to braising, but the vegetables need to be cut into very small pieces or thin strips, and stirred in a large, roomy pan (preferably a Chinese wok or stir-fry pan) over a high heat until they are part-cooked. A few tablespoons of water are then added to create a lot of steam which helps to soften the vegetables. A lid may then be put over the pan for a short time. Stir-frying is faster than braising. Brown rice can be made delicious by stir-frying in olive oil with some spring onion and garlic. Add chopped herbs, turmeric and a few dashes of tamari sauce.

Soups

Soups are a wonderful way to get all the goodness out of vegetables, since nothing is thrown away. A thick, chunky soup can be a meal in itself.

Baking

Especially if chopped very small (as in a food processor) vegetables can be mixed with chopped nuts and with cooked grains such as brown rice or buckwheat, and then oven-baked. Flavoured with herbs or soya sauce, this deliciously moist dish complements any main item on the menu; or it could be served as a lunchtime snack, on its own or with a sauce.

"Intuitive" cooking

To avoid extra shopping, I only follow recipes when I am cooking a special meal. Intuitive cooking is when you whip up a meal using the ingredients you already have. Forget sausages, fish fingers, oven chips and canned baked beans—give me fresh potatoes, fresh (or chopped frozen) vegetables, garlic, rice noodles, olive oil, tofu, soya yoghurt and the home-frozen brown rice and beans already mentioned, and I can produce quick and delicious meals with very little effort. Here are my secrets. All you need is some basic cooking techniques and plenty of herbs and spices for different flavours. You never need eat a bland boiled vegetable again!

Home-made Indian curries

I make a lot of curries, and they are incredibly simple. Here are the basic steps involved. You will need a spice grinder filled with your favourite

Refined Foods

Foods made from white flour (e.g. bread, pasta, cookies and cake)

Sugar and syrup of all types

White (polished) rice

Most breakfast cereals

Most cooking oils and margarines.

Foods are refined for various reasons, often to extend their shelf life. Refining means removing part of the food (often the nutrient-rich outer layer) or extracting from the whole food only the part you want (such as sugar or pure oil), leaving up to 90 per cent of the vitamins and minerals behind. The manufacturers may then try to sell you back the wheatgerm or bran removed from the cereals, or the vitamin E extracted from the oils.

By law, refined foods often have to be "fortified" with added vitamins as they are so depleted. Unrefined foods don't need added vitamins since they can be up to ten times more nutritious.

mixture. I like cloves, cardamom (remove the shells first), black pepper, fennel, coriander seeds and chopped cinnamon pieces. These are good for intestinal health and help prevent gas formation too.

1. Heat some oil in a saucepan and add finely chopped onion and garlic. I also like to add some cashew nuts sometimes.
2. When beginning to sizzle gently, grind in some of your spice mixture. Heat for a few seconds until you can smell the aroma.
3. Then for a bean curry just add some of your home-frozen beans. Or you could add cooked lentils instead. For a vegetable curry add any mixture of vegetables:
   - Diced potatoes and torn cabbage leaves or diced aubergine with coriander leaves
   - Frozen chopped mixed vegetables
   - Cauliflower or broccoli florets, diced courgettes and tomato
4. Sprinkle on some powdered turmeric if you are treating your liver, plus enough water to just cover the ingredients. Stir and season with potassium salt. You could also add some tomato puree or coconut cream.
5. Simmer gently for about one hour. If there is too much liquid, boil rapidly with the lid off until reduced. Serve with brown rice. I also like to spoon some thick soya or sheep's yoghurt over the top—or see the sour cream recipe in Part V.

Home-made Thai curry

This is even simpler. You will need some Thai curry paste and coconut cream. Coconut cream is sold in blocks and is easily available in supermarkets. Thai curry paste ingredients are usually free of major allergens although they may contain a little salt. If you are vegetarian, watch out for brands containing minced prawns.

You will also need some tofu. The silken variety of tofu is not suitable for this recipe.

1. Cut the tofu into bite-sized chunks, coat with rice flour seasoned with cayenne pepper, onion granules and potassium salt, and fry in olive oil for about two minutes on each side. Leave to drain on a piece of kitchen paper.
2. Put mixed chopped vegetables in a saucepan, add enough water almost to cover, and bring to a simmer. Stir in Thai curry paste and pieces of coconut cream to taste. Leave to simmer for about 30 minutes then stir in the fried tofu pieces.
3. Serve poured over rice vermicelli.

Stir-fried fish with rice noodles

You can use any fish fillets, or frozen peeled prawns. You will also need the flat rice noodles which you can buy in Chinese groceries or in larger supermarkets. Cut the fish into bite-sized chunks and place on top of chopped frozen vegetables and olive oil in a stir-fry pan. Sprinkle with your choice of dried herbs and some potassium salt. Add a few tablespoons of water and cook over a low heat with the lid on until the vegetables are tender and the fish pieces opaque all the way through—about 15 minutes. You can go away and do something else in the meantime.

Soak the noodles for 2-3 minutes in boiling water and drain. If there is any liquid remaining in the stir-fry pan, turn up the heat until it has evaporated. Put the contents of the stir-fry pan in a bowl. Replace the pan on a medium heat, and add another tablespoon of olive oil plus some chopped garlic. When just beginning to sizzle, add the drained noodles and stir-fry over a high heat for half a minute, ensuring that the noodles are coated with oil. Season with potassium salt. Then add back the fish and vegetables. Mix well and serve immediately.

Baked potatoes with braised vegetables

While potatoes are baking in the oven, finely chop some onion and add to a stir-fry pan or saucepan with some olive oil over a medium heat. Add the chopped vegetables of your choice: cabbage, carrots, courgettes, green beans, cauliflower florets are all good. Add garlic too if you like it. Cut the vegetables into different shapes to make the mixture more attractive, e.g. carrots into thin strips, French beans left whole, cauliflower florets really small. Stir into the onion, add a few tablespoons of water, and after bringing the water to the boil, cover tightly and cook on the lowest heat setting for 30 minutes. Stir from time to time and check that the vegetables have not dried out. Add a little more water if necessary.

Cut open the baked potatoes and top with the vegetable mixture and a dollop of soya yoghurt (or see the delicious sour cream or garlic crème recipes in Part V).

Vegetable soup

Another great standby is a thick vegetable soup, especially if you are trying to lose weight. Soups fill you up and satisfy you without loading you with calories. Just throw in diced potatoes and every vegetable you can think of, plus a few handfuls of cooked frozen beans, split peas or lentils, a can of organic chopped tomatoes, lots of herbs and garlic and some potassium salt. Thicken the soup by whizzing it with the blender just for 20 seconds or so. You want it to be part blended and part chunky. Finish it off by stirring in a tablespoon of soya cream if you want a cream soup.

A soup made with loads of dark green cabbage or spring greens is an easy and tasty way to eat these vitally important vegetables.

Part V

Gourmet recipes

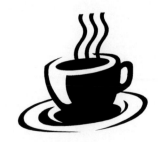

Breakfast

Always eat breakfast, even if you are trying to lose weight.

During the night your body slows down its metabolism (burns calories more slowly) to conserve energy. Only when you start eating again does it speed things up.

A carbohydrate-only breakfast will leave you feeling hungry again quite quickly[269], so make sure you include some protein and oils in your breakfast to keep your blood sugar even.

Nuts, fish and avocados are ideal.

Yoghurt with Almonds and Apple Compote

Makes one serving

Instructions

Swirl 4 tbsp sheep's milk or soya yoghurt into a generous serving of apple sauce (see page 255).

Sprinkle liberally with toasted flaked almonds.

Variations

Apricots or prunes (soaked in water overnight) gently poached until tender also go well with yoghurt.

For a very filling breakfast, put a cup of sheep's yoghurt in a sieve lined with kitchen paper, and allow to drain into a bowl for one hour. Discard the watery liquid, then put the thickened yoghurt in a dish, and add sliced banana, chopped dates, raisins and crushed walnuts. This is guaranteed to keep you going until lunchtime!

Sheep's (and cow's) yoghurt has a sharper flavour than soya yoghurt.

What It's Good For

Both sheep's and soya yoghurts are rich in protein. It's a good idea to start your day with some protein because this is the time of day when your body can best assimilate it.

Protein is also more filling than carbohydrate. An all-carbohydrate breakfast can leave you feeling hungry again within two hours.

Breakfast Corn Pancakes and Waffles

Ingredients to make 4 pancakes

2 heaped tbsp each of

Finely ground yellow polenta meal

Buckwheat flour

Soya (soy) flour

(adding up to a combined quantity of about 115 g/4 ounces/½ cup)

250 ml/8½ fluid oz/generous ¾ cup water

½ tsp potassium baking powder

NB: Waffles use more batter than pancakes.

Instructions

Mix the ingredients well together to form a smooth, runny batter. It should be able to quickly spread to the edges when poured into a pan. Heat a lightly oiled frying pan (skillet) over a medium to high heat. When hot, pour in enough batter to cover the bottom of the pan and quickly tilt the pan so that the batter can run to the edges, forming a pancake shape. Cook for about one minute, or until small holes form and the top is just set. Turn the pancake over with a spatula (or toss it if you're brave!) and cook the other side for about the same time. Oil the pan again and stir the batter before making the next pancake. Stack the pancakes and keep them warm until you are ready to eat them. Spread with apple butter (see page 255) and cinnamon or ground cardamom, or with all-fruit blueberry jam, and roll them up.

The pancake batter will keep in the fridge for a few days, so you can make just one or two pancakes very quickly. Stir well before cooking.

Waffles

Make a thicker batter, using less water, and spoon it into an oiled, preheated waffle iron. Cook for 2-3 minutes. Turn the waffle upside-down before serving, and spread with pure peanut, cashew or almond butter and/or all-fruit blueberry jam or orange marmalade.

What It's Good For

Yellow polenta flour is rich in anti-cancer carotenes (similar to beta carotene). Buckwheat flour is rich in molybdenum—a mineral needed by the liver for detoxification work. Soya flour is a rich source of hormone-balancing isoflavones which help to prevent problems relating to excess or insufficient oestrogen and excess testosterone. In clinical trials women with menopausal symptoms have reversed them by eating a diet rich in soya flour.

Authentic Swiss Muesli with Flaked Nuts and Sweet Apricots

Ingredients for one serving

<u>3 tbsp medium or fine ground oatmeal</u>

<u>Water</u>

<u>Soya or almond milk* to taste</u>

<u>1 tbsp flaked nuts</u>

<u>1 unsulphured dried apricot, chopped small</u>

*See page 273

Dried apricots are orange in colour if treated with sulphur dioxide. This additive is an intestinal irritant and can cause bloating and gas. Unsulphured apricots (from health food shops) are dark brown and much sweeter in flavour.

Instructions

Did you know that the Swiss never eat muesli straight out of the packet? They know that raw grains should always be soaked (or cooked) before eating them, because this breaks down mildly poisonous chemicals they contain, known as enzyme inhibitors, that can upset your intestines.

Soak the oatmeal overnight in water. The amount of water you need will depend on how much the oatmeal can absorb—about three times its volume for medium oatmeal, and more for fine oatmeal. If you find after an hour or so that the mixture has become too solid, add more water. No milk is necessary since the oats create their own milk. In the morning check the consistency and add a little soya or nut milk if you wish, to achieve your preferred consistency. If you use fine oatmeal, the result will be very creamy. Stir in the dried apricot pieces and sprinkle with flaked nuts.

What It's Good For

Oats and oatmeal are one of the best possible sources of magnesium and B vitamins. These nutrients are often lacking in diets which rely on convenience foods. A magnesium deficiency can reduce your liver's ability to get rid of toxins and can be responsible for a lot of the symptoms listed on page 21, especially those related to anxiety and stress. Magnesium is rapidly used up in stress situations[23]. Muscles have difficulty relaxing when they are short of magnesium.

Fried Herring Cakes

Ingredients for 2 servings

2 medium herrings, scaled, trimmed and gutted

2 tbsp olive oil

2 dessertspoons chick pea (gram) flour

Potassium salt

Freshly ground black pepper

Instructions

Poach the herrings in a few tablespoons of water in a lidded pan over a low heat for ten minutes, until the fish comes apart easily. Allow the fish to cool, then slit it open lengthwise and carefully remove all the bones.

Using a fork, mash the fish with the chick pea flour and seasonings, then, using your hands, divide it into four balls and form each ball into a fairly thin patty. Dust the outside of the patties with more chick pea flour.

Heat the oil in a frying pan (skillet) over a fairly high heat, then put the patties into the pan and fry for 1-2 minutes on each side or until brown. The patties can be prepared the night before for cooking in the morning.

Serve hot with home-made tomato ketchup (see page 263).

You could also serve these herring cakes cold as a starter, on a bed of shredded lettuce with lemon wedges. Or tuck them into a folded round of unleavened bread and top with salad ingredients and a squeeze of lemon juice.

What It's Good For

Herrings are rich in omega 3 oils which help prevent heart attacks. They discourage red blood cells from clumping and blocking arteries. If foods were priced according to how healthy they are, few of us would be able to afford herrings. They are probably the best value fish you can get, and very beautiful with shiny, silvery scales. Herrings are also an excellent source of zinc. A zinc deficiency can lead to skin and immunity problems, a poor sense of taste or smell, and to prostate problems in older men.

Sultana and Sunflower Seed Porridge with Milk and Cream

Ingredients for one serving

<u>250 ml/9 fluid oz/generous ¾ cup soya (soy) milk</u>

<u>3 tbsp rolled oats or medium oatmeal</u>

<u>2 tsp raisins</u>

<u>2 tsp sunflower seeds</u>

<u>Soya (soy) cream</u>

Special Tip

Add a few drops of natural vanilla extract to soya milk to make it taste more like cow's milk. Vanilla is very similar to coumarin, a substance which gives cow's milk its flavour of new-mown hay. Coumarin actually comes from new-mown hay.

Instructions

Put the milk and oats in a small, heavy-bottomed saucepan (enamelled cast iron if you have one) over a medium heat.

Bring to the boil, stirring constantly, then turn down the heat to a simmer and add the raisins and sunflower seeds.

Keep stirring for a minute or two until it thickens. Add a little more soya milk if you prefer a more runny porridge. Serve with a little soya cream poured over the top.

This is a delicious and satisfying breakfast, especially on a cold winter's day. If you prefer extra sweetness, use a variety of soya milk which has been sweetened with a little apple juice.

This recipe takes only 5 minutes to make.

What It's Good For

See page 143 for the benefits of oats and oatmeal. Sunflower seeds are rich in essential polyunsaturated oils, calcium, magnesium and methionine, which is normally not found in large amounts in plant foods. Methionine is turned into glutathione in your liver, which, together with the trace element selenium, makes an important free radical fighting enzyme known as glutathione peroxidase. Unlike animal fats, the omega 6 oils in natural sunflower seeds are very beneficial to health.

Granola

Ingredients for 2 servings

6 tbsp rolled oats

3 tbsp chopped mixed nuts

2 tbsp sunflower seeds

1 tbsp groundnut oil

1 tbsp raisins

1 tbsp unsulphured dried apricots, diced

A few drops of natural vanilla extract

Instructions

Mix all the ingredients except the dried fruit thoroughly together.

Put a dry frying pan (skillet) over a low heat. When hot, add the ingredients and cook for 20 minutes, stirring occasionally.

Remove from the heat and stir in the dried fruit. Once cool, store in an airtight container.

To serve, pour into a bowl and add soya milk. You could also add prunes, apple compote or fresh fruit such as bananas, pears or strawberries.

What It's Good For

This delicious, nutty cereal can be eaten for breakfast or as a snack at any time of day. See pages 143 and 145 for the benefits of oats and sunflower seeds. Dried fruit is rich in the mineral potassium. Groundnut oil has been used in this recipe because it has to be heated. Like olive oil, groundnut oil contains mainly monounsaturated fatty acids, which are less easily damaged by heat than most other oils. Groundnut oil also has little flavour of its own, and so is ideal for recipes like this.

Avocado Smoothie with Banana and Strawberries

Ingredients for 2 servings

One avocado pear

600 ml/1 pint/2 cups soya milk

Half a banana, broken into pieces

One handful of sweet strawberries

1 tsp natural vanilla extract

Instructions

Probably the fastest breakfast in the universe!

Open the avocado and remove the stone. Cut the flesh into pieces.

Liquidize all the ingredients together and drink immediately.

Small, ripe avocados with a good flavour are best for this recipe. Liquidized avocado turns brown quickly, so don't let this hang around before drinking it.

What It's Good For

Described as one of nature's most perfect foods, creamy, buttery avocado pears are so nutritious that they are practically a whole meal in themselves. They are rich in protein, omega 6 polyunsaturated oils, vitamin B6 and other B vitamins, vitamin E, iron and copper, and provide three times as much potassium as bananas. They are also easy to digest. The rough-skinned Hass avocado has a particularly good flavour. The protein in this drink will help to keep you going until lunchtime.

Hi-Nutrition Smoothie

Ingredients for 2 servings

One avocado pear

600 ml/1 pint/2 cups rice milk

One banana, broken into pieces

Half an orange, peeled but with
some white outer pith
remaining

2 tbsp sheep's yoghurt or thick
soya yoghurt or silken tofu

10 Brazil nuts or 2 tbsp ground
almonds

Special equipment if using
Brazil nuts

Rotary drum grater with handle

Instructions

If using Brazil nuts, wash and dry them, then grate finely using the rotary drum grater. Add the grated Brazils or ground almonds to the rice milk and leave to soak for at least two hours or overnight to improve the digestibility of the nuts.

Open the avocado and remove the stone. Cut the flesh into pieces.

Liquidize all the ingredients together and drink immediately.

Small, ripe avocados with a good flavour are best for this recipe. Liquidized avocado turns brown quickly, so don't let this hang around before drinking it.

What It's Good For

This smoothie can be consumed at any time of day and is ideal for invalids who need a healthy meal replacement formula. The avocado, yoghurt (or tofu) and nuts all provide protein. The avocado and nuts also supply nutritious oils and the vitamin C in the orange helps you to absorb iron from the ingredients. Bananas provide glucose, potassium and vitamin B6. It is well worth using Brazil nuts if you can because they are one of the few good sources of selenium, needed by your liver for detoxification.

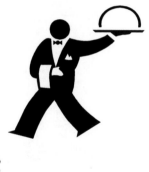

Lunches, suppers snacks & starters

A really cool way to serve a family meal or a dinner for guests is to make it a sit-down buffet meal. It's similar to a high tea-the traditional mix and match evening meal in Northern England-or to a Chinese or Eastern European meal, where people help themselves from a variety of hot or cold dishes.

Try arranging a selection of the following dishes in the centre of the dining table:

◊ Eggplant Caviar
◊ Frittata with Ginger and Courgettes
◊ Potato Wedges Roasted with Olive Oil and Garlic
◊ Guacamole
◊ Falafel
◊ Mini Rainbow Salads
◊ German Potato Salad
◊ Pumpernickel, and rye crispbread.

Or put out the ingredients for Danish Open Sandwiches and let people build their own.

And of course buffets are great for parties and the cold items for packed lunches too!

Russian Borscht

Ingredients for 6-8 servings

1.7 litres/3 pints/6 cups water

¼ head small to medium green cabbage, coarsely shredded

2 medium potatoes, cut into four lengthwise, then thinly sliced

3 medium beetroot (beets), boiled whole, peeled, cooled and coarsely grated

2 medium carrots, coarsely grated

1 medium onion

1 small can tomato purée (paste)

4 cloves garlic, peeled

2 tbsp extra virgin olive oil

Potassium salt

Instructions

Put the potatoes and shredded cabbage in a large saucepan with the water and potassium salt and bring to the boil. Simmer for 15 minutes then add the grated carrot and simmer for a further 5 minutes.

Meanwhile cut the onion into 8 pieces and process with the garlic cloves in a food processor with the "S" blade.

Heat the oil in a stir-fry pan or sauté pan, and stir the onion and garlic mixture over a medium heat until softened but not brown.

When the cabbage, potato and carrot are tender, stir in the tomato purée then add the softened onion and garlic mixture, followed by the grated beetroot. Gently heat through until just simmering, then serve in bowls topped with a dollop of sour cream (see page 253).

What It's Good For

Beetroot is a wonderful herb-like food which stimulates your liver cells and is one of the richest plant sources of iron in a well-assimilated form. Cabbage is a great anti-cancer vegetable, since it helps your liver to process toxins into more harmless substances. It is also rich in a powerful antioxidant flavonoid known as quercetin which has been found to help prevent cataracts and allergic problems. Use the darkest green cabbage you can find.

Eggplant Caviar

Ingredients for 2-4 servings

1 medium aubergine (eggplant), washed and dried

1 small onion, finely chopped in a food processor

2 medium tomatoes, skinned, deseeded and roughly chopped

2 tbsp lemon juice

Extra virgin olive oil

1 tbsp parsley, finely chopped

Potassium salt

Black pepper

Parsley or coriander leaf (cilantro) to garnish

Instructions

Steam the aubergine whole (or cut in half to fit the pan) for 15 minutes until soft. Sweat the onion over a medium heat for 5 minutes with 2 tbsp olive oil. When the aubergine is ready, dice it finely and add it to the pan with the onions. Stir, cover the pan and continue cooking very gently for another 5 minutes, then turn off the heat. Stir in the chopped tomatoes, parsley, potassium salt and pepper, lemon juice and another tablespoon of olive oil. Mix and incorporate thoroughly. Allow to cool, then chill and garnish with a sprig of parsley or coriander (cilantro) before serving on a bed of shredded iceberg lettuce. Serve as part of a buffet meal or put teaspoonfuls on cucumber slices or pieces of mini-poppadoms, or on small squares of wheat- and yeast-free pumpernickel bread and top with a dollop of sour cream (see page 253).

This dish is better if made the day before and kept cool before serving.

Variation

Can also be made with raw onion or spring onion (scallion) instead of cooked.

What It's Good For

Russians really do eat this dish, and call it caviar. Many prefer it to the real thing. In Ayurvedic medicine aubergine is considered a potent food to support a woman's hormonal processes. Aubergines are also known as eggplants because of their creamy texture when cooked. They do not contain "bitter juices" and do not need to be treated with salt before cooking. If you throw away their juice you will throw away a lot of their nutritional value.

Frittata (Italian Omelette)
with Ginger and Courgettes

Ingredients for 6 servings

115 g/4 ounces/½ cup chick pea (gram) flour, sieved

250 ml/9 fluid oz/1 cup water

1 medium courgette (zucchini) fairly thinly sliced

4 spring onions (scallions) including the green part, very thinly sliced

4 cloves garlic, finely chopped

1 tbsp finely grated fresh ginger

Extra virgin olive oil

Tip

Cut any hard bits off a big piece of ginger then grate it all and freeze teaspoonfuls in the individual wells of ice cube trays. (The skin is so delicate you don't need to peel it.)

Instructions

Stir the water into the gram flour a little at a time, until it is all incorporated and the mixture is smooth. Stir in the grated ginger. Don't be alarmed at how watery the mixture is—it will puff up nicely.

Fry the courgette slices in 2-3 tbsp olive oil over a medium heat on each side for 2 minutes until golden, using a frying pan (skillet) with a 9½ inch diameter. Remove from the pan, then add the onion and garlic. Stir and fry gently for 2 minutes until soft but not brown. Replace the courgettes in the pan and arrange the contents of the pan evenly over the bottom. Give the gram flour, ginger and water mixture a final stirring, then pour it carefully into the hot frying pan. Scramble the ingredients at the bottom of the pan very gently and briefly with a spoon, then cover the pan tightly and leave over a low to moderate heat for 15 minutes, until the sides and bottom of the frittata are golden brown and the top is set.

Slide the frittata on to a large plate, put another plate over the top, invert, then slide the frittata back into the frying pan to cook the other side for 5 minutes.

Serve the frittata warm or cold, cut into wedges and garnished with watercress.

What It's Good For

Gram (chick pea) flour is very rich in protein, and in this dish makes a delicious replacement for eggs, which are normally used to make frittata (a type of thick, round omelette). It is also a good source of many other nutrients, including calcium, magnesium, iron, copper and some of the B vitamins. Ginger is a wonderful aid to digestion. In Chinese medicine it is considered to warm the circulation and to combat catarrh and bronchitis.

Detoxification Soup

Ingredients for 6 servings

1.7 litres/3 pints/6 cups water

225 g/½ lb white fish, cut into chunks

1 long, white (mooli) radish, cut into matchsticks

1 medium onion, chopped

2 boiled, peeled beetroot (beets), diced

225 g/½ lb brussels sprouts, sliced

1 small can of tomato purée (paste)

2 tbsp extra virgin olive oil

1 tbsp gelatine

2 tsp turmeric (yellow oriental spice)

1 tsp Glaubers Salts (sodium sulphate - ask your pharmacist)

Instructions

Sweat the chopped onion gently in the olive oil, in the bottom of a large saucepan. When softened, stir in the turmeric until it is thoroughly incorporated. Pour in the water and bring almost to the boil. When nearly boiling, remove from the heat, sprinkle in the gelatine powder and whisk until dissolved, then stir in the Glaubers salts and tomato purée. Finally, add the fish and vegetables, except the beetroot.

Bring back to the boil and simmer gently for 20 minutes. Gently stir in the diced beetroot and serve.

What It's Good For

This recipe is medicinal, with four sets of ingredients to help your liver (i) Clear toxins from your blood (brussels sprouts, beetroot, protein, glycine (gelatine), sulphate); (ii) Neutralize toxic free radicals produced in your liver: (quercetin (onions), vitamin C (brussels sprouts), lycopene (tomato purée); (iii) Help the flow of bile to flush wastes from liver and gallbladder into intestines and stools (radish, turmeric); (iv) Help protect your liver cells against toxic damage (turmeric).

Potato Wedges Roasted with Olive Oil and Garlic

Ingredients for each serving

1 medium potato, scrubbed

1 clove garlic, chopped

2 tbsp extra virgin olive oil

1 tsp potassium salt

Cayenne pepper

Instructions

Preheat the oven to 200°C/400°F/gas mark 6.

Pound the chopped garlic with the salt until smooth, using a mortar and pestle, then stir in the olive oil and cayenne pepper. Put this mixture in a shallow, oven-proof dish large enough to hold the potato wedges.

Bring one inch of water to the boil in a saucepan with a steamer basket.

Leave the skins on the potatoes. Cut each potato into half lengthwise and each half into four long wedges. Put the potato wedges in the steamer and steam over a medium heat for five minutes. Remove the wedges and brush each one with the oil and garlic mixture, ensuring it is thoroughly coated.

Arrange the wedges peeled side down in the dish and roast for 30 minutes. Baste after 15 minutes by dipping a basting brush into the oil, and brushing the wedges with it before returning the dish to the oven.

Serve as a snack dipped in hummus (page 155) or eggplant caviar (page 151).

What It's Good For

Potatoes are rich in potassium and many other nutrients. They also contain a small amount of vitamin C. Cooking them in this way, with a little olive oil, is an excellent way to make them crunchy and get all their goodness without the excessive fat of deep-frying

Hummus

Ingredients for 4 servings

In this recipe a cup means an ordinary teacup

1½ cups freshly cooked
    chickpeas (still warm)*

½ cup cooking liquid from the
    chickpeas

2 heaped tbsp sesame seeds

4 tbsp extra virgin olive oil

1 tbsp lemon juice

1 clove garlic, crushed

½ tsp potassium salt

Cayenne pepper to taste

*See page 129

Instructions

Blend all the ingredients together in a food processor, adding more cooking liquid if necessary, until the mixture achieves the consistency of a thick dip.

Use as a dip for crudités (page 175) or roast potato wedges (page 154) or combine with alfalfa sprouts (page 130), peanuts, green pepper strips and grated radish and tuck into a folded round of unleavened bread (page 260).

What It's Good For

Chickpeas are very rich in protein, and are also a good source of many other nutrients, including calcium, magnesium, iron, copper and some of the B vitamins. Sesame seeds are one of the best available sources of calcium and magnesium, and also provide protein and zinc. They are one of the few good plant sources of the amino acid methionine. Research shows that they can help to lower cholesterol levels in the body.

Plum and Spring Onion Sushi

Ingredients to make 32 pieces

2 sheets of nori* approx 19x20 cm/7½x8 inches, cut in half

Approx 16 tbsp short-grain brown rice boiled for an extra 5 minutes until it is a little sticky

4 ready-to-eat (firm) prunes which have been marinaded for 2 hours in 3 tbsp tamari sauce and 1 tbsp rice wine vinegar (or cider vinegar)

2 spring onions (scallions), cut into 1-inch segments then finely shredded lengthwise

1 tsp wasabi sauce or ½ tsp wasabi powder

*Thin but strong and flexible sheets of pressed seaweed. It can be bought from health food stores or by mail order from Clearspring (see page 294).

Instructions

Remove the prunes from the marinade, cut them into thin strips, and mix the wasabi with the rest of the marinade.

Place a half-sheet of nori on a clean tea towel, with the long edge towards you, and spread 2 tbsp of the cooked rice in a line along the centre from left to right. Lay a quarter of the prune strips on top of the rice followed by a quarter of the spring onion shreds. Carefully spread 2 more tbsp of rice over the top. Sprinkle with some of the marinade.

Now press the rice mixture down as firmly as you can with a fork. Roll the nori around the filling just like pastry round a sausage roll. Moisten one edge so that the edge of the nori will stick to the other edge. It may take a little practice to get the quantity of rice filling just right so that it all fits in the nori sheet.

Put the sushi roll to one side, resting on its seam, while you make the others. When you are ready to serve the sushi, cut the roll into 8 or more bite-sized segments, using a very sharp knife.

Alternative filling

Sticky rice plus cucumber and cooked carrot strips flavoured with umeboshi plum sauce (from Clearspring, page 294).

What It's Good For

Like most seafood, seaweed is rich in iodine, a trace mineral needed by your thyroid gland. Iodine is no longer routinely added to salt in the UK and most people get it from dairy produce; iodine is used to sterilize the teats of cows before milking! Iodine deficiency is linked with higher rates of breast diseases. Japanese women, who eat a diet very rich in iodine (including sushi) have always had a very low rate of breast cancer. Iodine deficiency may also cause damage to nerves required for hearing.

Miniature Baked Omelettes with Four Fillings

Ingredients for 4 servings

1 x 250 g pack/8½ ounces/generous 1
cup standard firm tofu

4 tbsp soya milk

Tamari sauce

Potassium salt & freshly ground black
pepper

**For the parsley and mushroom
filling**

3 medium white mushrooms, finely
chopped and fried in a little olive
oil for 1-2 minutes

1 tsp fresh, finely chopped parsley

For the shallot filling

1 medium shallot, finely diced and
gently fried in olive oil until soft
but not brown.

**For the carrot, ginger and
seaweed filling**

1 tbsp carrot grated into fine shreds

2 inch square piece of nori seaweed

1 tsp fresh grated ginger

**For the sun-dried tomato and
basil filling**

3 large basil leaves, finely shredded

1 medium piece sun-dried tomato,
finely shredded

Instructions

Preheat the oven to 200°C/400°F/gas mark 6, and oil 12 wells of a mini-muffin tin.

Toast the nori sheet quickly under a hot grill (broiler) until it lightens in colour and turns crispy. Break into small pieces.

Using the S-blade of your food processor, whizz the tofu with the soya milk, potassium salt and a few dashes of tamari sauce until creamy-smooth. This may take a few minutes. Scrape down the sides with a spatula from time to time.

Divide the mixture equally between four small bowls. To each bowl, add the ingredients for each of the fillings, plus a little black pepper, and stir together well.

Using two teaspoons, drop the mixture in the wells of the oiled mini-muffin tin and smooth down the surface. Bake in the oven for 20-25 minutes or until firm and springy and beginning to turn golden on top. Serve hot or cold on a bed of shredded lettuce, with some fruit chutney.

What It's Good For

The main ingredient in this recipe is tofu, a protein-rich soya product. See page 142 for some of the health benefits of soy. Unlike ordinary omelettes, this recipe is low in saturated fat but the taste and texture is remarkably like the real thing.
Try inventing some more fillings of your own.

Speciality Pâtés

The Basic Mixture

Makes 4 Servings

<u>115 g/4 ounces/½ cup dried butterbeans (lima beans)</u>

<u>75 ml cold-pressed, unrefined sunflower oil</u>

Instructions

Cover the beans with four times their volume in boiling water and leave to soak overnight. Drain and place in a pressure cooker over a high heat with plenty of water to cover the beans generously. Put the lid on and bring the pressure cooker up to full steam. Cook for 6 to 10 minutes, depending on the age of the beans, then turn off the heat and immediately plunge the base of the pressure cooker into a sink of cold water. Once the pressure has reduced and you can open the lid, check that the beans are soft and tender by eating one. Do not allow the beans to become cold before you carry out the next stage.

Transfer the warm beans to a food processor. Using the S blade, process them with the sunflower oil until smooth and creamy. This may take several minutes. Scrape the sides down with a rubber spatula from time to time.

This basic mixture is flavoured by adding other ingredients

- Either to the food processor while blending
- Or to the oil, to flavour it before processing it with the beans
- Or to the finished product, by mashing them in roughly.

What It's Good For

The basic ingredients of these pâtés are butterbeans and sunflower oil. Like all pulses (members of the bean and lentil family), they are rich in protein, especially in the amino acid lysine, which is hard to get from other plant foods. Try to use a cold-pressed, unrefined sunflower oil rather than supermarket oils, which are usually bleached and chemically treated to improve their shelf life. Unrefined oils should be as fresh as possible since they do not keep as well as chemically treated oils.

Poached Salmon and Dill Pâté

Ingredients for 4 servings

1 quantity of basic pâté mix

60 g/2 ounces fresh filleted
    salmon

1 tsp fresh dill, chopped

2 tsp fresh lemon juice

Potassium salt

Freshly ground black pepper

Instructions

Stir the lemon juice and seasoning into the basic pâté mix and incorporate thoroughly. Poach the fish in a few tablespoons of water for 5 minutes in a small covered pan. The salmon is cooked when it flakes easily. Drain the salmon and flake it, then mash it roughly into the basic pâté mix together with the chopped dill.

Mushroom and Garlic Pâté

Ingredients for 4 servings

One quantity of basic pâté mix

115 g/4 ounces/1 cup
    mushrooms, chopped

½ clove garlic, chopped

Extra virgin olive oil

Tamari sauce

Freshly ground black pepper

Instructions

Use mushrooms which have developed some black gills, as this helps to give this pâté a good colour.

Fry the chopped mushrooms in olive oil until golden. Whizz the mushrooms and garlic with the pâté mix and a few dashes of tamari sauce in a food processor until smooth. Stir in the black pepper.

How to serve the speciality pâtés

Spread on pumpernickel, rice cakes, oatcakes or wheat-free rye crispbreads such as Ryvita.
Mix with salad ingredients such as alfalfa sprouts, spread on warm pancakes (see page 142) and roll up like a Swiss roll. Keep warm until ready to serve.
Make canapés by squeezing the pâté from an icing bag on to cucumber slices. Top with half an olive.

(Continued on page 160)

Italian Herb Pâté

Ingredients for 4 servings

1 quanity of basic pâté mix

2 tbsp chopped fresh basil or pesto sauce (page 225)

Potassium salt

Freshly ground black pepper

Instructions

Whizz these ingredients together in a food processor.

Garlic, Chilli and Tomato Pâté

Ingredients for 4 servings

One quantity of basic pâté mix

1 tbsp tomato purée (paste)

½ clove garlic

½ tsp cayenne pepper

Potassium salt

Instructions

Stir the ingredients together until thoroughly incorporated.

Make polenta as described on page 216. Spread it out in a well-oiled large dish or tray so that it makes only a thin layer. When cold, cut out small rounds of polenta with a pastry cutter, fry in hot olive oil until golden, then top with pâté and a sprinkling of fresh herbs or finely diced sweet peppers. Serve immediately.
Fill ramekin dishes with the pâtés and serve as a starter for spreading on crudités (pieces of raw carrot, celery, radish etc.).
The pâtés are liable to discolour slightly if left exposed for too long. You cannot entirely prevent this but it helps to whizz a tablespoon of fresh lemon juice into the basic mix.

Delicious Dips

You can also make dips with your basic pâté mix. Serve these with:
- Mini-poppadoms
- Crudités (carrot and celery sticks, radishes etc.—page 175)
- Corn chips
- Potato wedges (page 154)
- As a dressing for salads
- As a topping for baked potatoes.

Avocado Dip

Ingredients for 4 servings

1 quanity of basic pâté mix

1 avocado pear, roughly chopped

2 tsp fresh lemon juice

Freshly ground black pepper

Instructions

Whizz all the ingredients together in a food processor until smooth.

Carrot and Coriander Dip

Ingredients for 4 servings

One quantity of basic pâté mix

2 tbsp coriander (cilantro) leaves, finely chopped

½ tsp cayenne pepper

Potassium salt

Instructions

Stir the ingredients together until thoroughly incorporated.

Try Some Ideas of Your Own

Lots of vegetables can be used to make delicious dips. Broccoli is especially delicious. Just peel the stem of a small head of broccoli, cut into small pieces and separate the head into small florets. Then steam until tender and whizz into the basic pâté mix. Try it with olives, onions or shallots, asparagus, artichokes, or roasted sweet peppers. Add herbs and spices to taste. Dips are made using added ingredients with a fairly high water content and so are softer than pâtés.

Spiced Bean Röstis

Ingredients for 2 servings

225 g/½ lb/1 cup cooked black-eyed beans (see page 129)

½ small onion, finely chopped or grated

3 medium-sized starchy (i.e. non-waxy) potatoes

½ tbsp thick soya yoghurt (such as Sojasun brand)

½ tsp curry powder

Olive oil

Potassium salt

Ground black pepper

Instructions

Peel and grate the potatoes, putting the gratings into a bowl of cold water. Mash the beans thoroughly and mix or blend in a food processor with the remaining ingredients except the olive oil and potato. Form the bean mixture into 4 patties. Using your hands, squeeze out the excess water from the grated potato and lay it on a clean tea towel. Fold the tea towel over and press the potatoes again to dry them as much as possible. Put the grated potatoes on a large plate. Place the bean patties on top of the potatoes, and press down gently. Cover the tops of the potatoes with as much grated potato as you can and press gently again. The potato will create quite a ragged covering, but this will adhere to the mixture when you start to cook the patties. Put a heavy-bottomed frying pan (skillet) over a moderate heat and add a few tbsp olive oil. Slide a spatula under each rösti to transfer it to the pan, and cook for about 5 minutes each side or until the potato is brown and crisp. Serve immediately with a mixed salad and a spoonful of Cacik (page 262) or Garlic Crème (page 254).

Recipe by Carolyn Gibbs

What It's Good For

These little Röstis are delicious and packed with protein from the beans. (Leftover basic pâté mix works just as well). Beans are rich in an amino acid known as lysine, which is lacking in most plant foods. In the human body, lysine is also converted into carnitine, an amino acid which helps to transport fat and convert it into energy. Vegetarians and vegans should eat beans and lentils regularly to avoid developing a lysine deficiency.

Creamy Butternut Soup

Ingredients for 4 servings

1 medium butternut squash

1 litre/1¾ pints/4 cups soya (soy) milk

1 large onion, finely chopped

2 tbsp extra virgin olive oil

Freshly ground black pepper

Instructions

Preheat the oven to 180°C/350°F/gas mark 4.

Cut the squash in half lengthwise, and remove the seeds with a spoon. Lay the squash pieces cut side down on a greased baking tray and bake in the preheated oven for 30 minutes or until soft.

Meanwhile sweat the onion in the olive oil in a large, heavy-bottomed saucepan over a low heat.

When the squash is ready, peel off the outside skin, chop the flesh and add it to the pan of onions, stir and heat through then add the soya milk. Bring almost to the boil, stirring from time to time.

Using a hand blender, whizz the ingredients together until smooth and creamy.

If you find the soup a little too thick, you can add some water to correct the consistency.

Reheat if necessary, stir in some freshly ground black pepper and serve immediately. I find that this soup does not need any salt, but you can add a little potassium salt if you wish.

What It's Good For

Like carrots and orange sweet potatoes, butternut squash are rich in cancer-preventing carotenes.

The best thing about this soup is that it tastes like something made with lavish amounts of cream, yet it is quite low in calories

Danish Open Sandwiches (Smørrebrød)

Open sandwiches are made with only one slice of bread (in this case pumpernickel), piled high with delicacies, and eaten with a knife and fork. Prepare ingredients according to how many people you are catering for.

Salmon and Potato Salad Topping

Ingredients

Wheat- and yeast-free
  pumpernickel bread*

Fresh salmon, filleted

Potato salad (see page 224)
  made with finely diced
  potatoes

Mayonnaise (see page 258)

Cucumber, finely diced

Dried dill herb

*This is a black rye bread with a strong, sweet flavour, ideal for open sandwiches. It is easily available from supermarkets and delicatessens.

Instructions

Poach the salmon fillet by putting it in a small saucepan with a few tablespoons of water and cooking with the lid on for about 10 minutes over a gentle heat until the fish is opaque throughout and flakes easily.

Remove the fish with a slotted spoon and allow to cool. Separate into large flakes. Gently fold the salmon flakes into the potato salad.

Spread a spoonful of mayonnaise on to a slice of pumpernickel, then add a large dollop of the potato salad and salmon mixture. Cover with a tablespoon of diced cucumber and finish with a sprinkling of chopped chives.

Recipe by Carolyn Gibbs

What It's Good For

Dianne Onstad's *Whole Foods Companion* tells us that the basic bread of mediaeval Britain consisted of coarsely ground rye and pea flours, sometimes with a little barley flour mixed in. Rye is most popular in Russia, as it tolerates the severe climate better than other grains. Wholegrain rye is rich in B vitamins, magnesium, iron and zinc, and as its fibre absorbs water well, it is excellent for bowel health. Black rye breads are made by cooking the bread at a relatively low temperature for a long time.

Hummus and Rainbow Salad Topping

Ingredients

Wheat- and yeast-free
  pumpernickel bread*

Hummus (see page 155)

Baby new potatoes

Mayonnaise

Gherkins, drained, well-rinsed and
  finely sliced

Grated carrot

Grated raw beetroot

Cherry tomatoes, sliced

Red sweet (bell) pepper, very finely
  diced

Yellow sweet (bell) pepper, very
  finely diced

Lettuce leaves, finely shredded

Spring onion (scallion), finely sliced

Fresh flat-leaf parsley, chopped

*See note on previous page

Instructions

Steam the baby new potatoes in their jackets until tender. Allow them to cool, then cut them into slices about ½cm/¼ inch thick.

Spread a generous layer of hummus on a slice of pumpernickel. Cover with a layer of sliced potato then spread with mayonnaise. Follow with sliced gherkins, grated carrot and beetroot, cherry tomato slices and a sprinkling of the diced peppers. Finish with a little shredded lettuce and a sprinkling of spring onion and chopped parsley.

If you are only making a couple of sandwiches, you may want to cut down on the number of different ingredients, since only a tiny amount of each one will be needed.

Recipe by Carolyn Gibbs

What It's Good For

Why not make up some open sandwich toppings of your own? The Speciality Pâtés and Crab Terrine also make a delicious base and can be topped with chopped gherkins, capers, spring onion, (scallion), pickled garlic, alfalfa sprouts (see page 130) and Sour Cream (page 253) or Garlic Crème (page 254).

Guacamole

Ingredients for 2-4 servings

1 small, ripe avocado

1 medium tomato, skinned, deseeded and finely chopped

½ green chilli pepper (seeds removed), very thinly sliced

2 tbsp mayonnaise (see page 258)

1 tbsp fresh lemon juice

½ clove garlic, crushed

Potassium salt

Instructions

Scoop the flesh out of the avocado and, using a fork, immediately mash the lemon juice into it.

Keep mashing until no large lumps remain, then stir in the crushed garlic and potassium salt until thoroughly incorporated, followed by the mayonnaise and then the chopped tomato and chilli pepper.

Serve as a starter or as part of a buffet meal, with tortilla chips or wheat-free crispbread or crackers to dip in the guacamole, or put spoonfuls on to little squares of warm unleavened bread (see page 260).

What It's Good For

Described as one of nature's most perfect foods, creamy, buttery avocado pears are so nutritious that they are practically a whole meal in themselves. They are easy to digest, and rich in protein, omega 6 polyunsaturated oils, vitamin B₆ and other B vitamins, vitamin E, iron and copper, with three times as much potassium as bananas. The rough-skinned Hass avocado has a particularly good flavour. The raw garlic in this recipe will help people with dysbiosis.

French Onion Soup

Ingredients for 2 servings

2 medium onions, peeled, cut in half vertically then thinly sliced

2 tbsp extra virgin olive oil

560 ml/1 pint/2 cups boiling water

1 heaped tbsp wheat-free miso

Herbs to taste: thyme, bay leaves and parsley are all suitable

Freshly ground black pepper

Instructions

Heat the oil in a large saucepan over a medium heat, then add the onions and stir-fry for about 20 minutes until beginning to caramelize.

Add the water followed by the miso and the herbs. Stir well to dissolve the miso.

Bring the liquid back to the boil, cover, and simmer over a low heat for 30 minutes. Season with freshly-ground black pepper before serving.

What It's Good For

The therapeutic value of the humble onion is often forgotten in favour of its famous cousin garlic. Onions are a rich source of the anti-allergy flavonoid quercetin, which is very similar to the drug disodium chromoglycate given to switch off allergic symptoms. Like the drug, quercetin can inhibit the release of histamine, the cause of allergic symptoms, inflammation and asthma attacks. Quercetin has also been investigated for its virus-fighting properties[250].

Falafel (chickpea patties)

Ingredients to make 8-9 small patties

115 g/4 ounces dried chickpeas which have been covered with four times their volume in boiling water and soaked overnight

1 medium onion, cut into 8 pieces

2 tbsp fresh coriander (cilantro) leaves, finely chopped

2 cloves garlic, roughly chopped

1 tsp coriander seeds

1 tsp cumin seeds

¼ tsp potassium baking powder

Potassium salt

Cayenne pepper

Olive oil for frying

Instructions

Drain the soaked chickpeas, and, using the S blade, whizz them in a food processor with the onion and garlic until they become a smooth paste which clumps together. Roughly crush the coriander and cumin seeds with a mortar and pestle then dry-roast them in a medium-hot frying pan for about half a minute to release the aromas. Stir the spices, seasonings and baking powder into the chickpea mixture and mix thoroughly.

Preheat a frying pan (skillet) over a medium heat and pour in olive oil to coat the bottom of the pan. Take tablespoons of the chickpea mixture, and, using your hands, form them into little patties measuring about 2 inches in diameter. When the oil is hot, gently lower the patties into it and cook for about 5 minutes on each side. Handle them gently when turning them over—I use a pair of flat tongs such as those used for turning fried fish. Drain the falafels on absorbent kitchen paper and serve hot or cold as a starter, snack, packed lunch or light supper dish with Cacik (page 262) and a green salad, or tucked into a folded round of unleavened bread (page 260) and topped with shredded lettuce and Garlic Crème (page 254).

What It's Good For

Chickpeas are very rich in protein, and are a good source of many other nutrients, including calcium, magnesium, iron, copper and some of the B vitamins. Falafels are a Middle Eastern dish and are often served stuffed into pitta bread and topped with salad and yoghurt. Always buy pulses/legumes (members of the bean and lentil family) with the longest "sell-by" date you can find. Lengthy storage makes them tough and they will take longer to cook.

Cream of Mushroom Soup

Ingredients for 2 servings

115 g/4 ounces/1 cup fresh mushrooms, roughly chopped

1 medium onion, roughly chopped

1 pint boiling water

2 tbsp extra virgin olive oil

1 rounded tbsp wheat-free miso

1 rounded tbsp brown rice flour

1 tbsp fresh parsley, finely chopped

1 tbsp soya (soy) cream

Freshly ground black pepper

Instructions

Heat the oil in a large saucepan over a medium heat and sweat the onions for a few minutes until translucent. Add the mushrooms, turn up the heat and stir-fry briskly for about 3 minutes. Sprinkle the brown rice flour over the mushrooms and onions, and stir it in thoroughly.

Dissolve the miso in the boiling water and pour over the mushrooms and onions. Stir well, bring back to the boil then turn the heat down to low, cover the pan and simmer for 20 minutes.

Remove the pan from the heat, and whizz the soup in the pan with a hand blender until you achieve the consistency you want. Stir in the soya cream and chopped parsley, season with freshly ground black pepper and serve immediately.

What It's Good For

The main benefit of common (white) mushrooms is their vitamin and mineral content. They are rich in B vitamins, iron, copper, zinc and chromium.

Some varieties of mushroom, especially the shiitake, are now known to have special medicinal properties due to their content of *lentinan*, a substance with anti-cancer properties.

Spinach and Lentil Soup

Ingredients for 6 servings

1.2 litres/2 pints/4 cups water

115g/4 ounces/½ cup brown
    lentils or Puy lentils*

250 g/9 ounces fresh spinach

1 large onion, chopped

2 tbsp miso

1 tbsp tomato purée (paste)

1 tbsp fresh lemon juice

Freshly ground black pepper

*These are small green speckled lentils.
They are best for this soup as they retain a
slightly chewy texture which contrasts well
with the smoothness of the spinach.

Instructions

Put the water, lentils and chopped onion in a large saucepan and bring to the boil, then cover the pan and simmer gently for 30 minutes.

Meanwhile, wash the spinach in a sinkful of cold water and drain in a colander. Twist off any tough, fibrous stalks from the spinach leaves, then take bundles of leaves, and shred them coarsely with a knife. Turn the shredded spinach bundles round 90 degrees and shred crosswise so that the spinach ends up roughly chopped.

When the lentils are ready, stir in the miso and tomato purée (paste), and incorporate thoroughly, then stir in the spinach. Put the lid on and leave over a low heat for 5 minutes or until the spinach has wilted and softened.

Using a hand blender, briefly whizz the soup while still in the pan, so that most of the lentils are still a little chewy, while the rest of the soup is thick and smooth. Stir in the freshly ground black pepper. If you wish, you could also pour in a little soya cream before serving.

What It's Good For

Spinach and lentils are good sources of an important B vitamin known as folic acid. This is likely to be in short supply in a diet consisting mostly of convenience foods because it is easily destroyed by food processing and lengthy storage. Spinach is also an excellent source of iron, but remember that iron from plant foods is not well absorbed unless the meal also contains vitamin C. The lemon juice in this recipe will help you absorb the iron, and you could also finish the meal with some fresh fruit.

Red Lentil and Chestnut Soup with Cumin and Parsley

Ingredients for 2 servings

150 ml/¼ pint/½ cup red lentils measured in a measuring jug

600 ml/1 pint/2 cups water

8 vacuum-packed chestnuts*

1 medium onion, chopped

2 tbsp olive oil

1 tbsp miso

1 tbsp chopped fresh parsley

½ tsp cumin seeds, roughly crushed with a mortar and pestle

Potassium salt

Freshly ground black pepper

*You could also use dried chestnuts. They will need prior soaking overnight followed by boiling until they are tender. Fresh chestnuts will need to be boiled until tender and then peeled while hot.

Instructions

Put the water and lentils in a saucepan and bring to the boil. Squash the chestnuts gently with the heel of your hand so that they will break up a little when cooking.

Meanwhile in a separate pan fry the onions in the olive oil over a medium heat until beginning to soften. Add the cumin and stir-fry until the aroma is released.

Add the contents of the pan to the lentils along with the chestnuts and simmer together for 45 minutes. Just before serving, add the seasoning and parsley.

What It's Good For

I like to use red onions for this recipe. The red colour is anthocyanin, a good antioxidant. Chestnuts are low in oil and are nutritionally quite similar to grains such as corn or rice. They are a good source of potassium, magnesium and iron. If lentils make you "windy" (as they do with most people), add more spices to the onions along with the cumin, especially cinnamon, cloves and cayenne pepper. Alternatively follow your meal with Digestive Tea (page 266).

Potato Pancakes with a Spinach, Mushroom and Goat's Cheese Filling

Ingredients to make 1 pancake

2 medium-sized waxy potatoes

55 g/2 ounces/½ cup
mushrooms, thinly sliced*

25 g/1 ounce hard goat's cheese,
finely grated

50 g spinach, washed and
shredded

Olive oil

Freshly ground black pepper

*You could use some of the more unusual
varieties of mushrooms such as shiitake if
you would like a change.

Instructions

Preheat a 25 cm/9½ inch diameter frying pan over a medium heat until very hot, then add 2 tbsp oil.

Coarsely grate the potatoes as quickly as you can to prevent browning, then transfer them to the hot frying pan. Using the tip of a spatula, distribute them evenly in the pan and press down to flatten. Cover the frying pan and leave the pancake to cook for one minute then turn the heat down low-medium and leave it to cook for a further 9 minutes.

Remove the pan from the heat and carefully slide the pancake on to a large plate. Cover the pancake with a second plate, then invert the plates, thus turning the pancake over. Replace the pan over a medium heat. When hot, add another tbsp oil, then carefully slide the pancake back into the pan to cook the other side and replace the lid. Turn the heat down again after one minute and then cook for a further 5 minutes. Remove from the pan and keep warm.

While the pancake is cooking, stir-fry the mushrooms in 2 tbsp hot olive oil until golden. Stir in the shredded spinach and toss until wilted. Remove from the heat and spoon on to one half of the potato pancake. Cover with grated cheese, season with freshly ground black pepper then fold the other half of the pancake over the filling and serve.

What It's Good For

Waxy potatoes allow you to make a deliciously succulent pancake without the need for egg. Potatoes are rich in potassium, and also lysine, a protein constituent (amino acid) which is low in most plant foods except beans and lentils, and is especially needed by herpes sufferers. Goat's cheese is also a good source of protein (including lysine). Spinach is a wonderful source of iron and other minerals, and mushrooms provide B vitamins and chromium.

Potato Pancakes with a Mexican Stuffing

Ingredients to make 4-8 portions

2 potato pancakes made as described on page 172

2 avocado pears

1 quantity of refried beans made as described on page 189

1 tsp lemon juice

Potassium salt

Freshly ground black pepper

Instructions

Preheat the oven to 200°C/400°F/Gas mark 6.

Peel and mash the avocados with the lemon juice. Season with potassium salt and pepper. Spread one of the potato pancakes with this mixture.

Spread the other potato pancake with the warm refried beans.

Sandwich the pancakes together, with the fillings in the middle.

Place on a baking tray and heat in the oven for 10-15 minutes.

Serve cut into wedges on a bed of lettuce.

What It's Good For

Delicious buttery avocadoes are rich in protein, omega 6 essential polyunsaturated oils, vitamin B6 and other B vitamins, vitamin E, iron and copper, and provide three tiems as much potassium as bananas. They are also easy to digest. Beans are also a good source of protein—one of the few good plant sources of the amino acid lysine, needed for your body to produce carnitine which helps you metabolize the fats and oils in your diet and turn them into energy.

Spring Greens Braised with Potatoes and Red Onions, with a Sour Cream Topping

Ingredients to make 2 servings

2 large potatoes, diced small

4 large leaves from a head of spring greens, cut crosswise into thin ribbons

1 medium red onion, cut in half lengthwise then thinly sliced

1 inch piece of root ginger, shredded (optional)

Spice mixture to taste (e.g. any combination of ground black pepper, cardamom, fennel, cloves, coriander seeds (optional)

A quantity of sour cream made as described on page 253

Fresh chives, finely chopped

2 tbsp olive oil

Potassium salt

Instructions

Using a large saucepan or sauté pan with a heavy base, fry the onion in the olive oil over a medium heat. When beginning to soften, add the spices (if using), heat through, then the potatoes and ginger (if using). Stir-fry together for one minute. Stir in the spring greens. Add 3 tbsp water, and season with potassium salt.

Cover the pan tightly, and cook over the lowest heat for 30 minutes, checking from time to time that there is enough moisture to prevent the contents from burning. If necessary add a little more water.

When all the ingredients are tender, all remaining moisture should be boiled off by removing the lid and turning up the heat. Turn out on to a plate and top with sour cream sprinkled with fresh chives and ground black pepper.

What It's Good For

Spring greens are a rich source of folic acid, magnesium, iron and lutein—the carotene which plays an important part in your eyesight.

Without enough folic acid you can become depressed because your body cannot turn the amino acids tyrosine and tryptophan into adrenal hormones and serotonin, respectively. Many psychiatric patients are found to have a folic acid deficiency[233].

Crudités

Ingredients for 2 servings

1 large carrot

1 large green (bell) pepper

1 large sweet red (bell) pepper

2 stalks of celery

Half a mooli* radish

Half a cucumber

*Mooli radishes are long, white radishes about twice the size of carrots. They are often used in Oriental cookery, and can be found in larger supermarkets. If you cannot obtain one, use ordinary radishes.

Instructions

Cut the radish and carrot into 6 cm/3 inch segments then slice these lengthwise first one way and then the other to make sticks.

Cut around the stalk of the peppers and remove it, then cut the peppers into eight pieces lengthwise. Discard the seeds but retain as much of the white pith as possible.

Using a sharp knife or vegetable peeler, peel the outside of the celery stalks so that the tough fibres are stripped away, then cut the stalks in half.

Cut the cucumber into 6 cm/3 inch segments then cut each segment into four pieces lengthwise.

Arrange the crudités on a plate, with a selection of dips for people to help themselves.

Suitable dips from this book are those on page 141 and also:

- Sour cream (page 253)
- Hummus (page 155)
- Garlic crème (page 254).

What It's Good For

Delicious crunchy raw vegetables are an ideal party snack. Among other this, this dish provides: Carrots—beta carotene; Peppers—vitamin C and flavonoids; Celery—organic sodium (unlike sodium from salt, this is not harmful) and coumarins, which help to release fluid retention; Cucumber—silicon (good for bone and skin strength); Mooli radish—sulphur compounds, which are highly beneficial for the liver.

Crab Terrine

Ingredients for 4-6 servings

1 medium-sized crab, dressed*

115 g/4 ounces silken tofu (see page 134)

2 tbsp sunflower oil

15 g/½ ounce gelatine powder

Soya or sheep's milk yoghurt as required†

1 tbsp fresh lemon juice

3 tbsp water

Potassium salt

Freshly ground black pepper

*You can either buy the crab ready-dressed, or, for a better flavour, dress it yourself just before making this recipe (see next page).

†If using soya yoghurt, choose a thick variety such as Sojasun. Sheep's yoghurt is sharper than soya yoghurt, so use it if you prefer a slightly more acidic flavour.

Instructions

Put the 3 tbsp water in a small dish, and sprinkle the gelatine powder over it to soften.

Whizz the silken tofu, brown crab meat, sunflower oil, potassium salt and lemon juice until smooth, in a food processor using the S blade. If you are using a firm variety of silken tofu such as Sanchi Organic Tofu, you will also need to add 2 tbsp of water to soften the consistency.

Heat 2 tbsp water in a small saucepan over a moderate heat until it is boiling vigorously, then remove it from the heat, empty out the water and immediately put the softened gelatine into the hot pan. If the pan retains heat well, the gelatine should then dissolve and quickly become runny when stirred. (If it does not, you will need to boil some water in a larger pan and then put the smaller pan inside it so that you can heat the gelatine to the runny stage without scorching it).

Pour some of the whizzed crab mixture into the pan of gelatine and stir thoroughly, then pour this mixture back into the food processor with the rest. Process again briefly until the gelatine has been thoroughly incorporated, scraping down the

What It's Good For

As they grow larger, crabs have to grow a new (soft) shell inside the old one. This soft shell can be scraped out and is not only delicious but extremely nutritious and full of the bone-nourishing minerals calcium, magnesium and zinc. Crabs are also an exceptionally good source of iodine and selenium, trace elements which are very depleted in British crops. Both are important for your thyroid gland, which governs your metabolism. Low iodine levels can increase the risk of breast disease in women.

Dressing a Crab

Ask the fishmonger to prise it open for you if you don't know how to do this, and to remove the inedible "dead men's fingers" (contrary to popular belief, they are not poisonous). Ask for a male crab if you want one with more white meat.

Dressing a crab just means prising the meat out from every little nook and cranny of the crab. It can take up to an hour. Keeping the white meat separate from the brown meat (which is also known as the "cream" of the crab) use strong kitchen scissors to cut through the internal body shell and up the small leg segments before prising them open, and a skewer to ease out the meat. Crack the large claws with a hammer.

sides with a rubber spatula half-way through.

Then, using the same spatula, scrape the crab mixture into a measuring jug with a capacity of at least one pint (570 ml) and fold in the shredded white crab meat. Season with freshly ground black pepper. If the contents of the jug do not reach the 1 pint mark, top them up with soya or sheep's yoghurt.

Mix well, then pour into a small loaf tin or long plastic mould which has been lined with clingfilm. Chill for several hours before serving.

Serving suggestions

- Cut into slabs and serve as a starter on shredded lettuce with wheat-free crispbread or crackers,
- Dollop on to warm Potato Cakes Grand Prix as a delicious topping.

More About Selenium

Scientists now know that people who eat a selenium-rich diet have a much lower risk of getting a heart attack or cancer. Selenium should be absorbed from the soil into our cereal crops, but the soil in most areas of the UK, New Zealand, Finland and parts of China are very poor in selenium. So we have to make up for it by consuming more Brazil nuts, seafood and selenium supplements. Selenium also helps to activate thyroid hormone and to make an antioxidant enzyme, glutathione peroxidase.

Potato Ravioli

Ingredients for about 24 small ravioli (2 servings)

<u>One quantity of Potato Gnocci dough (see page 229)</u>

<u>2 tbsp pesto sauce (page 225)</u>

<u>25 g/1 ounce finely grated goat's cheese* for filling plus 55 g/2 ounces for topping</u>

*Choose a hard variety that grates easily

Instructions

Divide the potato dough in half and form each half into a ball. Using a rolling pin, roll out the dough ball into a sheet about ½ cm/¼ inch thick.

Using a glass tumbler or pastry cutter with a diameter of about 5 cm/2½ inches, cut out as many rounds from this sheet as you can.

Bring a large saucepan of water to the boil.

Dot the centre of each round with a small blob of pesto sauce and a pinch of grated cheese, then fold the rounds over and, using the very tips of your fingers, carefully pinch the edges together to form a tiny "pasty".

You should not have trouble getting the edges to stay together if your pinches are tiny enough, but if you do you could dampen the edges of the rounds with a little water before pressing together.

As you prepare the ravioli, put them on a plate then gently slide them off the plate into the gently boiling water. Cook for 60-80 seconds then remove them from the water with a slotted spoon. Serve immediately, sprinkled with the rest of the grated cheese.

What It's Good For

Based on my experience, I would say that about half of all people with a food intolerance have problems with cow's milk products. As with other food intolerances, these problems can be anything from headaches to eczema, joint pains or digestive problems. Substituting goat or sheep's milk, cheese and yoghurt is not the answer for everyone but go ahead and enjoy an occasional recipe like this if it does not cause you any symptoms.

Lamb's Liver Terrine with Onions and Thyme

Ingredients for 4-6 servings

300 g/10 ounces organic lamb's liver, roughly cut into chunks

150 g/5 ounces onions, finely chopped

2 walnut-sized knobs of coconut oil

1 tsp dried thyme

Potassium salt

Freshly-ground black pepper

Instructions

Heat one knob of coconut oil in a frying pan (skillet) over a medium heat, add the onions, and sweat them for 5 minutes until translucent.

Keeping the pan hot, remove the onions from the pan with a slotted spoon into the bowl of a food processor fitted with the S blade, then add the second knob of coconut oil followed by the chunks of lamb's liver. Stir and fry for about 5 minutes, until cooked, then add the liver to the onions in the food processor. Season with potassium salt.

Scraping down the sides with a rubber spatula from time to time, whizz the liver and onions until the mixture is finely ground and clumps together.

While still warm, empty the mixture into a terrine dish with a capacity of about half a litre/¾ pint and smooth down the surface with a fork. Allow to cool and when cold cover the dish with a piece of absorbent kitchen paper (to prevent condensation dripping on the contents) followed by a lid or a sheet of clingfilm, and place in the fridge for at least 3 hours. Serve slices of the terrine on wheat– and yeast-free crackers, crispbread or pumpernickel, or on a bed of lettuce with salad and mayonnaise.

What It's Good For

Poisonous amounts of vitamin A are only found in intensively-reared animals—their feed contains artificially large amounts of vitamin A added as a growth-promoter. Their liver can end up containing 20 times the normal amount of vitamin A. Organic liver does not have this problem. Liver provides protein, vitamin A, B vitamins and many minerals including chromium and zinc. It is worth consuming it occasionally; not everyone is efficient at making vitamin A from beta carotene.

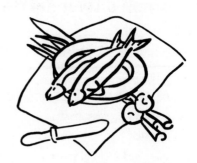

Main Meals

Lots of people are confused about how much they should eat at different meals.

The truth is, a heavy meal eaten late in the day is much more easily turned into body fat. This is because you would normally be sleeping at night and cannot use it up like your other meals.

The old maxim "Breakfast like a King, lunch like a prince and dine like a pauper" is absolutely true!

Balkan Peppers Stuffed with a Bean Medley

Ingredients for 4 servings

2 capsicum peppers, washed

1 x 400g can/10 ounces/
  1 generous cup cooked mixed
  beans (haricot beans, pinto
  beans, chick peas etc.)

1 large onion, thinly sliced

1 stick celery, finely chopped

4 cloves garlic, chopped

200 ml water

2 tbsp olive oil

1 dessertspoon rice flour

1 heaped tsp (sweet) paprika
  powder

1 tbsp fresh chopped parsley

Potassium salt

Freshly ground black pepper

Instructions

Preheat the oven to 180°C/350°F/gas mark 4.

Cut the peppers in half, remove the stalks and centres, and stand the peppers open side up in a close-fitting deep dish. (If necessary cut a little off the bottom so that they can stand without falling over.)

Using a stir-fry pan or a large saucepan with a heavy base, fry the onions, celery and garlic over a medium heat for five minutes or until beginning to brown. Stir in the paprika, rice flour, parsley and seasonings. Add the water a little at a time, stirring to form a gravy. When all the water has been incorporated, fold in the beans.

Spoon the bean mixture into and around the half peppers. Cover the dish and place in the oven for one hour. By this time the peppers should be tender.

Serve with creamed potatoes and a green salad.

Variation

Try adding chopped mushrooms instead of celery.

What It's Good For

A hearty dish for a winter's day, this brings you all the goodness of carotene from the peppers and protein from the beans. Paprika powder—used to make Hungarian goulash—is simply dried and powdered sweet capsicum peppers. These are a very popular crop in Eastern Europe. Housewives preserve and bottle peppers to last throughout the winter, and there are many wonderful and unusual preserving recipes combining different ingredients.

Organic Chicken Sauté with Vegetables and Garlic

Ingredients for 2 servings

2 medium portions organic chicken

1 x 400 g/14 ounce can chopped plum tomatoes

4 medium potatoes, peeled and cut in half

1 large onion, roughly diced

1 large carrot, cut into 1-inch segments

115 g/4 ounces/1 cup white mushrooms, thickly sliced

4 cloves garlic, peeled and roughly chopped

2 tbsp extra virgin olive oil

2 tbsp rice flour

1 tbsp soya cream

Potassium salt

Black pepper

Instructions

This is a one-pot meal made in a pressure cooker. Season the chicken portions with potassium salt then coat thoroughly with rice flour. Heat the olive oil in the pressure cooker with the lid off then add the chicken pieces. Fry over a high heat until golden and crisp on both sides (this seals in the juices), then stir in the onion and garlic, and continue stirring until they begin to soften. Pour in the chopped tomatoes, stir, put the lid on and bring the pressure cooker up to full steam. Maintaining a steady pressure, cook for 20 minutes.

Put the pressure cooker in a sink of cold water to bring the pressure down and enable you to remove the lid. Stir the contents, then add the remaining vegetables to the pan, fitting them neatly around the chicken and ensuring they are all coated with the sauce. (If necessary add a little water to the pan to enable this). Replace the lid and heat again to full steam. Once again maintaining a steady pressure, cook for a further 12 minutes.

Put the pressure cooker in cold water again and once it is safe to do so, remove the lid, check

What It's Good For

Even free-range chickens may be fed standard commercial feed which contains antibiotics, chicken dung and other unsavoury items. We do not know what residues remain in the bird's meat and fat, and how they affect our health. Eating organic chicken overcomes all these dilemmas. And the flavour is far better. Chicken is an excellent, low-fat source of protein—even with its skin left on. Protein is essential for all body processes, including the important detoxification work of your liver.

Special Equipment

A pressure cooker

that the vegetables are tender, and remove the chicken and vegetable pieces to a heated serving dish with the aid of a slotted spoon. Keep warm. Replace the pressure cooker on the stove, without putting the lid on, and turn up the heat until you can fast-boil the sauce remaining in the pan. Keep stirring and reduce to about 2-3 ladlefuls of thick sauce. Remove from the heat and add 1 tbsp soya cream, plus some freshly ground black pepper. Stir through and pour the sauce over the chicken and vegetables. Serve immediately.

This is a dish rich in many nutrients. Most notably Italian plum tomatoes, with their deep, rich red colour are the best source of lycopene, a type of carotene which due to its powerful antioxidant properties has been found to help prevent prostate cancer and also breast cancer. A similar antioxidant, beta carotene is found in carrots. The body can also convert beta carotene into vitamin A.

Onions are a good source of the flavonoid quercetin, which helps to fight allergies. Mushrooms are one of the few natural good sources of chromium, a trace element needed for sugar and carbohydrate metabolism.

Baked Potatoes with Salmon and Sour Cream

Ingredients for 2 servings

2 baking potatoes, well scrubbed

115 g/4 ounces fresh salmon, filleted

1 spring onion (scallion), finely sliced

Soya milk

1 tsp fresh dill, chopped

Potassium salt

Freshly ground black pepper

Instructions

Preheat the oven to 200°C/400°F/Gas mark 6.

Prick the potatoes all over with a fork, and bake them for 45 minutes or until they feel soft when you squeeze them. Poach the salmon in a few tablespoons of water in a lidded pan over a low heat for five minutes, until the fish flakes easily.

Remove the potatoes from the oven and slice in half lengthways. Scoop out the potato flesh, leaving the skins intact. Mash the potato flesh with a little soya milk and seasoning, then gently fold in the spring onion and salmon flakes, trying not to break them up too much, and pile the mixture into the potato skin halves. Return to the oven for 15 minutes to heat through, then serve with a generous topping of sour cream (see page 253) and a sprinkling of dill.

More ideas for baked potato toppings

- Chickpeas and guacamole (page 166)
- Pesto (page 225)
- Onion marmalade (page 215)
- Avocado and tomato in vinaigrette with chopped coriander (cilantro)

What It's Good For

Like herrings (see recipe on page 144, salmon is a so-called "oily" fish, rich in omega 3 oils which help prevent red blood cells from clumping together and causing heart attacks. You may not know that these oily fish themselves are a far richer source of omega 3 oils than fish oil supplements. Salmon is also an excellent source of protein, which is needed by your liver to process toxins.

Baked Potatoes with Green Cabbage Courgettes and Red Onion

Ingredients for 2 servings

2 baking potatoes, well scrubbed

4 large leaves from a head of green cabbage, shredded cross-wise into ribbons

1 large courgette, cut lengthwise into little sticks (use a julienne cutter if you have one)

1 red onion cut in half lengthwise and thinly sliced

4 tbsp sheep's milk yoghurt or thick soya yoghurt

2 tbsp olive oil

1 tbsp fresh chives, chopped

Potassium salt

Freshly ground black pepper

Instructions

Preheat the oven to 200°C/400°F/Gas mark 6.

Prick the potatoes all over with a fork, and bake them for 45 minutes or until they feel soft when you squeeze them.

Meanwhile make the topping. Stir the chives into the yoghurt and season with potassium salt and black pepper. Leave to one side.

In a large heavy-bottomed saucepan, gently stir-fry the onion slices in the olive oil for a minute or so until beginning to soften. Add the cabbage and courgette sticks, and stir-fry together for half a minute. Add 3 tbsp water, then cover the pan tightly and turn down the heat to the lowest setting. Cook for 15 minutes, checking occasionally that there is enough moisture in the pan to prevent burning.

Remove from the heat and season with potassium salt and black pepper. Keep warm until the potatoes are ready.

Remove the potatoes from the oven and cut into quarters, but not all the way through. Open out the potatoes and pile on the vegetables. Top with the yoghurt and chive mixture.

What It's Good For

Dark green cabbage is one of the best sources of lutein, a type of carotene which helps to protect your eyesight. Lutein is hard to get from your diet unless you regularly eat deep green leafy vegetables. These are also a good source of magnesium, which is often lacking in the average diet.

Red onions contain anthocyanin—a powerful antioxidant with a blue colour that can also look red or purple in certain plants.

Stuffed Sweet Peppers with Wild Rice and Porcini Mushrooms

Ingredients for 2 servings

2 medium to large sweet peppers (red, green or yellow)

125 g/4½ ounces/½ cup firm tofu

4 tbsp cooked brown rice, to include 1 tsp cooked wild or red rice

1 small to medium onion, finely chopped

1 small handful dried porcini mushrooms which have been soaked in boiling water for half an hour and then finely chopped

4 cloves garlic, finely chopped

2 tbsp soya (soy) milk

2 tbsp extra virgin olive oil

1 tsp fresh basil, finely chopped

Potassium salt

Freshly ground black pepper

Instructions

Preheat the oven to 180°C/350°F/gas mark 4. Blanch the peppers for two minutes in a pan of boiling water then remove and drain. Sweat the chopped onion slowly in the olive oil over a low heat, with the lid on the pan. Cut the tops (with stalks) off the peppers and save them to make lids. Remove the seeds with a teaspoon.

In a blender or food processor (with S blade), whizz the tofu and soya milk, scraping the sides down with a spatula from time to time, until smooth and creamy.

When the onions are soft, add the garlic, chopped mushrooms, cooked rice, basil and seasoning. Stir-fry together in the pan for half a minute, then fold in the creamed tofu. Remove from the heat, and keep folding with a spoon to ensure that all the ingredients are thoroughly incorporated.

Stuff the peppers with this mixture and press it in firmly. Replace the tops of the peppers. Stand the peppers up in an oiled oven-proof dish (or lay them down if they won't stand), brush with olive oil, and bake for 45 minutes or until tender.

Using a sharp knife, cut each pepper across into 4-6 slices and serve with Ratatouille (page 217) or Garlic Potatoes Corfu Style (page 214).

What It's Good For

The main ingredients of this dish are tofu and sweet peppers. See page 142 for the benefits of tofu and other soya products. Sweet peppers are an excellent source of vitamin C and flavonoids. Many of the flavonoids are concentrated in the white pith, so try not to throw it away. Green sweet peppers are simply an unripe version of red ones, and contain less carotene.

Red Thai Curry with Pan-Fried Tofu

Ingredients for 1 serving

<u>3 thick slices from a block of firm tofu</u>

<u>1 cm/½ inch piece cut from a block of creamed coconut</u>

<u>½ cup mixed frozen vegetables (e.g. carrots and red sweet [bell] peppers diced small, peas, sweetcorn [corn])</u>

<u>1 portion uncooked vermicelli rice noodles or 1 portion cooked brown rice</u>

<u>150 ml/¼ pint/½ cup water</u>

<u>2 tbsp groundnut oil for frying</u>

<u>1 tbsp brown rice flour</u>

<u>2 tsp red Thai curry paste (more if you like it stronger)</u>

<u>Potassium salt</u>

<u>Cayenne pepper</u>

Instructions

Cut the tofu into bite-size pieces, pat dry with kitchen paper, sprinkle with potassium salt and cayenne pepper and coat well with brown rice flour. Heat the oil in a frying pan (skillet). When hot enough for the tofu to sizzle, carefully put the pieces in the pan and fry on each side for 1-2 minutes or until golden. Drain on absorbent kitchen paper.

Heat the water in a saucepan. Add the curry paste and coconut cream, stirring until dissolved. Add the frozen vegetables, put the lid on the saucepan and simmer for a few minutes.

Place the vermicelli rice noodles in a bowl. Boil a kettleful of water and pour the water generously over the noodles, leaving them plenty of room to swell. Leave for 2 minutes then run some cold water into the bowl before draining the noodles thoroughly in a large sieve. If using rice, heat the rice in a tightly lidded pan over a medium heat with 2 tablespoons of water.

When the vegetables are heated through, stir in the fried tofu pieces and coat with the sauce. Serve the rice or noodles with the vegetables and tofu on top and a little of the sauce spooned over.

What It's Good For

Tofu, with its richness of hormone-balancing compounds, and coconut cream, with the anti-viral properties of the coconut oil it contains, are key ingredients here, with mixed vegetables providing a rich balance of antioxidant nutrients, and cayenne pepper (found in the curry paste) helping to warm the circulation and improve the digestion. This is a delicious meal which can be put together in only 10 minutes.

Mexican Tortillas with Garlic, Lime and Refried Beans

To make 4 lazy tortillas

90 g/3 ounces/3 heaped tbsp finely ground yellow polenta meal

20 g/1 ounce/1 heaped tbsp buckwheat flour

200 ml/generous 6 fluid oz/¾ cup water

Instructions

When cooked, these tortillas look just like the real thing—on one side only. On the other side they look like pancakes! Needless to say, hide the pancake side with your filling and no-one will notice the difference.

Mix the ingredients thoroughly. Depending on your flours, you may need a little more or a little less water, so don't be afraid to experiment a bit. Heat a dry non-stick frying pan (skillet) over a medium to high heat. Stir the mixture then pour in a ladleful and gently shake the pan so that it quickly spreads out on all sides to the thickness of a pancake. Try to keep the shape circular, and aim to make the tortillas about 12 cm/6 inches in diameter.

After about one minute, when the top has set and the edges start to curl upwards, flip the tortilla over and cook the other side. Press down with a spatula and cook for another minute or until the bottom is looking slightly floury with brown specks.

Make the other three tortillas in the same way, and stack them, separated by a layer of absorbent kitchen paper, until you are ready to fill them.

What It's Good For

It would be very difficult to pack any more nutrients into a meal than you can get from this lovely dish. Here are just a few examples of what it provides. Beans and polenta flour: high-class protein combination. Tomatoes: anti-cancer carotene lycopene. Raw garlic: blood sterilizing, anti-candida and anti-cancer action. Onion: anti-allergy, anti-virus and anti-cancer flavonoid quercetin. Lime: vitamin C and blood vessel strengthening flavonoids.

To make the filling

450 g/1 lb/2 cups cooked pinto
    beans (see page 129),
    mashed roughly with a
    potato masher or fork

4 fresh tomatoes, skinned and
    chopped

1 large onion, chopped

The flesh of 1 small lime, cut in
    four and sliced

Plus 1 tsp grated lime zest

2 green hot chilli peppers, cut
    into long, thin strips

4 cloves garlic, crushed

2 tbsp fresh coriander leaf
    (cilantro) chopped

2 tbsp extra virgin olive oil

1 tsp black mustard seeds

Tamari sauce

Potassium salt

Shredded iceberg lettuce and
    Garlic Crème (page 254) to
    garnish

Instructions

Heat the olive oil over a medium heat in a deep frying pan (skillet), or preferably a stir-fry pan, and add the mustard seeds. When they begin to pop, add the chopped onion, 3½ cloves of the crushed garlic, and the chilli pepper strips.

Stir-fry until they are beginning to soften, then add the lime flesh and zest and fry for another two minutes, gently turning occasionally with a spoon without breaking up the lime pieces.

Fold in the chopped tomatoes and allow to cook for a further 2 minutes, occasionally turning the mixture, until the tomatoes are soft. Add the mashed beans, chopped coriander, the rest of the chopped garlic, a few dashes of tamari sauce and some potassium salt, fold in gently, turn down the heat to low and cover the pan. Leave for 5 minutes to heat through, occasionally turning the ingredients gently with a spoon. The beans will soften and blend with the other ingredients.

Meanwhile heat up the tortillas under the grill (broiler) and keep warm. When the filling is ready, hold a tortilla "pancake side up" in your hand and pile filling into it, squeezing the sides slightly together. Cover the top of the exposed filling with a handful of shredded iceberg lettuce and pour over a few spoonfuls of Garlic Crème.

More Ideas

You can also make enchiladas by rolling the refried bean filling up in the corn pancakes described on page 142, laying the rolls seam-side down, and topping with a tomato, garlic and chilli sauce and a dollop of Garlic Crème.

Make a tomato salsa to go with either of these dishes, using finely chopped tomatoes, diced avocado pear, chilli pepper, coriander leaf and capers plus a squeeze of lemon juice and a dash of Tabasco chilli sauce.

Rejuvenation Soup (a one-pot meal)

Ingredients for 6 servings

1 organic chicken or duck
   carcass

The giblets (liver, neck and heart
   only)

1.7 litres/3 pints/6 cups water

Approx 200 g/7 ounces rice
   vermicelli

4 dark green cabbage leaves,
   shredded

2 carrots, sliced

2 tomatoes, roughly chopped

1 large onion, chopped

2 tbsp brown miso

Black pepper

Special Equipment

A pressure cooker

Instructions

You would normally use the remains of a roast chicken or duck for this soup, but any small bones will do, for instance those left after filleting a chicken.

Cut any greeny-yellow marks off the liver (these are bitter and come from bile). Put the bones in a pressure cooker with the giblets and water and press down on the carcass to ensure it is covered with water. Bring to full steam and cook for 45 minutes. Cool the pressure cooker in a sink of cold water until you can open the lid, then strain the stock through a sieve into a large saucepan. Dissolve the miso in the stock, season with black pepper and add the vegetables.

Once the contents of the sieve have cooled, use your hands to pick the remains of any meat off the neck and bones, and put them in the saucepan. Crumble the liver and thinly slice the heart, and put these in the pan too. Discard the remains of the carcass.

Now bring the pan to the boil and simmer for 30 minutes. Add the rice vermicelli and leave to soak in the soup for 2 minutes before stirring and serving. This soup makes a complete meal and can be refrigerated once cool and reheated as needed.

What It's Good For

A great way to use the giblets from a chicken or duck, plus the bones which normally get thrown away. In effect, you are getting a couple more meals out of the bird. Liver is rich in vitamin A, folic acid, iron, copper, zinc and B vitamins. Bones are rich in calcium, magnesium and many other minerals, as well as glycine, which helps your liver to process toxins. With antioxidants in the dark green cabbage leaves, and all the vitamins in the miso, eating this soup regularly could seriously rejuvenate you!

Plaice Meunière with Mustard, Lemon and Parsley Sauce

Ingredients for 2 servings

2 large plaice fillets

3 tbsp extra virgin olive oil plus 2 tbsp for frying

Juice of half a lemon

1 dessertspoon fresh or 1 tsp dried parsley, chopped

Brown rice flour

½ tsp arrowroot powder

½ tsp yellow mustard powder

Potassium salt

Black pepper

Instructions

Combine the 3 tbsp oil in a small saucepan with the lemon juice and heat very gently. Blend the arrowroot and mustard powders with a tablespoon of water and stir into the mixture in the saucepan. Stir until it thickens, then remove from the heat and season with potassium salt and black pepper. Stir in the parsley.

Heat 2 tbsp oil in a frying pan. Season the plaice fillets and coat thoroughly with rice flour. When the oil is hot, put the fillet in the pan, skin side up. Cook for 2 minutes or until the bottom is beginning to crisp and turn golden. Turn over and cook the other side for 1-2 minutes, pressing down a little with a spatula as the fish will curl up slightly. Drain the fish on absorbent kitchen paper and keep warm. Repeat with the other fillet if it did not fit in the same pan.

When ready to serve, whisk the sauce, and pour over the fish. A good vegetable accompaniment would be Diced New Potatoes and Courgettes with Pesto Coating (see page 225).

Variation

This sauce can also be served with poached halibut.

What It's Good For

Fish is not just an excellent source of good quality protein, but is easy to digest and contains little or no saturated fat. This makes it ideal for someone whose liver is under stress. Olive oil contains fatty acids which help to combat the yeast *Candida albicans*. Extra virgin olive oil is also now known to help preserve our mental powers as we age. Many people who find it hard to digest fats seem to have much less of a problem with olive oil.

Hot Spicy Prawns with Rice Noodles and Mixed Vegetables

Ingredients for 1 serving

115 g/4 ounces rice noodles

115 g/4 ounces/½ cup frozen mixed vegetables diced small (e.g. peas, carrots, peppers, [sweet]corn)

1 handful frozen peeled prawns*

1 tsp tamari sauce* or Thai fish sauce*

4 tbsp extra virgin olive oil

Potassium salt

Cayenne pepper

*Caution: These contain salt

Special Equipment

A stir-fry pan

Instructions

Put the frozen prawns and vegetables in a small lidded saucepan with 2 tbsp olive oil and heat gently until thawed. Continue cooking gently for 5 minutes with the lid off to allow the juices to evaporate. Remove from the heat, sprinkle with cayenne pepper and stir.

Follow the instructions on the rice noodles packet with regard to soaking them in hot water, although you may find that halving the soaking time indicated on the packet produces a better result (ideally they should still be definitely "al dente" because stir-frying will finish cooking them). I like to use thin noodles—slightly thicker than vermicelli—which take only 2 minutes to soak.

As soon as the noodles have finished soaking, drain them quickly in a large sieve and put them in a bowl. Pour cold water over them, strain them again (throw the water away) and suspend them over the empty bowl to catch any drips.

Heat a stir-fry pan over a medium heat. When hot, add 2 tbsp olive oil and then the rice noodles. Stir-fry for about 20 seconds, then add potassium salt and tamari sauce or fish sauce and stir-fry for

What It's Good For

When cooked in this way, frozen vegetables are rich in vitamins and minerals. The vegetables are frozen soon after harvest and do not then lose nutrients like those which hang around in shops and then at home for several days. But if you defrost frozen vegetables and then throw away their defrost liquid, you will be throwing away most of their vitamins. Likewise if you boil them and then throw away the cooking water.

another 20 seconds. By now the noodles should be soft. Add the prawns and vegetables and stir-fry together briefly until thoroughly incorporated. Pile on to a plate and eat immediately.

Variations

Instead of prawns I often use fish fillets (salmon, whiting, haddock etc.) which can be poached in a few tablespoons of water in a lidded pan over a low heat for five minutes, then flaked and added to the cooked vegetables. My favourite variation is to use finely shredded green cabbage instead of frozen vegetables. Use a mandolin-type appliance to shred it, then briefly stir-fry it in olive oil in the stir-fry pan, add 2 tbsp water, cover the stir-fry pan tightly, and leave it over a low to medium heat to steam for 5 minutes. Stir the cabbage into the noodles as you did with the frozen vegetables.

You could also use small pieces of leftover steamed vegetables such as broccoli and carrots. Just add them to the noodles then put a lid over the stir-fry pan and leave to heat through for 2 minutes over the lowest possible heat before serving.

This is delicious and satisfying dish for the kind of person who often arrives home late, tired and hungry, and would rather order a take-away or pizza than start cooking. Now you will never need another take-away. Making this dish takes less time than waiting for your take-away, and costs a fraction of the amount.

Like other seafood, prawns are rich in nutrients from the sea, including zinc and iodine.

Baked Salmon Parcels with Lime and Dill

Ingredients for each serving

One salmon fillet weighing
about 115 g/4 ounces

Limes (one for each 3-4 fillets),
thinly sliced

Olive oil

Fresh dill weed, roughly
chopped

Potassium salt

Freshly ground black pepper

Instructions

Preheat the oven to gas mark 4

Brush the salmon fillets with olive oil then season with potassium salt and freshly ground black pepper. Sprinkle a pinch of chopped dill over the fish, then lay 3 overlapping slices of lime on top. Place each fillet carefully in the centre of a piece of baking foil, and fold the foil around the fish, tucking in the edges to make a parcel. If you wish to avoid aluminium, it is possible to make the parcels with baking parchment or grease-proof paper instead. Use a stapler to hold the edges of the parcel together. Lay the parcels in an open oven-proof dish or tray and bake in the oven for 25 minutes or until the fish is opaque throughout. Never overcook fish - it is at its best when only just done.

Serve immediately, with Sour Cream (page 253) and mixed vegetables, or with a Baked Rice dish (pages 210 and 211).

What It's Good For

Like herrings (see recipe on page 144), salmon is a so-called "oily" fish, rich in omega 3 oils which help prevent red blood cells from clumping together and causing heart attacks. You may not know that these oily fish themselves are a far richer source of omega 3 oils than fish oil supplements. Salmon is also an excellent source of protein, needed by your liver to process toxins.

Pasta Spirals Baked with a Sauce of Tomatoes Mushrooms and Olives Topped with Sour Cream

Ingredients for 4 servings

700 g/1½ lb/3 cups fresh tomatoes, skinned and chopped (you could also use good quality plum tomatoes canned in natural juice)

225 g/8 ounces/1 cup onions, finely chopped

225 g/8 ounces/4 handfuls pasta spirals made from rice or corn

225 g/8 ounces/1 cup mushrooms, finely diced

2 tbsp tomato purée (paste)

6 black olives, stoned and cut in four

(not ones preserved in lemon or vinegar)

4 cloves garlic, peeled and chopped

Extra virgin olive oil

1 tbsp fresh basil, chopped

1 tbsp fresh chives, chopped

Potassium salt

Freshly ground black pepper

Instructions

Preheat the oven to 180°C/350°F/gas mark 4. In a large saucepan, gently fry the chopped onion in 4 tbsp olive oil until soft but not brown. Stir in the chopped garlic and cook for half a minute, then stir in the chopped tomatoes. Put a lid on the pan and cook over a medium heat for 15 minutes to break down the tomatoes. Fry the diced mushrooms in 3 tbsp olive oil until golden.

Remove the lid from the saucepan, add the tomato purée, mushrooms, olive pieces and potassium salt, and continue to boil for 45 minutes over a medium heat without the lid until the sauce is reduced to a thick consistency. Stir in the chopped basil.

Put the pasta spirals in a large pan of fast boiling water and cook according to the directions on the packet until they are just "al dente". Do not overcook them. Run some cold water into the pan as soon as they are ready, drain them, put them in an oven-proof dish, and thoroughly mix them with 2 tbsp olive oil. Add the pasta sauce and stir together.

Cover the dish and bake in the oven for 45 minutes. Serve with Sour Cream (see page 253) spooned on top and a sprinkling of chives.

What It's Good For

There are lots of goodies in this recipes, including chromium and B vitamins from the mushrooms, anti-cancer lycopene from the tomatoes, soya in the Sour Cream, and methionine in the pasta spirals (if made from rice). Methionine is turned to glutathione in your liver, and used to help it detoxify pollutants. Extra virgin olive oil is useful in the treatment of candidiasis, and is now known to help you retain your brainpower in older age.

Brown Beans in a Spicy Tomato Sauce with Creamed Potatoes

Ingredients for 4 servings

450 g/1 lb/2 cups cooked borlotti beans* (see page 129)

450 g/1 lb/2½ cups tomatoes, skinned and roughly chopped

4 cloves garlic, peeled and crushed

2 tbsp extra virgin olive oil

2 tbsp tomato purée (paste)

1 tbsp wheat-free miso

1 tsp porcini mushroom powder

Dried or fresh chopped herbs according to taste: thyme, parsley, tarragon, basil

Cayenne pepper

*Borlotti beans are mainly used in Italian cooking. They look a little like kidney beans but are fatter, with a rich brown colour. If you cannot find them, use red kidney beans.

Instructions

Heat the olive oil in a large saucepan over a medium heat, then add the tomatoes. Crush them with the back of a kitchen spoon until they begin to release their juice, then dissolve the miso in the juice. Add herbs, seasonings, cooked beans and porcini mushroom powder, stir to incorporate thoroughly, then put the lid on the pan and simmer gently for 1 hour, stirring occasionally.

At the end of this time, remove the lid. Break some of the beans up by roughly mashing them with a fork or potato masher. The beans should end up just covered by sauce, so if necessary turn up the heat to fast boil away any excess liquid.

Serve with Creamed Potatoes (next page) and a topping of Sour Cream (see page 253) or Garlic Crème (see page 254).

What It's Good For

This is another rich and satisfying dish, especially on a winter's evening. Beans are rich in protein, especially the anti-herpes amino acid lysine. Miso is rich in B vitamins. Tomatoes, especially when cooked and concentrated, are loaded with the anti-cancer carotene known as lycopene.

If you have any difficulty with digesting beans, try using the Digestive Tea on page 266 to accompany your meal.

To make the Creamed Potatoes

Allow one large floury potato for each serving

Cold-pressed sunflower oil

(or soya (soy) cream)

Potassium salt

Freshly ground black pepper

Special Equipment

A potato press

It is difficult to make really good creamed potatoes without a potato press—a metal press shaped like a very large garlic press. Cooked potato chunks are pressed through it, and emerge mashed through small holes, which eliminates all lumps.

N.B. Do not try to make creamed potatoes in a food processor—they will not have a good texture.

Cut the potatoes into chunks and boil them in one inch of water until tender. Remove from the heat. Put the potato press and a large bowl under the hot water tap to warm them so that they will not cool the potatoes too much. Using a slotted spoon, remove a spoonful of potato pieces at a time and put them through the press into the bowl. Using a wooden spoon, stir a few tablespoons of sunflower oil and potato cooking water into the potatoes. Add the seasoning. Keep stirring in the hot water until you have the consistency you want.

Alternatively you could omit the oil, and add soya cream instead. Serve immediately.

What It's Good For

Potatoes are often thought of as a "fattening" food, but in fact are not at all high in calories. A medium-sized potato provides only about 110 Calories.

It is the butter and sauces potatoes are served with, and the oil they are fried in which can make them fattening.

Potatoes are rich in potassium and also contain some protein and a little vitamin C.

German Erbsensuppe (pea soup) with Carrots and Miso
A one-pot meal

Ingredients for 4 servings

225 g/8 ounces/1 cup dried marrowfat peas

115 g/4 ounces/firm, low-fat sausage (optional) such as cabanos, cut into large chunks

2 medium potatoes, diced

3 medium carrots, cut into chunks

1 large onion or 1 leek, cut into chunks

1 tbsp pale miso*

Potassium salt

Freshly ground black pepper

*See page 132

Special Equipment

A pressure cooker

Instructions

Pour boiling water over the peas, allowing plenty of room for them to swell, and soak them overnight.

Discard the soaking water, then put the peas in a pressure cooker and cover with cold water. Bring up to full steam then cook for 5 minutes*. Plunge the pressure cooker into a sink of cold water to prevent further cooking and reduce the pressure enough to allow you to open the lid. The peas should be well-softened, and some of them quite mushy.

Stir in the miso then the vegetable and sausage pieces (if used). Pour in just enough water to cover the ingredients, stir well, then bring back to the boil and simmer over a low heat for one hour, stirring occasionally. Season with potassium salt and freshly ground black pepper and serve in large shallow stew plates.

Variations

In Germany all types of vegetables are thrown into this soup and it is very good for using up leftovers. You can also cook it with yellow split peas instead of marrowfat peas, or, instead of sausage, add some lean chunks of cooked ham to heat through just before serving.

*Older peas may need longer cooking times

What It's Good For

Like beans, marrowfat peas are rich in protein, and this dish makes a substantial and highly nutritious complete meal. Sausages are mentioned as an optional ingredient because it is traditional to cook this dish with them. Some types are not particularly fatty and a little goes a long way.

But do remember that sausages and ham contain preservatives and often quite a lot of salt.

Curried White Beans with Aubergine and Tomato

Ingredients for 2-3 servings

3 handfuls cooked white haricot (navy) beans (see page 129)

1 small aubergine (eggplant), diced

1 medium potato, diced

2 large tomatoes, chopped

1 medium onion, chopped

2 cloves garlic, chopped

½ tsp chilli paste or 2 tsp red Thai curry paste

2 tbsp groundnut oil

1 tsp fresh ginger, chopped

Potassium salt

Instructions

Using a stir-fry pan, fry the onion in the oil until it turns translucent, then stir in the chopped garlic and ginger, the curry paste and then the beans and stir-fry for half a minute.

Add the diced potatoes and aubergines and stir everything well together.

Stir in the chopped tomatoes and potassium salt. Add water to almost cover the ingredients in the pan.

Cover tightly and leave to simmer over a low heat for 20 minutes. Then turn up the heat to moderate and continue cooking with the lid off, stirring regularly to prevent the ingredients from sticking to the bottom of the pan, for another 20-25 minutes or until the sauce is well reduced and just coats the beans and potatoes.

Serve garnished with fresh coriander (cilantro), accompanied by brown rice or a piece of warm unleavened bread.

To vary the bland flavour of brown rice, try stir-frying it with a little olive oil and some chopped spring onion and garlic. Sprinkle in the herbs of your choice and a few dashes of tamari sauce. It will become instantly delicious.

What It's Good For

Beans are a good source of B vitamins and protein, especially the amino acid lysine, which is lacking in most other plant foods. Aubergines—hailed in Ayurvedic medicine for their beneficial effects on female hormones—provide flavonoids and many vitamins and minerals. They are deliciously creamy although they contain no fat or oil. Tomatoes, especially when cooked, are a good source of lycopene, an anti-cancer carotene. Chilli peppers contain ingredients which help to relieve intestinal flatulence.

Pancake Pizza

Ingredients for 2 medium-sized pizzas

For the batter (dough)

55 g/2 ounces/1 tbsp fine oatmeal

55 g/2 ounces/1 tbsp spelt flour*

55 g/2 ounces/1½ tbsp soya (soy) flour

250 ml/9 fluid oz/1 cup water

1 rounded tsp potassium baking powder

For the topping

Extra virgin olive oil

1 x 400 g can of chopped Italian plum tomatoes

110 g/4 ounces/1 cup grated hard goat or sheep's cheese

*See page 134

Instructions

Preheat the oven to gas mark 8. Also preheat a lightly oiled frying pan (skillet) over a medium-high heat. Put the tomatoes in a sieve over a bowl to drain off the liquid.

Mix the batter ingredients and beat until smooth. The batter has the right consistency if it settles into a round of about ½ cm/¼ inch in thickness when poured into the pan.

When the pan is hot, pour in half the batter and tilt a little if necessary to get a round shape. Cook for 1-2 minutes, or until the top of the pancake has set and the bottom is beginning to brown. Turn it over and cook the other side.

Put the cooked pancakes on an oiled baking sheet. Brush them liberally with olive oil, then spread with the chopped tomato flesh (and other topping ingredients if you wish). Cover well with the grated cheese then put on the top shelf of the oven to cook for 10-15 minutes, or until golden and bubbling. Serve immediately.

Variation

Add some finely grated carrot and grated goat or sheep's cheese to the pizza base batter, make the pancake then cut it into wedges and eat plain as a snack or accompaniment to a meal, or add toppings and bake as above.

What It's Good For

This recipe is particularly useful for allergic children, since it is quite similar to real pizza, especially if you can find a really nice goat or sheep's cheese that grates well and melts nicely. The oatmeal in this recipe provides magnesium, and the tomatoes provide the anti-cancer carotene known as lycopene.

Protein is provided by the combination of the three types of flour and the cheese.

New England Real Baked Beans

Ingredients for 4 servings

450 g/1 lb/2 cups cooked pinto*
beans (see page 129

4 tbsp tomato purée (paste)

4 tbsp blackstrap molasses

600 ml/1 pint/2 cups water
which has been saved after
steaming vegetables

4 bay leaves

Potassium salt

A pinch of cayenne pepper

*You could use white haricot (navy) beans if
you prefer.

Instructions

Preheat the oven to 140°C/275°F/gas mark 1.

Place the ingredients in a saucepan and bring
to the boil, stirring well to dissolve the molasses.
Transfer to a casserole dish and cover it tightly.

Place in the oven and cook for 4 hours. It will
not spoil if left a couple of hours longer, though
you should check occasionally to ensure that the
beans are still covered with liquid.

Before serving, transfer the beans to a warm
dish and fast-boil the sauce in a saucepan for a
few minutes to concentrate it until it reaches your
preferred consistency.

Serve the beans with Southern Sweet Potato
Bread (see page 208) or with creamed potatoes
(page 197).

What It's Good For

Beans are an excellent source of protein, especially when combined with grains
(e.g. cornmeal, rice, oats, rye). They are also rich in B vitamins.

Blackstrap molasses is a thick residue left from sugar processing, and contains all the
minerals of the sugar cane or sugar beet that were left behind when white or brown
sugar was produced: calcium, magnesium, iron, zinc and manganese to name just a
few.

Fillets of Red Mullet Fried Cajun-Style

Ingredients for 2 servings

4 red mullet fillets*

2 tsp paprika (not the hot variety)

2 tsp onion powder

2 tsp garlic powder

2 tsp dried thyme or oregano

1 tsp cayenne pepper

1 tsp ground black pepper

1 tsp potassium salt

Groundnut oil for frying

*If your fishmonger does not sell them ready-filleted, ask him to fillet them for you.

Instructions

Using a mortar and pestle, grind the thyme or oregano to a powder, then mix thoroughly with the other dry ingredients. Spread the resulting powder out on a plate.

Dry the fish fillets with absorbent kitchen paper, then press both sides of them firmly into the powder until they are thickly coated.

Heat 4 tbsp groundnut oil in a frying pan (skillet) over a high heat. When the oil is very hot, add the fish fillets, flesh side down, and cook for one minute. Turn over and cook the other side for half a minute, pressing down if necessary to prevent the fillets from curling up.

Drain briefly on absorbent kitchen paper then serve immediately with a vegetable or salad accompaniment. This dish goes very well with German Potato Salad (see page 224).

What It's Good For

Cajun cookery is hot and spicy and comes from New Orleans and other parts of the Southern United States. Cayenne pepper has two special benefits: it is warming and great for the circulation, and it also has a soothing effect on the digestive system, with the ability to combat intestinal flatulence.

Thyme and oregano contain antibacterial and antifungal ingredients and so are useful as part of an anti-candida diet.

Queen Scallops with Rice Noodles and Spring Greens

Ingredients for 2 servings

225 g/8 ounces of queen scallops[1] (excluding shells)

200 g/7 ounces spring greens (collards)

200 g/7 ounces thin rice noodles[2]

¼ pint/150 ml/½ cup cold water

Olive oil

2 tbsp soya (soy) cream

1 tsp fresh parsley, chopped

1 rounded tsp pale miso dissolved in ¼ pint/150 ml/ ½ cup hot water

1 rounded tsp arrowroot powder dissolved in 1 tbsp water

Potassium salt

Freshly ground black pepper

1. These are the very small variety
2. See page 133

Instructions

Trim and wash the greens. Cut them across into thick ribbons. Put a large stir-fry pan or saucepan over a medium heat. When hot add 2 tbsp olive oil and the greens. Stir well, then add the cold water and cover the pan. Turn the heat down to medium-low, cook for 5 minutes then season with potassium salt, stir and check that the water has not all evaporated. (If it has, add a little more). Replace the lid, cook for another 5 minutes then fast-boil away any remaining liquid. Remove from the heat; keep warm.

Bring a kettle of water to the boil then pour it over the rice noodles and leave to soak for 2 minutes. Drain then cover with cold water and drain again.

Put a frying pan (skillet) over a medium heat; when hot add 2 tbsp olive oil. Briefly sear the scallops on either side in the hot oil and remove. Pour the miso and hot water into the pan, stir in the dissolved arrowroot, return the scallops to the pan and simmer for about 5 minutes. Stir in the parsley and soya cream and remove from the heat. Keep warm.

Heat 2 tbsp olive oil in a stir-fry pan over a high heat, then add the soaked rice noodles. Stir-fry for about 20 seconds then add the greens, combine gently and pour into a warm serving dish. Pour the scallops and their sauce on top, and use two forks to combine the scallops with the other ingredients. Season with black pepper and serve immediately.

What It's Good For

Greens are a member of the cabbage family, and contain ingredients which help your liver to break down pollutants in your body, helping to lower your cancer risk. Greens are rich in chlorophyll (which helps to neutralize toxins in your intestines), and in calcium, iron and lutein, a carotene type of antioxidant which has a protective effect on your eyesight. The calcium in green vegetables is easy to assimilate, making greens a better source of calcium than milk.

Moroccan Couscous with Seven Vegetables

Ingredients for 2 servings

Millet grains measured up to the 120 ml/4 fluid oz/½ cup mark in a measuring jug

200 ml/7 fluid oz/generous ¾ cup water

1 cup of cooked chickpeas

½ cup raw cashew nuts, washed and drained

1 large courgette cut into chunks

1 medium onion, quartered

1 medium carrot, quartered

1 sweet (bell) pepper cut into 8 pieces

2 x 1 inch chunks of white mooli radish

4 chunks of pumpkin, squash, or vegetable marrow, each about 1 inch square

1 large tomato, sliced

2 tbsp olive oil

1 tsp turmeric

Instructions

Nowadays the grain product sold as couscous is usually made from crushed wheat, but traditional North African couscous can be made with crushed millet grains. The grain is soaked and then cooked by steaming over a "tagine", a meat and vegetable stew which imbues it with flavours. The simplified version here uses whole millet grains and omits the steaming process, but if you have a pan in which you can suspend a colander- or sieveful of cooked millet grains while the tagine cooks underneath, you could transfer the millet there to stay hot in the steam and absorb the flavours.

To cook the millet

Toast the millet grains in a dry frying pan over a medium heat for about 10 minutes or until they give off a roasted aroma and begin to change colour. Transfer them to a saucepan, add the water, cover, bring to the boil and simmer over a low heat for 30 minutes.

Remove from the heat. Remove the lid, add 1 tbsp water, stir briefly, then replace the lid and leave undisturbed for five minutes. You can time the tagine to be ready now for serving with the millet, or transfer the millet to a colander set over the tagine as described above.

What It's Good For

What a delicious way to get your daily vegetables. This dish is very versatile, and is a good way to use up any seasonal vegetables, especially white mooli radish, which is not a traditional vegetable in this dish, but is perfect for it. Radishes are said to balance the production of thyroid hormones, to dry up congestion and eliminate cold symptoms, and to stimulate the flow of bile, thus aiding digestion. Other traditional vegetables include quartered artichokes, white turnips and green beans. Instead of

Cayenne pepper

Bouquet garni: a stick of celery tied up with parsley, thyme and rosemary

Spices: whole peppercorns, cloves, cinnamon and crushed cumin seeds tied up in muslin*

Potassium salt

Harissa (hot pepper) sauce to serve

*If you have trouble finding muslin, you could use a wire mesh "tea infuser" suspended in the pan instead.

To make the tagine

Using a large saucepan with a heavy base, brown the onion and carrot pieces in the olive oil over a medium heat. Sprinkle with cayenne pepper. Next add the turmeric and all the other ingredients except the remaining herbs and spices. Stir together and pour in just enough water to cover them. Then add the bouquet garni and remaining spices.

Bring to the boil and simmer gently for one hour.

Using a slotted spoon, remove the vegetables from the pan and arrange them on top of the millet. Keep hot. Remove the bouquet garni and the muslin bag from the pan and reduce the sauce to about 300 ml/½ pint/1 cup by fast-boiling. Serve the sauce separately. Harissa, a fiery hot pepper sauce, is also traditionally served with couscous.

Variation

If you wish, you could also add some chicken pieces to this dish. Just brown them at the same time as the onion, and proceed in exactly the same way.

cashew nuts you could use almonds, and instead of a tomato you could use an apricot. Millet is a very ancient grain and has been cultivated for longer than rice, wheat and rye. It is a rich source of many vitamins and minerals and is one of the best sources of the mineral silicon, which is needed for strong bones and teeth. People with food intolerances rarely have a problem with millet, as it is gluten free and easy to digest. It can safely be added to any hypoallergenic diet. Millet is also said to have anti-fungal properties and therefore may be able to help people with intestinal candidiasis.

Grilled Chicken Nuggets Marinated in Ginger and Garlic

Ingredients for each serving

One medium-sized chicken breast, boned and skinned

1 tbsp olive oil

2 tbsp tamari sauce

1 tsp fresh ginger, finely chopped

1 tsp fresh garlic, finely chopped

Instructions

Cut the chicken breast into strips about half an inch wide. Whisk together the other ingredients in a bowl large enough to hold all the chicken.

Place the chicken in the bowl and ensure it is well coated with marinade.

Leave for several hours (preferably overnight), turning the chicken occasionally.

Remove the grid from the grill (broiler) pan. Line the pan with foil, then preheat the grill to its highest setting.

Roll up the chicken strips and thread them close together on a flat skewer. Lay the skewer over the grill pan and place under the hot grill.

Cook for about 5 minutes on each side or until the chicken is cooked through. Serve with salad in a piece of folded unleavened bread, or with rice or millet.

The remaining marinade can be poured over some cold, cooked rice or millet in a hot stir-fry pan. Simply toss and stir over a medium heat, with a little extra water if necessary, until the grains are heated through.

What It's Good For

Chicken is a good source of protein, and low in animal fat. While some therapeutic diets restrict protein, remember your liver cannot detoxify your blood unless it gets enough protein to manufacture essential enzymes. People with chronic fatigue syndrome especially need to avoid very low protein diets. When grilling meat and chicken, cut off and discard any charred, blackened pieces as they contain toxic compounds. Avoid barbecuing, because toxic smoke settles on the meat.

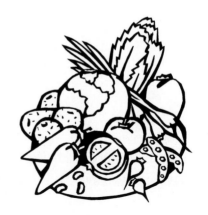

Side dishes and accompaniments

If you have children who dislike vegetables, this could be simply because they don't like them boiled.

After all, most children like canned vegetable soups, so it could simply be a matter of how they're served.

Here are plenty of ideas for making them tasty and succulent-e.g. chopped small and baked with rice and onion, or made into a colourful rainbow salad.

Southern Sweet Potato Bread

Ingredients for 6-8 servings

1 medium-to large orange sweet
potato, cooked and peeled

100 g/3½ ounces soya (soy)
flour

100 g3½ ounces finely-ground
yellow polenta meal

100 ml/3½ fluid oz soya (soy)
milk

2 tbsp sunflower oil

1 heaped tsp potassium baking
powder

Instructions

Preheat the oven to gas mark 5.

All sweet potatoes have a purplish skin. The only way to tell if the flesh is orange is to scrape one gently with a fingernail. When preparing for this recipe, leave the potato whole, prick it all over with a sharp knife or fork, then steam for about 45 minutes or until soft. Or you could steam it for 20 minutes in a microwave instead.

Roughly chop the cooked, peeled sweet potato and put it in a food processor with all the other ingredients. Using the blade attachment, whizz the mixture until smooth, then transfer it to a small oiled loaf tin and bake for 40 minutes or until beginning to brown on top.

Serve cut into hunks with New England Baked Beans (page 201) and other bean dishes.

What It's Good For

Both yellow polenta and sweet potatoes with orange-coloured flesh are rich in powerful antioxidants known as carotenes (similar to beta-carotene) and so can help to prevent cancer.

This delicious sweet moist bread is best served freshly made and warm. Any leftovers can be wrapped in foil once cold. Reheat in the foil in a moderate oven for 10 minutes.

Warm Salad of Grilled Vegetables with Lemon Zest

Ingredients for 4 servings

2 medium onions, cut in four

2 sweet (bell) peppers, one red one green, deseeded and cut in four

4 medium tomatoes, halved

1 lemon

1 green chilli pepper, deseeded and finely chopped

1 handful Greek olives (black)

2 tbsp capers

1 tbsp coriander leaves (cilantro), coarsely chopped

Extra-virgin olive oil

Instructions

Preheat the grill (broiler) to its highest setting.

Thread the onion quarters, sweet pepper pieces and tomato halves on skewers, brush liberally with olive oil and place under the grill (broiler) for 10 minutes, turning and brushing again with oil occasionally until the vegetables are beginning to tinge brown.

Meanwhile grate the zest off the lemon, then make a dressing by juicing the lemon and whisking the juice with 4 tbsp olive oil.

Add the zest to the dressing, together with the finely chopped chilli pepper and the capers.

When the vegetables are ready, slip them off the skewers, pour the dressing over them and ensure they are thoroughly coated.

Serve warm or tepid, sprinkled with the Greek olives and chopped coriander.

What It's Good For

One of the major cancer-fighting flavonoids found in onions is quercetin, which also helps to fight allergies and prevent cataracts. Lemon peel has the flavonoid hesperidin, which fights varicose veins and fluid retention by preventing blood vessel walls from getting thin and leaky, and nobiletin, which is anti-inflammatory and helps the liver process toxins. Lemon juice and peppers are rich in vitamin C. Vitamin C is also needed for strong, healthy skin and blood vessels.

Baked Rice Dishes

Lemon Baked Rice

Ingredients for 4 servings

300 ml/½ pint/1 cup organic brown rice (pour the rice into a measuring jug to measure the quantity) soaked for 6 hours or more in 600 ml/1 pint/2 cups water

Half a fresh lemon (preferably unwaxed*)

2 medium onions thinly sliced into half-rings

1 handful sunflower seeds

8 tbsp extra virgin olive oil

Potassium salt

Black pepper

*If not unwaxed, scrub the lemon in very hot water with detergent to remove as much pesticide-treated wax as possible.

Instructions

Leaving the rice in its soaking water, bring to the boil in a lidded saucepan then simmer very gently for 20-25 minutes, until just tender. Quickly tip the rice into a large sieve to drain off any remaining water (save it for soup or stock as it is very rich in vitamins) then tip the rice straight back in the pan, replace the lid and leave the rice undisturbed for at least 5 minutes.

Preheat the oven to 190°C/375°F/gas mark 5.

Heat the oil in a large frying pan or stir-fry pan and fry the onions over a high heat until they are beginning to turn brown and crispy. (You will probably need to do this in two batches to avoid overcrowding the pan, which will create too much steam.)

Cut the half lemon into four pieces and pick out all the pips. Whizz the lemon pieces in a food processor until finely chopped. Fold the cooked onions, chopped lemon and the sunflower seeds into the brown rice, and season with potassium salt and pepper.

Put the rice in a casserole dish with a well-fitting lid, and bake for 40 minutes.

What It's Good For

This dish is very rich in cancer-fighting flavonoid antioxidants. One of the major flavonoids found in onions is quercetin, which reduces histamine and helps prevent cataracts. Lemon peel is rich in the flavonoid hesperidin, which fights varicose veins and fluid retention by preventing blood vessel walls from getting thin and leaky, and nobiletin, which has anti-inflammatory action and helps the liver to process toxins. Brown rice is an excellent source of B vitamins.

Walnut and Mushroom Baked Rice

Ingredients for 3-4 servings

In this recipe a cup is an ordinary teacup

2 cups cooked brown rice

1 medium carrot, grated

50 g/2 ounces/½ cup walnuts coarsely ground in food processor

1/4 lb mushrooms, diced

1 onion, cut in four

2 sticks celery, roughly cut into segments

1 green (bell) pepper, cut into 8 pieces

4 tbsp olive oil

A few leaves of fresh basil, chopped, or 1/2 tsp dried basil

Tamari sauce

Ground black pepper

Instructions

Preheat the oven to 190°C/375°F/gas mark 5.

Process the onion, celery and green pepper together in a food processor until finely chopped. Place a large saucepan, or preferably a stir-fry pan, over a moderate to high heat, and when hot, add 2 tbsp olive oil, followed by the onion, celery and green pepper mixture and the grated carrot. Stir-fry for five minutes until the mixture begins to soften, then take off the heat and transfer the contents to a bowl.

Clean and dry the pan then replace over a medium-high heat and add the chopped mushrooms. Stir-fry without oil for a minute to dry them out a little, then add the oil and continue to stir-fry until golden brown.

Take off the heat, replace the vegetables in the pan, and mix in the chopped walnuts, basil, pepper and a few dashes of tamari sauce. Finally fold the grains in gently, ensuring that they do not break up.

Transfer the contents to an oiled loaf tin, smooth and press down evenly with a fork, cover with foil and bake for about 40 minutes.

Variations

Use cooked buckwheat or millet instead of brown rice, or include a tablespoon of wild rice.

What It's Good For

The combination of walnuts with brown rice in this recipe yields substantial amounts of protein, so this dish could just be served with a salad or a portion of braised vegetables, and perhaps some garlic mushrooms. It provides a very broad spread of nutrients, from B vitamins (brown rice) to beta carotene (carrots), chromium (mushrooms), and vitamin C (peppers). Other beneficial items include fluid retention-fighting coumarin (celery) and allergy-fighting quercetin (onions).

Baked Red Cabbage with Apple and Garlic

Ingredients for 4 servings

½ red cabbage, finely shredded

1 small, full-flavoured sweet apple, cored and thinly sliced

1 small onion, chopped

2 tbsp extra virgin olive oil

2 tbsp apple juice

1 tbsp raisins

2 cloves garlic, crushed or chopped

Black pepper

Instructions

Preheat the oven to 160°C/325°F/gas mark 3.

Heat the oil in a stir-fry pan or large, heavy-bottomed saucepan, and stir-fry the onion gently until softened.

Add the apple and garlic and then the shredded cabbage, stirring continuously until it has shrunk a little. Then remove from the heat, stir in the raisins, put the mixture in a casserole dish, pour over the apple juice, season with black pepper, cover tightly and cook for one hour.

Serve with roast organic chicken and Creamed Potatoes (page 197) or with a stuffed Potato Pancake (page 172).

What It's Good For

Members of the cabbage family are known to contain more anti-cancer substances than any other vegetables. And as a general rule, the more brightly-coloured a vegetable, the more free radical fighters it also contains in the form of flavonoids and carotenes. So, apart from being absolutely delicious, especially in this recipe, red cabbage is also extremely good for you! The red colour is anthocyanin, a flavonoid with powerful antioxidant action.

Vegetable Rösti Pancakes

Ingredients for 2 servings

1 medium waxy potato, cut in four

1 medium carrot, cut into several segments

1 medium courgette (zucchini), cut into several segments

3 tbsp olive oil

1 tbsp soya or buckwheat flour

Black pepper

Instructions

Grate all the vegetable pieces together, using a food processor, or coarsely grate them by hand. Season with black pepper. Do not add any form of salt to the vegetables, as this will make them release liquid.

The grated vegetables must be cooked immediately as potatoes discolour quickly when grated.

Heat the oil in a large frying pan (skillet) over a medium heat. Divide the grated vegetables into four portions. Form two portions into a round shape with your hands. Put them in the frying pan, and gently flatten them into thinnish pancakes, pressing with the edge of a spatula. (The edges can remain ragged.)

Cook for 1-2 minutes until the edges are turning golden and crispy, then remove the pancakes with a spatula and carefully slide them one at a time on to a small plate, put another plate on top, invert and slide back into the hot pan to cook the other side. Once cooked keep in a warm place until ready to serve. Repeat with the remaining portions.

Serve as a light snack with apple sauce (see page 255) or as a vegetable accompaniment, or cold as part of a buffet meal.

What It's Good For

Taking only a few minutes to make, these succulent little pancakes are a delicious and unusual way to serve vegetables. Carrots are rich in antioxidant carotenes, especially beta carotene. Potatoes and courgettes are a good source of potassium and many vitamins and minerals.

Garlic Potatoes Corfu Style

Ingredients for 4 servings

4 large potatoes, peeled

4 cloves of garlic, chopped

100 ml extra virgin olive oil

1 tsp chopped fresh rosemary

Boiling water

Potassium salt

Freshly ground black pepper

Instructions

Preheat the oven to 200°C/400°F/gas mark 6.

Cut the potatoes into large dice or thick slices and place in a shallow oven-proof dish. Sprinkle with seasoning, followed by chopped garlic and rosemary, then pour in the olive oil. Top up with enough boiling water to almost cover the potatoes, cover the dish with foil and place in the oven.

Cook for 45 minutes, then remove the foil and cook for a further 30 minutes uncovered, or until the water has evaporated and the potatoes are crisp and golden on top and tender in the middle. Drain off the excess oil, which is full of flavour and can be saved for another dish.

As the level of oil drops with the evaporation of the water, all the potatoes are coated with the oil and the wonderful flavours of the garlic and rosemary.

Variations

In Corfu, this dish is often made with a selection of different vegetables: courgettes (zucchini), carrots, onions and tomatoes, for example.

What It's Good For

Eating this dish, you won't be able to help dreaming of sun-drenched Mediterranean shores! Potatoes are rich in potassium and minerals, and although only raw garlic has anti-bacterial and anti-fungal effects in the intestines, cooked garlic still has many beneficial effects on arteries, blood pressure, cholesterol, diabetes and the elimination of toxic (heavy) metals from the body.

Onion Marmalade

Ingredients for 3-4 servings

450 g/1 lb onions, peeled

2 tbsp extra virgin olive oil

Potassium salt

Instructions

Using a mandolin type appliance (with a spiked holder for the onions so that you don't slice into your fingers!) slice the onions thinly, then place them in a stir-fry pan with the oil over a medium heat. Using a large spoon, break up the onion slices into rings, and stir-fry until well-coated. Put a lid on the pan, and leave the onions to sweat over a very low heat for 30 minutes. Remove the lid, add potassium salt and stir-fry the onions with the lid off for 10 minutes to reduce any excess moisture. The onions should be soft and melting.

Reheat before serving. This is especially good with fish and steamed potatoes.

What It's Good For

The therapeutic value of the humble onion is often forgotten in favour of its famous cousin garlic. Onions are a rich source of the flavonoid quercetin, which is similar to the drug disodium chromoglycate, given to allergy sufferers to switch off their symptoms. Like the drug, quercetin inhibits the release of histamine, which is responsible for allergic symptoms and asthma attacks. Quercetin is also being researched for its anti-viral properties[145,159,250].

Polenta with Olives and Sun-Dried Tomatoes

Ingredients for 4-6 servings

250 g/9 ounces yellow polenta meal, preferably coarse-ground

1½ litres/2½ pints/5¼ cups boiling water

50 g/2 ounces/1 cup white mushrooms, diced small and fried for 2 minutes in 1 tbsp olive oil

8 large green olives, stoned and cut in four

15 g/½ ounce/1 heaped tbsp sun-dried tomatoes, thinly shredded

Potassium salt

Freshly ground black pepper

To ensure that your polenta turns out right, these instructions should be followed even if the packet gives different quantities of water or cooking times.

Instructions

Pour the polenta meal and potassium salt into a saucepan containing the boiling water, whisking it rapidly as you do so to prevent lumps from forming. Turn the heat down to a gentle simmer and stir the polenta from time to time with a large wooden spoon, leaving the lid off the pan. The polenta is not ready yet even if it thickens and starts to sputter—keep turning the heat down until the sputtering is minimal. Keep stirring until the mixture is gelatinous and stiff. This takes about 40 minutes.

When the polenta is ready, combine the diced mushrooms, olive pieces and sun-dried tomato shreds and fold them evenly and very gently into the polenta. Spoon the polenta into an oiled shallow dish large enough to result in a layer 1-2 cm/half to one inch thick when the polenta is spread out in it. Spoon in the polenta and then use the back of a fork to get the layer as even as possible.

Cover the dish with a tea towel and allow it to cool, then refrigerate until chilled. When you are ready to serve the polenta, divide it into portions, carefully remove them from the dish, and fry on each side in hot olive oil until golden and crispy. Serve with Ratatouille (see page opposite).

What It's Good For

Polenta is yellow cornmeal, rich in anti-cancer carotenes, and also essential polyunsaturated oils, vitamin E and complex carbohydrates.

Polenta cooked in this way is very versatile, and In Italy it is often used as a substitute for pasta.

Ratatouille

Ingredients for 4 servings

1 medium-sized aubergine (eggplant) cut into large dice

1x400 g/14 ounce can of Italian plum tomatoes

2 medium-sized courgettes (zucchini) sliced about ½ cm/¼ inch thick

1 medium-sized green (bell) pepper, cut into about 20 pieces

4 cloves garlic, peeled and flattened with the side of a large knife

4 tbsp extra virgin olive oil

1 tsp mixed dried Provençale herbs

Potassium salt

Freshly ground black pepper

Instructions

Heat the oil in a large, heavy-bottomed saucepan over a medium heat. When hot, put all the vegetables in the pan. Stir, add the herbs and potassium salt, then cover the pan, bring to the boil, turn the heat down and sweat the vegetables over a low heat for one hour, stirring occasionally.

Remove the lid and check the consistency. If necessary, boil the ratatouille rapidly with the lid off to reduce the sauce until you have a thick consistency. The vegetables should not swim in liquid.

Stir in the freshly ground black pepper and serve hot or cold. This goes especially well with polenta (see page 216).

What It's Good For

This old southern French peasant dish could be one of the reasons why the Mediterranean peoples have a superior life expectancy. Rich in heart-disease preventing vitamin C and flavonoid and carotene antioxidants, this kind of food is just perfect for good body maintenance. Even the rosemary herb used in Provençale cookery contains antioxidants. I have recommended canned tomatoes here for their rich deep red, which indicates a good content of the anti-cancer carotene lycopene.

Cauliflower in Cream Sauce

Ingredients for 2-4 servings

1 medium head of cauliflower

425 ml/¾ pint/1½ cups water

2 tbsp groundnut oil

1 rounded dessertspoon brown rice flour

2 tbsp soya (soy) cream

Potassium salt

Special Equipment

A steaming basket

Instructions

Bring the water to the boil in a large saucepan which can be used for steaming. Divide the cauliflower into small florets. Wash thoroughly and place in a steaming basket inside the pan of boiling water. Steam over a medium heat with the lid on for 10-15 minutes, until tender.

Put the oil in another saucepan over a gentle heat and stir in the rice flour. When the cauliflower is cooked, drain the cooking water into a jug, add some potassium salt, and keep the cauliflower warm. Whisk the hot cooking water gradually into the oil and rice flour mixture until evenly blended and thickened. Simmer over a low heat for 5 minutes, stirring from time to time.

Add the soya cream and gently warm through without boiling. Pour the sauce over the cauliflower, toss so that it is well coated, and serve immediately.

What It's Good For

Like broccoli, cabbage and brussels sprouts, cauliflower belongs to the Brassica family of vegetables—famous for its ability to fight cancer-causing chemicals. The anti-cancer substances in these vegetables include indoles, phenols, coumarins and isothiocyanates. They provide raw materials for your liver to get rid of cancer-causing pollutants, and block the effects of cancer-causing compounds. They also help prevent many female problems, by assisting the liver to break down excess oestrogen.

Aromatic Carrots with Garlic and Shallots

Ingredients for 4 servings

4 medium carrots, cut into
    julienne strips

2 medium shallots, peeled and
    roughly diced

4 cloves garlic, peeled and
    crushed

2 tbsp extra virgin olive oil

A pinch of your favourite mixed
    dried herbs (e.g. tarragon
    and thyme)

Potassium salt

Freshly ground black pepper

Instructions

Heat the oil over a medium heat in a heavy-bottomed saucepan, and add the shallots. Cook until beginning to soften, then stir in the garlic and carrot strips. Ensure they are coated with oil.

Season with potassium salt and a sprinkling of herbs, then add four tbsp water, turn the heat down to its lowest setting, and cover the pan tightly.

Cook for 25 minutes, after which time the carrots should be tender.

If there are more than a couple of tablespoons of cooking juices in the bottom of the pan, turn up the heat to fast-boil it until reduced. Gently turn the carrots to moisten them with the juices, then season with freshly ground black pepper and serve immediately.

Variation

Try mixing the carrots with quartered brussels sprouts. This cooking method (braising) can also be used with shredded cabbage and dwarf green beans.

What It's Good For

This is a wonderful nutrient-conserving method of cooking carrots, and so delicious that you will never again want to cook them any other way. Carrots are rich in antioxidant carotenes, especially beta carotene. Because people who eat a lot of carrots get less lung cancer, scientists have carried out research giving beta carotene supplements to smokers to see whether supplements have the same effect. It appears that they are not nearly so effective as carrots themselves.

Potato Cakes *Grand Prix*

So called because they are so quick to make!

Ingredients

Allow 1 medium starchy potato
for each serving of 2 potato
cakes

Olive oil for frying

Potassium salt

Special Equipment

A round "cooking ring" or pastry
cutter with a diameter of about
3 inches for each potato cake.

Instructions

Peel and coarsely grate the potatoes, putting the gratings into a bowl of cold water. Using your hands, remove two handfuls of grated potato from the water, squeeze out the excess water and lay the grated potato on a clean tea towel. Fold the tea towel over and press the potatoes again to dry them as much as possible.

Put a large frying pan (skillet) over a medium heat and coat the bottom with a thin layer of olive oil. When the oil is hot, put the cooking rings into the pan, and drop grated potato into each ring, pressing down gently so that you get a cake with a thickness of about ½ cm/¼ inch. Drizzle a teaspoon of olive oil over the potato cakes, then sprinkle with a pinch of potassium salt. Cook for five minutes, or until the bottom of the cakes is crisp and golden, then carefully remove the rings, turn the cakes over with flat tongs and cook the other side without the ring.

Drain the cakes on absorbent kitchen paper and keep them warm while you cook the next batch. Serve with apple sauce or as a vegetable accompaniment.

What It's Good For

Potatoes are often thought of as a "fattening" food, but in fact are not at all high in calories. A medium-sized potato provides only about 110 Calories.

It is the butter and sauces potatoes are served with, and the oil they are fried in which can make them fattening.

Potatoes are rich in potassium and also contain some protein and a little vitamin C.

Vegetables with Garlic Crème
on a Crispy Potato Base

Ingredients for 2 servings

2 Potato Cakes Grand Prix as made on the previous page

2 tbsp Garlic Crème (page 254)

4 tbsp vegetables, e.g. braised onions and green beans or the carrot dish on page 219 or the warm salad on page 209

Instructions

Spoon the warm Garlic Crème on to the potato cakes and top with the vegetables.

An elegant but simple dish, especially suited to a dinner party. You could serve this with most of the fish dishes in this book, or with chicken, stuffed peppers (page 186), Potato Ravioli (page 178) or Miniature Baked Omelettes (page 157). Just add a little green salad to garnish.

Variation

Use Hummus (page 155) instead of Garlic Crème.

What It's Good For

Many people, especially children, say they don't like vegetables. But maybe they just don't like them boiled? Who could resist the succulent sweetness of carrots cooked slowly with onions, garlic and olive oil, especially when combined with the sort of crispy potato dish that everyone seems to love? Sometimes children find vegetables too bland because they have a zinc deficiency and cannot taste them. If your child only seems to like very salty or very sweet food, this could be the reason.

South Indian Vegetable Curry (Sambar)

Ingredients for 2 servings

2 cups (mugfuls) mixed vegetables* cut into 1 cm/½ inch pieces

1 large tomato, chopped

1 chilli pepper, deseeded, chopped

4 tbsp cooked red lentils**

2 tbsp olive oil

Potassium salt

Flavourings

A few dried curry leaves

1 tbsp chopped fresh coriander

1 tsp turmeric

½ tsp each of black mustard, fenugreek and cumin seeds, ground cinnamon, coriander, asafoetida, black pepper, cayenne pepper

*E.g. potato, mooli radish, courgette, aubergine, green beans, onion, carrot.

**To cook red lentils, simmer in 2¼ times their volume of water for 25 minutes.

Instructions

1. Using a large saucepan with a heavy base, heat the oil and the seeds.
2. When the mustard seeds begin to pop, add the chopped chilli pepper, stir briefly.
3. Add all the vegetables except the tomato and stir-fry for 2 minutes.
4. Stir in the ground spices and turmeric.
5. Add 2 cups water and the chopped tomato, curry leaves and potassium salt.
6. Bring to a gentle simmer and cook for 30 minutes.
7. Stir in the cooked lentils and chopped fresh coriander and simmer for 5 more minutes.

Serve hot with rice. Sambar is traditionally a fiery dish. If you find it too spicy, cut down on the cayenne pepper or add it at the end to gauge how much you can tolerate.

What It's Good For

Sambar is a staple dish in South India. It can also be thinned with water and eaten as soup. The traditional tamarind has been left out of this recipe because the Indian mystics do not recommend it. Always fiery, sambar owes its heat to the chilli (cayenne) pepper, which has great health benefits, especially for the circulation. This is just the dish to eat if you feel a cold coming on. Chillis also stimulate the digestion and help to prevent flatulence.

Braised Cornish Vegetables

Ingredients for each serving

1 medium potato

1 piece of swede (rutabaga) the same size as the potato

Half a medium onion

1 tbsp extra virgin olive oil

Potassium salt

Pepper

Instructions

These vegetables are the traditional filling inside a Cornish pasty, minus the meat. They make a succulent and delicious vegetable accompaniment which I find extremely more-ish!

Finely dice all the vegetables, then sweat them over a very low heat in a lidded pan with the olive oil for 45 minutes, stirring occasionally and adding a tablespoon of water if they show any sign of sticking to the bottom of the pan. Serve with grilled fish or spiced bean röstis or roast organic chicken.

What It's Good For

Swedes (known in Cornwall as turnips) are a sadly under-appreciated vegetable whose delicious sweetness perfectly complements potatoes and onions. Like cauliflower and cabbage, they are a member of the Brassica family which is famous for its anti-cancer benefits.

German Potato Salad

Ingredients for 4 servings

1 kg/2 pounds waxy potatoes

4 spring onions (scallions) finely sliced

6 tbsp extra virgin olive oil

4 tbsp mayonnaise (see page 258)

3 tbsp additive-free cider vinegar or white wine vinegar

1 tbsp capers, chopped

Potassium salt

Freshly-ground black pepper

Instructions

Steam the potatoes whole in their jackets until just tender (about 30-40 minutes).

Whisk together the oil, vinegar, salt and pepper in a large bowl, then stir in the spring onion slices and chopped capers. Leave to one side for the flavours to blend together.

When the potatoes are cooked, hold them on a fork (so that you don't burn your fingers) and peel them with a small knife.

Once peeled, cut them into medium-sized dice and, while still warm, put them them in the bowl containing the oil and vinegar dressing. (Whisk it again first if it has separated).

Gently turn the potatoes in the dressing until they are well coated. Leave to one side for at least one hour so that the potatoes can absorb the dressing.

Just before you are ready to serve the potato salad, spoon in the mayonnaise and turn the potatoes around in it gently until they are evenly coated.

What It's Good For

Potatoes gain a delicious flavour by soaking up vinaigrette and then only need a light coating of mayonnaise. Sometimes anti-candida diets forbid vinegar because it contains yeasts and most Candida sufferers have a yeast allergy. However, those in vinegar (and miso) are natural yeasts, and are much less likely to cause allergic reactions than the commercial yeasts found in wine, beer, bread, pizza dough etc. If it does, use lemon or lime juice instead.

Diced Fried New Potatoes and Courgettes with a Pesto Coating

Ingredients for 4 servings

4 medium-sized new potatoes, unpeeled, diced small

2 medium-sized courgettes, diced

1 large handful fresh basil leaves

25 g/1 ounce/1 small handful walnuts or pine nuts

4 tbsp extra virgin olive oil, plus

Ordinary olive oil for frying

1 clove garlic

Potassium salt

Instructions

Put enough olive oil to form a ½ cm/ ¼-inch layer in a large frying pan (skillet) over a medium to high heat. When hot, add the diced potatoes but do not overcrowd the pan. If necessary, cook them in two batches. Stir and turn over the potatoes occasionally to ensure that they cook as evenly as possible. When done, they should be golden and slightly crispy. This should take about 10 minutes. Remove the potatoes from the pan with a slotted spoon, drain them on absorbent kitchen paper and keep them warm.

Put the pan back over the heat and cook the diced courgettes in the same way, adding a little more oil if necessary. The courgettes should take about 5 minutes to cook. When done, remove them from the pan, drain them briefly on absorbent kitchen paper and keep warm.

Make the pesto coating by putting 4 tbsp olive oil in a blender with the garlic, fresh basil, walnuts or pine nuts and potassium salt. Whizz until smooth and creamy.

Combine the potatoes and courgettes in a bowl and spoon in the pesto sauce. Fold together until the vegetables are thoroughly coated and serve immediately. This goes well with the Plaice Meunière recipe on page 191.

What It's Good For

In herbal medicine, basil was traditionally used against nervous irritability. It is little used by herbalists today. It also has anti-fungal, anti-bacterial and anti-parasitic properties, which are useful for people suffering from candidiasis and other imbalances in their intestinal bacteria. Walnuts are sometimes known as "brain food", perhaps because they look like tiny brains! They are rich in essential polyunsaturated oils, protein, vitamin E, calcium, iron and zinc.

Mini Rainbow Salads

Ingredients

Any combination of the following, depending on how many people you are catering for.

Finely grated swede

Grated carrot

Grated raw beetroot or cooked beetroot cut into matchsticks

Tomatoes, thinly sliced

Grated mooli radish*

Sweet peppers (red, green, yellow) finely diced

Cooking rings

*Long, white "icicle" radishes

Instructions

Pile layers of contrasting coloured ingredients into cooking rings, ending with a slice of tomato. Press down gently.

Transfer to a bed of lettuce or alfalfa sprouts (or a mixture of both) and spoon vinaigrette dressing (see page 227) flavoured with thinly sliced spring onion (scallion) over the top. Remove the rings and serve as soon as possible.

What It's Good For

I have extolled the virtues of the humble swede elsewhere in this book, but most people don't know that it is truly delicious eaten raw. I discovered this when I travelled to Iceland and was given a simple but exquisite dish of poached white fish with onions sweated in butter and a salad of grated raw swede and vinegar. Raw grated carrot is good at preventing roundworm infestations. I feed it daily to my cat, who used to need worming regularly. Since the carrots he has been worm-free.

Vinaigrette Salad Dressing

Ingredients for
125 ml/4½ fluid oz/½ cup

6 tbsp extra virgin olive oil

2 tbsp cider vinegar or wine
vinegar

1 tsp English mustard powder

Potassium salt

Freshly ground black pepper

Instructions

Mix the mustard powder to a smooth paste with a little of the vinegar in a bowl, then, using a fork or small whisk, beat in a little oil followed by the rest of the oil and then the remaining ingredients.

This makes a basic vinaigrette. You can add any other ingredients you like, such as fresh or dried chopped herbs or gherkins, capers, raw garlic or finely sliced spring onion (scallion). Whisk the vinaigrette again just before serving.

If you are serving vinaigrette with a green salad, do not put it on the salad until the last minute.

What It's Good For

Extra virgin olive oil has been in the news recently since scientists found that it can help to prevent our brain processes from deteriorating as we get older. Sometimes anti-candida diets forbid vinegar because it contains yeasts and most Candida sufferers have a yeast allergy. However, those in vinegar (and miso) are natural yeasts, much less likely to cause allergic reactions than the commercial yeasts found in wine, beer, bread, pizza dough etc. If they do, use lemon or lime juice instead.

Three-Bean Salad

Ingredients for each serving

2 tbsp cooked chickpeas

2 tbsp cooked red kidney beans

2 tbsp cooked black-eyed beans

1 spring onion (scallion), thinly sliced

1 stick celery, sliced

1 tbsp fresh chopped parsley

Half a green pepper, thinly sliced

Half a red pepper, thinly sliced

2 tbsp vinaigrette dressing (see page 227)

Potassium salt

Freshly ground black pepper

Instructions

Combine all the ingredients and stir again just before serving.

This salad is ideal as part of a packed lunch together with German Potato Salad (page 224) and cold Falafel (page 168).

What It's Good For

Beans are rich in protein, filling, and delicious in salads. They are ideal in packed lunches because they contain a type of dietary fibre which slows down your absorption of carbohydrate from your meal. This helps to keep you feeling full for longer.

Sweet peppers are rich in vitamin C, and raw onion has some of the anti-fungal and anti-bacterial properties of raw garlic.

Potato Gnocci (Italian potato dumplings)

Ingredients for about 40 small Gnocci (2 servings)

400 g/14 ounces/4 medium waxy potatoes*

50 g/1¾ ounces/2 tbsp potato flour (potato starch)

Potassium salt

*You must use waxy potatoes for this or the gnocci will not hold together when cooked. If unsure, choose varieties sold as "salad" potatoes.

Special Equipment

A potato press

Instructions

Steam the potatoes in their jackets until tender (about 30 minutes). Hold them on a fork (so that you don't burn your fingers) and peel them with a small knife.

Put a large pan of unsalted water over a high heat and bring to the boil. Put the potatoes through a potato press then work the potato flour into them using a fork. Once the two ingredients are evenly blended, change to a rubber spatula and mash to a paste. Turn the paste out on to a board or worktop, and knead the mixture, using your hands, until it is smooth and pliable. Divide in half.

Again using your hands, roll this dough into a long sausage shape with a diameter of about 1 cm/ half an inch. Cut each roll into 10 segments, then briefly roll each segment between your hands to round it into an oval shape. Score the centre with the back of a fork to make little indentations which will help the gnocci to hold their sauce later on.

As you prepare the gnocci, put them on a small plate then gently slide them off the plate into the gently boiling water.

These small gnocci should rise to the surface after about 40 seconds of boiling. After they have risen, count another 20 seconds, then remove them from the water with a slotted spoon. You can also make larger gnocci and they will take a little longer to rise.

What It's Good For

Topped with tomato, mushroom and olive sauce (page 195) and a dollop of Garlic Crème (page 254). Folded gently into braised vegetables. Warmed through then coated with pesto sauce (page 225). Lightly coated with olive oil then sprinkled with a liberal topping of grated goat's or sheep's cheese and placed under a hot grill (broiler) until golden and bubbling.

Millet with Crunchy Salad Vegetables and Fruit Pieces

Ingredients for 2 servings

Millet grains measured up to the 120 ml/4 fluid oz/½ cup mark in a measuring jug

200 ml/7 fluid oz/generous ¾ cup water

2 tbsp each of chopped, finely diced and/or grated salad vegetables: carrots, celery, sweet (bell) peppers, watercress, cucumber, mint, radishes, spring onion (scallion)

One apple or orange

4 tbsp vinaigrette dressing (see page 227)

1 tbsp lemon juice if using apple

Instructions

Toast the millet grains in a dry frying pan (skillet) over a medium heat for about 10 minutes, or until they give off a roasted aroma and begin to change colour. Transfer them to a saucepan, add the water, bring to the boil and simmer over a low heat for 30 minutes.

Remove from the heat. Remove the lid, add 1 tbsp water, stir briefly, then replace the lid and leave undisturbed until cool.

Cut the apple into small dice, and place in a bowl of water with the lemon juice (to prevent discolouring).

Alternatively, if using an orange, cut into segments as described on page 237.

Shortly before serving, fluff up the millet with a fork, whisk the vinaigrette and stir it into the millet with the vegetables. Finally fold in the fruit pieces. This dish is excellent in a packed lunch.

Variation

You could use cooked brown rice or buckwheat instead of millet.

What It's Good For

Millet is a very ancient grain, and has been cultivated for longer than rice, wheat and rye. It is a rich source of many vitamins and minerals and is one of the best sources of the mineral silica, which is needed for strong bones and teeth. People with food intolerances rarely have a problem with millet, as it is gluten free and easy to digest. It can safely be added to any hypoallergenic diet. Millet is also said to have anti-fungal properties and therefore may be able to help people with intestinal candiasis.

Super sweets

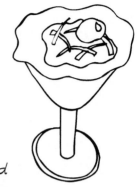

I guarantee you will be amazed at how easy it is to make delicious sweet dishes without sugar.

Those who try to sell us sugar insist there's no difference between the stuff in packets and the natural sugars in fruits. As far as your body is concerned, this is not true. Sugar bound up with the dietary fibre in fruit is absorbed much more slowly into your blood than added sugar, resulting in a more gradual rise in the hormone insulin.

But packet sugar (as well as honey and syrups) can produce high insulin levels in your body very quickly. Too much insulin encourages fatty deposits on artery walls, fluid retention, and is also stressful to your kidneys.

Little Castagnacci (Italian chestnut cakes)

Ingredients to make 12

200 g/7 ounces/1 cup chestnut flour

260 ml/scant ½ pint/1 cup water

Extra virgin olive oil

40g raisins

40g washed and dried brazil nuts, roughly chopped

1 tbsp fresh rosemary, chopped

Instructions

Preheat the oven to 190°C/375°F/gas mark 5.

Stir the water into the chestnut flour a little at a time until you have a smooth paste with a "soft dropping" consistency. Stir in the raisins and chopped brazil nuts, and 2 tbsp olive oil. Drop a teaspoon of olive oil into each of the wells of a well-oiled shallow bun or muffin tin, followed by tablespoons of the chestnut mixture to a depth of no more than half an inch. Smooth the tops flat with a fork, then sprinkle on a little chopped rosemary and olive oil. Bake for 25 minutes or until cracked on top, then allow to cool for at least 30 minutes before serving. These cakes do not keep well and are best eaten within a day or two.

Variation

This recipe is best made with chestnut flour, but it is possible to make something similar with boiled, peeled chestnuts, or with dried chestnuts which have been soaked in hot water overnight and then boiled until soft. Blend the chestnuts in a food processor with enough water to achieve a slightly stiff consistency before adding the other ingredients.

What It's Good For

This is an adaptation of an ancient Italian recipe—crunchy on the outside, sweet and moist in the centre. Chestnut flour is available from health food stores, or see page 294. Selenium-rich brazil nuts can help to prevent heart attacks and cancer, and to protect you against many pollutants. Always wash brazil nuts thoroughly before use, as they are prone to develop mould soon after shelling. Chestnuts are low in oil, and rich in potassium, magnesium and iron. They are nutritionally similar to grains.

Chewy Chocolate Truffles

Ingredients to make 15 truffles

115 g/4 ounces dried dates

40 g/1½ ounces cocoa powder

55 g/2 ounces coarsely-chopped nuts

Instructions

Put the dates in a small saucepan, add just enough water to cover them and bring to the boil. Simmer on the lowest heat with the lid on for 15 minutes or until soft, then transfer the dates to a bowl.

Stir in some of the cocoa powder and mash it into the dates with the back of a tablespoon. Repeat until most of the cocoa powder has been incorporated, and you have a stiff, dough-like consistency. Tip half the chopped nuts plus the remaining cocoa powder on to a board, scrape out the dough and add it to them, then, using your hands, knead these remaining ingredients into the dough.

Roll the dough into a long sausage about 1 cm/half an inch or less in diameter, and cut it into 15 segments. (If necessary dust with more cocoa powder to prevent it sticking to the board.) Using your hands, roll each segment into a ball, flatten slightly, place in a fondant case and sprinkle with more chopped nuts.

Alternatively, make a slightly stickier mixture (using less cocoa powder), and roll the truffle balls in the chopped nuts so that they cling to them.

What It's Good For

Chocaholics will love this recipe, which contains none of the fat and sugar which makes overindulgence in ordinary chocolate so harmful. Cocoa powder is rich in iron and magnesium. But do not use it if you suffer from breast lumps, cysts or tenderness. Cocoa and chocolate contain caffeine-like compounds which encourage breast problems in some women, and also migraine. Dates provide good quality dietary fibre, so these truffles can even help to keep your bowels working smoothly!

Gourmet Marzipan

Makes enough to cover 2 standard-size fruit cakes or to make 48 bouchées (mouth-size nibbles)

115 g/4 ounces dried dates

300 g/10½ ounces ground almonds/almond flour*

½ tsp natural vanilla essence

*For this recipe, commercially ground almonds produce a smoother result than those home-ground in a food processor.

Instructions

Put the dates in a small saucepan, add just enough water to cover them and bring to the boil. Simmer on the lowest heat with the lid on for 15 minutes or until soft. Transfer the dates to a bowl. Stir in the vanilla essence and some of the ground almonds. Mash them into the dates with the back of a tablespoon. Repeat until you have a stiff, dough-like consistency. Tip the remaining ground almonds on to a board, add the dough, then, using your hands, knead the remaining ground almonds into the dough.

The dough can be rolled out to the required dimensions for a cake (use more ground almonds to prevent the dough sticking to the board). First spread the cake with all-fruit apricot or cherry spread to hold the marzipan in place.

To make mouth-sized marzipan balls, roll the dough into sausages, cut off bite-size portions, and roll these into balls. These bouchées are delicious as they are or can be used to stuff prunes or dipped in melted bitter chocolate (with the aid of toothpicks to grip them). Place in fondant cases

Variation

Use unsulphured (dark brown) dried apricots or dried cherries instead of dates.

What It's Good For

Dates are an excellent source of good quality dietary fibre, so this wonderful marzipan can even help to keep your bowels working smoothly. Do not consume marzipan or any nut-rich recipes if you suffer from herpes, since nuts are rich in arginine, an amino acid which can cause flare-ups of the herpes virus. On the other hand arginine is very good for high blood pressure. Almonds are rich in calcium and magnesium and are a good source of protein.

Baked Rice Pudding with Coconut Cream

Ingredients for 4-6 servings

115 g/4 ounces/scant 1 cup unpolished sweet rice which has been soaked in water overnight then drained

1 litre carton soya (soy) milk

1 knob creamed coconut

1 handful raisins

2 tbsp almonds or cashew nuts, well-washed and finely chopped

Use cashew nuts instead of almonds if you prefer a sweeter flavour.

Instructions

Preheat the oven to 175°C/325°F/gas mark 3.

Place the ingredients in a saucepan and bring to a gentle simmer, stirring until the creamed coconut has dissolved. Pour into a casserole dish placed on a baking tray, cover and bake in the oven for 2 hours. Check that the pudding does not boil over, and if necessary turn the heat down a fraction to prevent this. Remove the pudding after one hour to give it a good stir then replace it in the oven to finish cooking. You could also try cooking this in a saucepan on top of the stove if you wish, with the gas or electric ring on its lowest setting, and a heat diffuser under the pan if necessary. In this case a cast-iron enamelled pan would be best.

Serve hot or cold

- On its own as a delicious breakfast dish, perhaps with prunes,
- Or as a dessert on a shallow plate beside one of the following garnishes:
  Sliced sharon fruit or persimmon and banana.
  Reconstituted Hunza apricots (small dried apricots which are pale and very sweet in flavour).
  A small chestnut cake (page 232).

What It's Good For

Sweet rice is also known as glutinous rice, and is an ingredient in many oriental sweet dishes. Unpolished sweet rice (a form of brown rice) is available from Infinity Foods (see page 294) in the UK. In this dish, the soya milk becomes condensed from long, slow cooking, giving you all the concentrated benefits of soy foods (see page 142). Creamed coconut contains coconut oil, which is good for people with post-viral chronic fatigue as it is rich in the anti-viral substance lauric acid.

Kiwi Fruit Slices in Apple Jelly with Strawberry Coulis

Ingredients for 4 servings

6 kiwi fruit, peeled and thinly sliced

200 g/½ lb/1½ cups sweet strawberries, chopped

275 ml/½ pint/1 cup apple juice plus 2 tbsp

1 rounded tbsp agar flakes

Instructions

Sprinkle the agar flakes on the apple juice in a saucepan. Do not stir. Place the pan over a medium heat and bring to a gentle simmer. Simmer for 3-5 minutes, stirring occasionally until dissolved.

Arrange the kiwi fruit as evenly as possible in overlapping layers in a shallow serving dish, saving the prettiest slices for the top layer. You could also place them in individual dishes or moulds. (First line the moulds with cling film to help you turn out the jellies without breaking.)

Spoon the apple juice gently over the fruit, until it is just covered with jelly. Sets quickly (about 30 minutes). Refrigerate once cool.

To make the coulis, place the chopped strawberries in a blender with 2 tbsp apple juice and whizz until smooth. Serve with the jelly and a dollop of sheep's yoghurt.

What It's Good For

Kiwi fruit is one of the richest known sources of vitamin C. It is very pretty when sliced. Agar is a flavourless natural gelling and thickening agent made from seaweed. While many brands of agar (or agar-agar) are available in oriental shops, some are made by methods involving chemical extraction and bleaching. Clearspring (see page 294) and other macrobiotic agars are made by a traditional process. Agar can be used in jellies and aspics, and as a thickener.

Banana Crème

Ingredients for 2 servings

1 banana

100 g/3½ ounces/½ cup firm tofu

100 ml/3½ fluid oz soya (soy) milk

55 g/2 ounces/½ cup raw cashew nut pieces, well washed and drained

1 tbsp tahini (sesame paste)

2 tsp lemon juice

1 tsp natural vanilla extract

Instructions

Whizz all the ingredients except the tahini in a food processor using the "S" blade, until they are well blended, then add the tahini and continue to whizz until the mixture is very smooth. (This could take up to 5 minutes processing).

Serve the Banana Crème on its own in small glass dishes, topped with peeled orange segments, or as a topping poured over pear slices or a banana cut in half lengthwise. Decorate with a sliced strawberry.

To peel orange segments

Cut the ends off a whole orange. Stand it up then cut the peel off in a downward direction, working all the way around the orange and removing the outer white pith and membrane as you cut.

Using the same knife, cut between each segment, on either side of the membrane separating it from the next segment. Go all the way around the orange like this. The V-shaped orange pieces should easily come out perfectly skinned.

What It's Good For

Soya milk and tofu provide hormone-balancing isoflavones which help to prevent problems from excess or insufficient oestrogen, and excess testosterone: menopausal hot flushes, breast cancer, prostate cancer. Cashew nuts are low in oil and rich in potassium and magnesium, iron and zinc. Raw cashews are liable to develop a little mould while in their packets, so should be washed before use. Bananas are rich in many vitamins and minerals, especially potassium.

Apple Custard

Ingredients for 2 servings

150 ml/¼ pint/½ cup soya (soy) milk

4 tbsp apple sauce made as described on page 255

Instructions

Put the apple sauce in a small saucepan over a medium heat and whisk in the soya milk. Keep whisking until the mixture thickens to the consistency of a thin custard.

Variation

Because of its higher pectin content, apple butter (see page 255) can be whipped with soya milk as described above, to make a slightly thicker, more frothy custard. The texture is slightly chalky, but you may enjoy it.

To make it, use only 1 tbsp apple butter to 150 ml soya milk and keep whisking until the result is thick and frothy.

What It's Good For

Apple peel contains amazing nutritional value. It is rich in quercetin and also pectin—a type of soluble dietary fibre. Pectin is used to set jam and is the reason why apple sauce can thicken soya milk in this recipe. Pectin can also help to treat constipation, and it binds to toxins in your intestines and helps your body eliminate them. Unfortunately, although the skin is the most nutritious part of the apple, it is also the part most liable to contain pesticides, so try to use organic apples if you can.

Oat and Treacle Wedges

Ingredients for 8 servings

<u>115 g/4 ounces/generous 1 cup rolled oats</u>

<u>55 g/2 ounces/scant half cup sunflower seeds</u>

<u>55 g/2 ounces/half cup raisins</u>

<u>50 ml/2 fluid oz/4 tbsp groundnut oil</u>

<u>2 tbsp date purée made as described on page 233</u>

<u>1 tbsp blackstrap molasses</u>

Instructions

Preheat the oven to 180°C/350°F/gas mark 4.

Mix the dry ingredients in a bowl. Warm the date purée in a saucepan then stir in the molasses and oil.

Add the dry ingredients to the saucepan and stir until thoroughly incorporated.

Press the mixture evenly into an oiled 19 cm/7½ inch diameter sandwich tin and bake in the centre of the oven for 25-30 minutes.

Cut into 8 wedges while still warm and allow to cool completely before eating.

What It's Good For

Oats and dates are a great source of soluble dietary fibre which helps you excrete cholesterol. Oats are also rich in B vitamins, and are one of the best sources of magnesium. Blackstrap molasses is a thick residue left from sugar processing, and contains all the minerals left behind when white or brown sugar is produced: calcium, magnesium, iron, zinc and manganese to name just a few. Sunflower seeds are also rich in magnesium, as well as essential polyunsaturated oils.

Fruity Almond Cookies

Ingredients for 20 cookies

115 g/4 oz unsulphured dried apricots

110 g/4 oz ground almonds

50 g/4 oz soya flour

50 g/2 oz chopped mixed nuts

50 g/2 oz mixed dried fruit with peel

1 level teaspoon potassium baking powder

1 teaspoon natural vanilla extract

Water as required.

Instructions

Preheat the oven to 180°C/350°F/gas mark 4.

Lightly oil a baking sheet. Dice the dried apricots, place them in a small saucepan and just cover with water. Bring to the boil and simmer very gently for 30 minutes. Add a little more water if necessary to prevent them drying out. Mix the dry ingredients together.

Once the apricots are cooked, purée them with a hand blender, adding a little more water if necessary to obtain a thick, smooth purée. Stir in the vanilla essence, then mix into the dry ingredients. Incorporate thoroughly, to achieve a thick, stiff paste.

Roll the paste into two long sausage shapes. Divide each roll into 10 segments. Roll each segment into a ball with your hands, press your hands together to flatten it, and place it on the baking sheet.

Bake in the preheated oven for 20 minutes. The cookies become stale after 24 hours but can be restored by gently warming under the grill (broiler).

What It's Good For

Dried apricots are orange in colour if treated with sulphur dioxide. This additive is an intestinal irritant and can cause bloating and gas. Unsulphured apricots (from health food shops) are dark brown and sweet. Apricots provide cancer-preventing carotenes, potassium and other minerals. Almonds are a great source of calcium and magnesium, iron, zinc and vitamin E and essential polyunsaturated oils. Due to their arginine content nuts are best avoided by people prone to cold sores and herpes.

Apple and Orange Mini-Muffins

Ingredients for 24 mini-muffins

175g/6 ounces/1 generous cup of fine maize flour or fine yellow polenta flour

55g/2ounces/¼ cup soya flour

2 large sweet eating apples

150 ml/¼ pint/½ cup sweet Florida orange juice

150 ml/¼ pint/½ cup sunflower oil

1 teaspoon potassium baking powder

a few drops of natural vanilla extract or a pinch of cinnamon

Special equipment

2 mini-muffin tins with 12 wells each, lightly oiled

Instructions

Preheat the oven to 180°C/350°F/gas mark 4.

Sift the dry ingredients into a bowl twice, to get as much air into them as possible.

Combine the liquid ingredients, then grate the apples into them. Stir, then pour the liquid into the dry ingredients and fold gently together until well combined. It is important not to use a mixer or to beat vigorously since this will reduce the air in the mixture.

Using a teaspoon, transfer the mixture to the wells of the mini-muffin tins and place on the middle shelf of the oven. Bake for 30 minutes or until a knife inserted into the muffins comes out clean.

This is a very adaptable recipe. You could experiment with adding chopped nuts, dried fruit, poppy seeds or other flavourings. You could also bake the mixture in a shallow cake tin and cut the resulting cake into squares to serve as a dessert with soya custard. For added sweetness and an unusual flavour, soak a piece of liquorice root in the orange juice for a few hours. Remove the liquorice before adding the juice to the mixture.

What It's Good For

Made only with fruit, unrefined flours and sunflower oil, you would not believe that these mini-muffins could taste so good and so sweet. Just one word of warning. If you suffer from coeliac disease or gluten intolerance, you ought to know that although sweetcorn and maize flour are assumed to be gluten free, in fact they are not. Gluten can be extracted from maize when it is processed into cornstarch, and sold as animal feed. If you cannot tolerate maize flour use rice flour for this recipe instead.

Exotic Warm Fruit Salad in Grape Juice

Ingredients for 4 servings

1 peach, thinly sliced

1 small mango, skinned and chopped

1 kiwi fruit, peeled and sliced

2 slices fresh pineapple (or canned pineapple in juice, drained)

2 tbsp fresh or frozen (defrosted) blueberries

2 tbsp red grape juice

Instructions

Preheat the oven to 180°C/350°F/gas mark 4.

Place the fruits in an oven-proof dish, pour the grape juice over them and cover with a well-fitting lid. Cook in the oven for 15-20 minutes then serve immediately.

Recipe by Carolyn Gibbs

What It's Good For

Vitamin C and cancer-preventing flavonoid antioxidants are the outstanding nutrients found in fruit. Flavonoids also help to keep the walls of blood vessels firm, so that they are less likely to leak water into the spaces between your cells, causing fluid retention. Like all yellow or orange fruits, peaches and mangos also contain carotenes. Fresh pineapple contains bromelain, an enzyme which can aid digestion by breaking down protein.

Blueberry and Apple Crispy Pancakes

Ingredients for 8-10 small pancakes

1 large sweet dessert apple*

115 g/4 ounces/4 tbsp fresh or frozen (defrosted) blueberries or bilberries

55 g/2 ounce chick pea (gram) flour, sieved

25 g/1 ounce ground almonds (almond flour) or ground sesame seeds

75 ml/2¼ fluid oz/5 tbsp apple juice

Groundnut oil

*Choose a variety with plenty of flavour, such as Cox's, Royal Gala, Braeburn or Worcester

Instructions

Combine the chick pea flour, ground almonds and cinnamon. Slowly add the apple juice, stirring all the time. beat with a wooden spoon until smooth. Grate the apple (including the skin) and add to the batter together with the blueberries. Stir well.

Place a heavy-bottomed frying pan (skillet) over a low to medium heat and add 2 tbsp oil. Once the oil is hot, drop dessertspoons of the batter into the pan, smooth down with a fork, and cook slowly until the bottom of the pancake has browned.

Flip over with a spatula and cook the other side. Re-oil the pan between batches. Serve immediately, with Coconut and Cashew Cream (see page 245) or Banana Crème (see page 237) and garnished with a few slices of fresh fruit such as oranges, pears or mangoes.

Variation

Use diced fresh pear and sliced banana instead of blueberries, and crushed or ground cardamom instead of cinnamon.

Recipe by Carolyn Gibbs

What It's Good For

This recipe provides high quality protein from the combination of ground almonds and chick pea flour, flavonoid antioxidants from the skins of the apple and blueberries, and buckets of vitamins and minerals. It is a common belief that we should not eat anything fried, and it is probably a good idea to stay off deep-fried foods, but in fact we do need to have some oil in our diet. The small amounts used in this book will ensure that you get that oil and are no cause for concern.

Black Forest Gelled Fruits

Ingredients for 4 servings

350 g/12 ounces frozen "Black Forest" fruits*

150 ml/5 fluid oz/¾ cup red grape juice measured out, plus extra as required

15 g/½ ounce/1 rounded tbsp powdered gelatine

*E.g. a mixture of blueberries, black cherries, blackberries, black grapes, strawberries, blackcurrants. This type of mixture is sold under various names in large supermarkets. You could also use the equivalent in fresh fruit.

Instructions

Place the fruit in a saucepan over a medium heat with the lid on and cook for about 3 minutes or until the fruits have softened a little and released some of their juice (if frozen, they do not have to defrost completely).

Remove from the heat. Put the 150 ml grape juice in a small saucepan and bring it to the boil. Take the pan off the heat and sprinkle the gelatine into it, whisking briskly until all the gelatine has dissolved.

Pour the fruit, with its juice, into a measuring jug. Add the dissolved gelatine and then top up with cold red grape juice to the 570 ml/1 pint/2 cup mark. Stir well.

Pour the mixture into a glass dish or mould and refrigerate until set (about two hours). Serve with Coconut and Cashew Cream (see page 245).

Recipe by Carolyn Gibbs

What It's Good For

The berries in this recipe contain a good mix of flavonoids. Flavonoids are the colourful pigments in their skins. The red and blue pigments are known as anthocyanins. Other flavonoids include catechins (found in grape seeds, cocoa powder and red wine) and quercetin (found in apple skins and onions). The medicinal actions of many herbs and plants (for instance Ginkgo biloba) are now known to be due to their flavonoids. Flavonoids can also help keep blood vessel walls healthy.

Coconut and Cashew Cream

Ingredients for 4 servings

<u>1 small tin coconut milk (165 ml/5.6 fluid oz)</u>

<u>85 g/3 ounces/raw cashew nuts, well washed and drained</u>

Instructions

Warm the coconut milk by putting the unopened can in a small saucepan of hot water for 10 minutes.

Open the can and put the coconut milk and cashews into a blender. Whizz until smooth and creamy, scraping the sides down occasionally with a rubber spatula. This process may take several minutes.

Set aside for one hour to thicken. Warm gently before serving or use cold.

What It's Good For

Most of us are used to eating salted cashew nuts, and do not realize how deliciously sweet these nuts are in their natural state. Raw cashews are low in oil and rich in potassium and magnesium, iron and zinc. Always wash raw cashews before use, as they can develop a little mould, which may affect the flavour as well as being harmful to health. The oils in coconut cream do not have a cholesterol-raising effect. They contain lauric acid, which combats the Epstein-Barr virus.

Blueberries in Yoghurt Layered with Soft Marzipan and Pear Slices

Ingredients for 4 servings

175 g/6 ounces fresh or frozen blueberries

1 ripe dessert pear (red-skinned if possible)

225 g/8 ounces plain soya (soy) or sheep's milk yoghurt

55 g/2 ounces ground almonds (almond flour)

55 g/2 ounces dried dates, chopped

4 tbsp red grape juice

Toasted chopped or flaked almonds

Instructions

Put the chopped dates in a small saucepan over a low heat with 6 tbsp water, cover and cook until soft. Remove from the heat and beat with a wooden spoon to a smooth paste. Stir in the ground almonds. The mixture should be the consistency of thick double cream—add a little more water if necessary.

Put the blueberries in a covered saucepan over a low heat until the juices run. Remove from the heat and leave to cool. Slice the pear thinly and put it in a saucepan over a low heat with the red grape juice to poach gently for 3-4 minutes or until tender. Remove from the heat then remove the pear slices from the pan with a slotted spoon.

Stir the yoghurt, pour it over the cooled blueberries, and fold in gently. Divide the pear slices between four individual glass serving dishes, then pour a layer of date and almond paste over them. Top with the yoghurt and blueberry mixture. Chill in the fridge for at least 1 hour and sprinkle generously with toasted chopped or flaked almonds just before serving.

Recipe by Carolyn Gibbs

What It's Good For

This recipe provides protein from the yoghurt (whichever type is used), flavonoids from the blueberries, and vitamin E, calcium, magnesium and other minerals from the almonds. It is also rich in vitamin C.

See page 142 for the benefits of soya products, and page 287 for information on flavonoids.

Baked Apples Filled with a Soft Cherry Marzipan

Ingredients for 4 servings

4 large dessert apples, washed and cored

75 g/2½ ounces dried cherries*

75 g/2½ ounces/½ cup ground almonds (almond flour)

2 tbsp toasted flaked almonds

Soya (soy) cream to taste

*Dried cherries and blueberries free of sugar and additives can be found in larger branches of Sainsburys supermarkets. Look in the baking department, near the raisins.

Instructions

Preheat the oven to 175°C/350°F/Gas mark 4. Put the cherries and just enough water to cover them in a small saucepan over a low heat. Cover and simmer for 10 minutes. Remove from the heat and liquidize the cherries with a hand blender in the pan then mash in the ground almonds.

Using a sharp knife, score a circle around the "waist" of each apple to allow it to expand on cooking, then place the apples in an oiled shallow oven-proof dish and stuff the marzipan into the centre of each apple. Place the dish in the centre of the oven and bake for 45 minutes or until tender. Remove from the oven, cut the apples vertically down the middle then turn them over and slice them thickly, trying not to dislodge the filling. Arrange overlapping apple slices on individual serving plates and serve warm with a topping of soya cream and toasted flaked almonds.

Variation

Use dried blueberries, raisins or apricots instead of cherries. Spoon the filling into peach halves instead of apples. Brush with groundnut oil and bake in a very hot oven for 15 minutes.

Recipe by Linda Lazarides and Carolyn Gibbs

What It's Good For

Do not consume marzipan or any nut-rich recipes if you suffer from herpes, since nuts are rich in arginine, which can cause flare-ups of the herpes virus. Almonds are rich in calcium and magnesium and are a good source of protein. Apple peel is very rich in cancer-preventing carotenes and flavonoids, as well as pectin. Pectin can help to treat constipation, and it binds to toxins in your intestines and helps your body eliminate them. Try to use organic apples, since pesticide collects in the skin.

Sweet Mango Pudding with Almonds and Cardamom

Ingredients for 4 servings

<u>300 ml/½ pint/1 cup soya (soy) milk</u>

<u>45 g/1½ ounces/1 rounded tbsp brown rice flour</u>

<u>1 tbsp ground almonds (almond flour)</u>

<u>1 tsp ground cardamom</u>

<u>1 extra-large or two small mangoes</u>

<u>Flaked almonds, toasted</u>

Instructions

Peel the mango, cut all the flesh off the stone and put it in a bowl. Using a blender or liquidizer, purée the mango flesh until smooth. (If it is not soft enough you can soften it by stewing in a pan for 20 minutes over a low heat with a tablespoon of water.)

Put the soya milk in a saucepan over a medium heat, and whisk the brown rice flour, ground almonds and ground cardamom into it. Bring to the boil, stirring, then turn the heat down low and continue stirring for another 6 minutes to thicken.

Remove from the heat, then stir the mango purée into the contents of the saucepan. Beat well until smooth and uniform.

Pour the pudding into individual glass dishes. Pour a little soya cream on top and swirl it. Can also be served cold, garnished with toasted almonds and some finely diced dried fruit such as dates or unsulphured apricots.

What It's Good For

Like brown rice, brown rice flour is a good source of B vitamins and also methionine, a protein constituent (amino acid) which your liver needs to make an important antioxidant enzyme. Mangoes are a good source of vitamin C and carotenes—antioxidants related to the beta carotene in carrots. Mangoes also contain flavonoids (more about these on page 287). Cardamom has anti-microbial properties and is good for dysbiosis and candidiasis sufferers.

Melon Balls in Ginger and Orange Sauce

Ingredients for 2 servings

1 chilled cantaloupe melon large enough to serve 2 people

275 ml/½ pint/1 cup orange juice* (freshly squeezed if possible)

1 tbsp shredded orange zest

1 rounded tsp arrowroot powder

1 tsp finely grated fresh ginger

*If you can get ruby red oranges, this makes a lovely colour contrast with the melon.

Special equipment

A melon baller

Instructions

Put one tbsp of the orange juice into a small bowl with the arrowroot powder and the rest in a saucepan over a medium heat. Stir the arrowroot powder and juice together until smooth, then add to the saucepan along with the ginger and zest. Stir until the mixture just begins to simmer then immediately remove from the heat.

Allow the sauce to cool.

Using a melon baller, make as many balls as you can from the melon. Place in individual serving dishes and spoon the sauce over them.

What It's Good For

Orange zest is rich in flavonoid antioxidants (see page 287). Orange juice, especially if very fresh, is a good source of the B vitamin folic acid as well as vitamin C and carotenes antioxidants (related to beta carotene in carrots. Folic acid is often in short supply in diets which rely on convenience food, because it is very vulnerable to heat and light. Ginger is a great aid to the digestion and helps to stimulate the circulation.

Yoghurt Cheesecake with Black Forest Fruits

Makes one 8 inch diameter cake

For the base

80 g/3 ounces/fine oatmeal

55 g/2 ounces raisins

55 g/2 ounces coconut oil, chilled

25 g/1 ounce spelt flour

For the topping

225 g/8 ounces frozen "Black Forest" fruits

450 g/1 pound/2 cups sheep's yoghurt

15 g/½ ounce gelatine powder

1 tsp natural vanilla extract

Red grape juice as required

*e.g. a mixture of blueberries, black cherries, blackberries, black grapes, strawberries, blackcurrants. This type of mixture is sold under different names in large supermarkets. You could also use the equivalent in fresh fruit.

Instructions

Preheat the oven to gas mark 5. Put the oatmeal, spelt flour and raisins in a food processor with the S blade, and process until the raisins are finely chopped and blended with the flours. Transfer to a bowl, add the vanilla extract and solid coconut oil and mash into the flour with a fork until the mixture resembles fine breadcrumbs. Press it evenly on to the base of an oiled 20 cm/8 inch diameter foil pie dish or sandwich tin (not one with a removable bottom). Bake for 10-15 minutes until golden then allow to cool.

Pour the yoghurt into a sieve lined with absorbent kitchen paper suspended over a bowl and leave it to drip for at least one hour.

Put the fruits in a covered saucepan over a low heat to cook gently in their own steam. Once they have released their juices, purée them in the pan with a hand blender. Bring the purée to the boil, then remove from the heat and sprinkle in the gelatine. Whisk briskly until it dissolves.

Combine strained yoghurt and fruit purée in a measuring jug. If the contents do not reach the 570 ml/1 pint/2 cups mark, top up with red grape juice. Whizz again with the blender until smooth, then pour into the sandwich tin over the pastry base and refrigerate until set.

What It's Good For

This is a protein-rich dessert, with all the flavour of cow's milk yoghurt, but much less likely to cause problems for food intolerance sufferers. Sheep's yoghurt is light and creamy, and if you like fruit and yoghurt combinations you will love this recipe. The berries contain a good mix of antioxidant flavonoids— the colourful pigments in their skins which can help to prevent many diseases by combating free radicals. The red and blue pigments are known as anthocyanidins.

Chocolate Mousse

Ingredients for 3 servings

250 g/9 ounces firm silken tofu

55 g/2 ounces dried dates

2 heaped tbsp cocoa powder

1 tsp natural vanilla extract

Soya (soy) milk as required

Soya (soy) cream and grated
    bitter chocolate to garnish

Instructions

Put the dates in a small saucepan and add just enough water to cover them. Cover, bring to the boil and simmer for 15 minutes or until soft.

Remove the dates with a slotted spoon (keep the cooking liquid) and put them in a food processor with the remaining ingredients. Whizz for half a minute, then scrape the sides down with a rubber spatula and check the thickness of the mixture. The firmer the tofu you have used, the more liquid it will need, so keep adding the date cooking liquid until you have a soft dropping consistency. If it still needs more liquid, add a little soya milk.

Keep whizzing until the texture is completely smooth and creamy. (This may take a few minutes).

Serve in glass dishes, decorated with a little soya cream and grated bitter chocolate.

Variations

For fruity mousses, use equal weights of silken tofu and all-fruit jam or spread (such as apricot). Thin with a little soya milk if necessary, and flavour with natural vanilla extract.

What It's Good For

Chocaholics will love this recipe, not realizing that it is made with protein from health-giving soya instead of the fats which can make overindulgence in ordinary chocolate so harmful. Cocoa powder is rich in iron, magnesium and antioxidant flavonoids. But do not use it if you suffer from migraine or breast lumps, cysts or tenderness. Cocoa and chocolate contain caffeine-like compounds which in some people seem to encourage these problems.

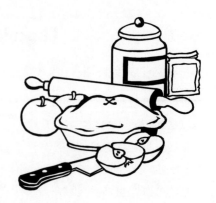

Little extras

Recipes for pastry, mayonnaise, ketchup, unleavened bread, apple sauce, and other useful extras.

If you really miss cheese, I hope you will enjoy the tasty cheese substitute on page 257. You can use it as a topping on hot food, or eat it with rice crackers and pumpernickel.

Sour Cream

Ingredients for 6 servings

250 g/9 ounces silken tofu*

2 tbsp apple juice

Up to 6 tbsp water

4 tbsp cold-pressed unrefined sunflower oil

2 tbsp fresh lemon juice

½ tsp natural vanilla extract

*Silken tofu has a creamy blancmange-like texture. It comes in soft, medium and firm varieties. The firmer the tofu, the more water you will need to blend into it for this recipe.

Instructions

Whizz all the ingredients except the water in a blender. If it is too thick, whizz in the water little by little until you reach the desired consistency. For savoury recipes you might also want to add a pinch of potassium salt.

Variations

Garlic Sour Cream

Add half a clove of chopped raw garlic and a pinch of potassium salt to the other ingredients in the blender before whizzing.

Mustard Sour Cream

Add a teaspoon of mustard powder to the other ingredients in the blender before whizzing.

What It's Good For

It is not widely known that the taste of cow's milk comes from a combination of lactose (milk sugar) and coumarin, a flavonoid-like substance found in hay and clover. Coumarin has a flavour almost identical to vanilla, which is why a little vanilla extract is used in this recipe.

See page 142 for the benefits of consuming soya products.

Garlic Crème

Makes 300 ml/½ pint/1 cup garlic crème

50 g/1¾ ounces/½ cup soya (soy) flour

275 ml/½ pint/1 cup boiling water

100 ml/3 fluid oz/⅓ cup cold-pressed unrefined sunflower oil*

1 tbsp flax seed oil (optional)

1 tbsp lemon juice

1 clove fresh garlic, roughly chopped

½ tsp potassium salt

*Can be replaced with extra virgin olive oil if you are a candidiasis sufferer.

Instructions

The flavours of soya and garlic complement each other perfectly in this delicious recipe, which is one of the best medicinal foods in this book.

Add the soya flour to the boiling water in a saucepan, and whisk to ensure no lumps remain. Simmer gently for 20 minutes, stirring from time to time and ensure it does not boil over. Remove from the heat and allow to cool.

Transfer to the goblet of a liquidizer and whizz with the lemon juice, salt, garlic and half the main oil. When smooth add the rest of the oil plus the flax seed oil (if you are using it) and whizz again for 1-2 minutes. This Garlic Crème will keep for a few days in the fridge, and you can also stir in other flavourings such as chopped herbs or mustard. Stir before use. Use cold as a topping or a dressing or as a sauce with fish.

What It's Good For

Raw garlic contains allicin, destroyed by cooking but with many health benefits. After consumption, it travels to all parts of your body, helping to sterilize them. Raw garlic has been used to treat bronchitis, dysentery, typhoid, cholera, food poisoning and worms, as well as cryptosporidial diarrhoea associated with AIDS. It can help to heal the bowels after amoebic dysentery and to combat the thrush-causing yeast *Candida albicans*. Flax seed oil is a good source of omega 3 essential polyunsaturated oils.

Apple Sauce and Apple Butter

Makes 570 ml/1 pint/2 cups apple sauce plus 275 ml/½ pint/1 cup of apple butter

2 kg/4½ pounds sweet apples with a good flavour, such as Cox's

150 ml/¼ pint/½ cup water

Special Equipment

A pressure cooker

Instructions

Core and segment the apples (this task is very quick if you use a coring/segmenting gadget) but do not peel them. Put the segments in a pressure cooker with the water, bring up to full steam and cook for 10 minutes.

Cool the pressure cooker and remove the lid. Put the contents in a food processor (with the S blade) and whizz until smooth. You will probably need to do this in two batches. It takes a few minutes to really pulverize the peel.

Return the apple purée to the pan, and leave over a medium heat for one hour, stirring from time to time. Turn the heat down to prevent violent sputtering. At the end of this time, use a ladle to spoon out 570 ml/1 pint/2 cups of the purée, which you can now use as apple sauce, and leave the rest to continue reducing over the heat for another 2-3 hours. At the end of this time you should have a very thick mixture which stiffens on cooling and becomes spreadable like butter.

Both apple sauce and apple butter can be frozen. You could freeze them in ice cube trays if you will only need to defrost a small amount at a time.

What It's Good For

Apple peel is rich in the cancer-preventing flavonoid quercetin, as well as the soluble fibre pectin. Pectin is used to set jam, and is the reason why this apple sauce recipe can thicken soya milk and turn it into custard (see page 238). Pectin can also bind to toxins in your intestines and help you eliminate them. The skin is the most nutritious part of the apple, but may harbour pesticides, alar (a chemical ripening agent), and pesticide-treated wax, so make this recipe with organic apples if you can.

Basic Tomato Sauce

Ingredients for 2 servings

2 x 400 g/14 ounce cans of chopped Italian plum tomatoes

3 cloves garlic, finely chopped

A few pieces dried porcini mushrooms, chopped small

1 tbsp capers, chopped

1 tbsp coriander (cilantro) chopped

2 tbsp extra virgin olive oil

Potassium salt

Freshly ground black pepper

Instructions

Put all the ingredients except the black pepper into a saucepan, bring to the boil, then simmer for one hour with the lid off or until reduced to a thick, glossy consistency. Stir in freshly-ground black pepper. This sauce can be served with wheat-free pasta, rösti recipes or grilled fish.

What It's Good For

Tomato sauce is very rich in a carotene known as lycopene, which is especially powerful in preventing prostate and breast cancer and is thought to be an even stronger neutralizer of free radicals than beta carotene.

This concentrated sauce is also an excellent source of potassium, vitamin C and minerals.

Melting Red Leicester

Ingredients to make 450 g/ 1 lb

280 ml/½ pint/1 cup water

2 tbsp agar flakes

Half a sweet red (bell) pepper

115 g/4 ounces/½ cup raw cashew nuts which have been soaked overnight and drained

2 tbsp miso (get a pale variety if you can)

1 tbsp fresh lemon juice

1 tsp onion granules

1 tsp garlic granules

1 level tsp potassium salt

½ tsp yellow mustard powder

Special equipment

A lightly oiled container to use as a mould

Instructions

Put the water in a small saucepan over a medium heat, sprinkle in the agar flakes without stirring, and bring to a gentle simmer.

Keep simmering for five minutes, stirring until all the agar has dissolved.

Put the mixture in a liquidizer or food processor together with the remaining ingredients, and process until smooth. This usually takes about five minutes. Keep scraping down the sides to ensure even processing.

Pour immediately into the mould and allow to cool. Cover and chill overnight. Can be served on rice crackers or with corn chips or mini-poppadoms. It will also melt on hot dishes like baked potatoes or wheat-free pasta.

What It's Good For

With a pleasantly cheesy flavour, this Red Leicester is low in fat and melts in the mouth with a light, pudding-like texture. The main ingredients are carotene-rich sweet red pepper (capsicum) and protein-rich cashew nuts providing potassium, magnesium, iron and zinc.

See page 294 for where to buy agar—a natural gelling agent made from seaweed.

Mayonnaise

Makes about 300 ml/½ pint/1 cup

100 g/3½ ounces silken tofu*

1 tbsp fresh lemon juice

100 ml/3½ fluid oz mild-flavoured extra virgin olive oil

Up to 100 ml/3½ fluid oz water

Potassium salt

*If you are using a soft silken tofu, you will need only a fraction of the water. If you are using an extra-firm silken tofu such as Sanchi Organic Tofu, you will need all of it.

Instructions

Using a blender, liquidize the tofu with the lemon juice, some or all of the water (depending on the softness of the tofu) and the potassium salt, then whizz in the olive oil.

This makes a thick basic mayonnaise. It can easily be thinned by whizzing in more water, or stretched by whizzing in more oil.

Variations

Mayonnaise can be flavoured with a teaspoon of pale miso (see page 132) which has been whisked into hot water and then allowed to cool, or with fresh garlic, dried garlic or onion granules, mustard, horseradish or fresh spring onion (scallion) among others.

What It's Good For

Tofu (made from soya) is a rich source of sex hormone-balancing flavonoids known as isoflavones. So a diet rich in tofu can help to prevent all kinds of problems, from menopausal hot flushes, to breast cancer and prostate cancer.

Extra virgin olive oil is an important part of the Mediterranean diet, which helps prevent health problems in old age and is also now known to help prevent a deterioration of mental faculties.

Short Crust Pastry

When rolled out makes 2 pastry rounds with a diameter of about 25 cm/10 inches.

100 g/3½ ounces/scant 1 cup
brown rice flour

100 g/3½ ounces/scant 1 cup
spelt flour[1]

100 g/3½ ounces/scant 1 cup
solid coconut oil at room
temperature[2]

120 ml/4 fluid ounces/scant ½
cup water

1. See page 134
2. See page 131

Instructions

Preheat the oven to 190°C/375°F gas mark 5.

Sift the dry ingredients into a large bowl, then add the solid coconut oil. Using a fork, mash the oil into the flours until the mixture resembles fine breadcrumbs. Add the water little by little, working it into the mixture with a rubber spatula until you can form a large, soft ball of dough with your hands. Knead briefly then refrigerate for at least half an hour.

Oil the tin (metal produces the best results) which will be in contact with the pastry while cooking. Remove the dough from the fridge, and knead only until you can roll the pastry out without it breaking up. If you find it hard to roll then you have not added enough water; try to work a little more water into the dough.

Roll out the pastry evenly, using brown rice flour to prevent it sticking, and turning it 90 degrees from time to time. Then use this pastry as you would any other shortcrust pastry: to make pasties, pies, pastry cases for flans, and so on. Bake for about 20 minutes or until golden.

If baking blind, prick the base with a fork before baking, to prevent air bubbles.

What It's Good For

This makes a very respectable shortcrust pastry with a good, light texture. The coconut oil does not make this pastry taste of coconut. Although solid at room temperature and so technically speaking a hard or saturated fat, the European Journal of Clinical Nutrition reports that consuming coconut oil does not cause increases in blood cholesterol levels. Coconut oil contains lauric acid, which combats "lipid-coated" viruses such as Epstein-Barr, common in chronic fatigue sufferers.

Unleavened Bread

Ingredients for approx 9 x 6-inch wide rounds of bread

10 oz/275 g wholemeal spelt flour*

2 tbsp thick soya (soy) yoghurt

100 ml/3½ fluid oz/scant ½ cup water

*See page 134

Instructions

Add the yoghurt and water to the flour and mix to a soft, pliable dough. Turn out on to a well-floured board and knead for about 8 minutes until the dough is smooth and elastic, using more flour if necessary to prevent sticking. Put in a bowl covered with a damp cloth for 30 minutes.

Break off egg-sized pieces of dough, and roll into rounds measuring about 12 cm/6 inches in diameter and ½ cm/¼ inch thick. Pre-heat an unoiled griddle pan or good quality frying pan (skillet) on a moderate heat for about 2 minutes. When the pan is hot, place a round of dough on it and cook for about a minute until the bread puffs up slightly. Briefly dab it all over very gently with a spatula to make it puff up more. Then immediately turn it over and repeat this on the other side. Turn and cook the other side. When both sides are cooked, turn the bread over again and .

Stack the rounds separated by absorbent kitchen paper. Keep warm until you are ready to serve them.

To Freeze

Slightly undercook the breads and omit the puffing up stage. Allow to cool, place them in polythene freezer bags and then in the freezer. To use, finish cooking the breads under a hot grill (broiler), but not too close to the heat as they will puff up.

What It's Good For

Spelt flour is sometimes known as "ancient wheat", but often does not provoke symptoms in wheat intolerance sufferers. It has all the goodness of wholemeal flour: B vitamins, vitamin E and minerals. But cooked without yeast, wholemeal spelt and wheat (and their bran products) can contain high levels of phytic acid, which binds to minerals in your diet and prevents you from absorbing them. This should not be a problem if your diet is varied and you eat this bread only in moderate amounts.

Pan-Baked Pea Bread

Ingredients for 8 thin rounds about 8 cm/4 inches wide

200g/7 ounces/1 cup chick pea (gram) flour

100 ml/3½ fluid oz/scant ½ cup water

2 tbsp arrowroot powder

1 tbsp groundnut oil

Brown rice flour for rolling out

Potassium salt

Instructions

Mix the dry ingredients then add the water and oil, and mix thoroughly, using the back of a spoon to work the ingredients together into a thick, stiff and sticky dough.

Divide the dough into 8 portions. Using brown rice flour to prevent sticking, roll the mixture into balls and flatten with your hand. Then, using a rolling pin, roll into thin rounds.

Preheat a dry griddle pan or good quality frying pan (skillet) over a medium heat until very hot. Put a dough round in the pan and cook for about one minute or until it puffs up and small brown spots appear on the bottom. Turn and cook the other side. These light and tasty breads are delicious served warm with soup, and can also be folded over and stuffed with salad ingredients plus any of the following:

- Grated hard goat's cheese,
- One of the Speciality Patés (pages 158-160),
- Guacamole (page 166),
- Hummus (page 155).

What It's Good For

Gram (chick pea) flour is very rich in protein. It is also a good source of many other nutrients, including calcium, magnesium, iron, copper and some of the B vitamins.

Cacik (yoghurt and cucumber sauce)

Ingredients for 4 servings

One standard tub of sheep's yoghurt (about 250 grams, or half a pint/1 cup in volume)

Half a cucumber, finely shredded or coarsely grated

1 clove garlic, crushed

2 tsp fresh mint, finely chopped, or 1 tsp dried mint

Potassium salt

Freshly ground black pepper

Instructions

Combine all the ingredients except the salt and mix well. Add the salt just before serving.

Use as a dip or as a sauce for Falafels (see page 168) or Spiced Bean Röstis (see page 162). For a thicker Cacik, first strain the yoghurt by draining it for an hour in a sieve lined with kitchen paper.

What It's Good For

Sheep's yoghurt, while rich in protein like cow's milk yoghurt, is often safe to eat for people with a cow's milk intolerance. Yoghurt is also rich in beneficial bacteria for the intestines. Cucumber is rich in potassium and other minerals, and is a particularly good source of bone- and tissue-building silicon. But do not peel your cucumbers, as these nutrients are mostly concentrated in the skin. Mint is used by herbalists as a remedy to help the digestion and soothe inflammation in the intestines.

Home-Made Tomato Ketchup

Makes 225 ml/8 fluid oz/¾ cup

<u>1 small can of tomato purée (paste) (140 g/5 ounces)</u>

<u>3 tbsp cider vinegar or wine vinegar</u>

<u>3 tbsp water</u>

<u>½ tsp English mustard powder</u>

<u>Freshly ground nutmeg</u>

<u>Potassium salt</u>

<u>Freshly ground black pepper</u>

Instructions

Mix the ingredients thoroughly and store in a jar in the fridge for up to four days.

Variations

Spice the ketchup up with cayenne pepper or some chopped gherkins or capers.

What It's Good For

No artificial preservatives, colourings or flavourings, no sugar or salt, this is quick to make but better than any commercial brand. Tomato purée is very rich in a carotene known as lycopene, which is especially powerful in preventing prostate and breast cancer and is thought to be an even stronger neutralizer of free radicals than beta carotene.

Sweet Chestnut Crust

When rolled out makes 2 x pastry rounds with a diameter of about 25 cm/10 inches.

100 g/3½ ounces/scant 1 cup chestnut flour[1]

100 g/3½ ounces/scant 1 cup spelt flour[2]

100 g/3½ ounces/scant 1 cup solid coconut oil, at room temperature

120 ml/4 fluid ounces/scant ½ cup white grape juice

20 g/¾ ounce soya (soy) milk powder[3]

½ tsp potassium baking powder

1. See page 131.

2. See page 134.

3. Available from health food shops.

Instructions

Preheat the oven to 190°C/375°F gas mark 5.

Sift the dry ingredients into a large bowl, then add the coconut oil, which should be in solid form. Using a fork, mash the oil into the dry ingredients until the mixture resembles fine breadcrumbs. Add the grape juice little by little, working it into the mixture with a rubber spatula until you can form a large, soft ball of dough with your hands. Knead briefly then refrigerate for at least half an hour.

Oil the tin (metal produces the best results) which will be in contact with the pastry while cooking. Remove the dough from the fridge, and knead only until you can roll the pastry out without it breaking up. If you find it hard to roll then you have not added enough liquid; try to work a little more grape juice into the dough.

Roll out the pastry evenly, using extra spelt flour to prevent it sticking, and turning it 90 degrees from time to time. Then use this pastry to make cases for sweet desserts, tarts and tartlets. Bake for about 25 minutes or until golden. To prevent air bubbles prick the base with a fork before baking blind.

What It's Good For

The main benefits of this recipe come from the chestnut flour, rich in potassium, magnesium and iron, and spelt flour, rich in B vitamins and vitamin E.

Although solid at room temperature, coconut oil does not seem to raise cholesterol levels like butter and other animal fats. It contains beneficial plant sterols, which help to prevent cholesterol rises. It also contains lauric acid, which combats the Epstein-Barr virus, known to be the cause of many cases of chronic fatigue syndrome.

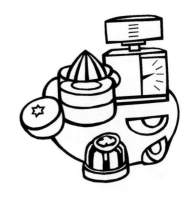

Drinks

Recipes for teas to help your digestion and prevent wind.

Nutrient-packed juices to combat arthritis and help your liver.

Alternatives to milk and commercial fizzy drinks.

Digestive Tea

Ingredients for 2 cup/mugfuls

600 ml/1 pint/2 cups very hot water

1 tsp fresh ginger, grated (or ½ tsp ground ginger)

1 tsp fennel seeds

½ tsp ground cinnamon

¼ tsp ground cloves

Instructions

Using a mortar and pestle, crush the fennel seeds and mix with the other spices. Put the mixture in a small teapot and pour the boiling water over it. Stir thoroughly, cover and leave for 5 minutes, then strain through a very fine strainer and drink.

What It's Good For

These spices are prescribed by medical herbalists to soothe the digestion after a meal and to treat flatulence. If you are not used to eating the foods in this book and have trouble digesting them, this tea will be very helpful while your body is adapting. Sip it slowly during and after your meal. If you'd like it to be even more effective, you could also add a pinch of cayenne pepper, but watch out for the extra bite!

Home-Made Apple, Celery, Parsley and Radish Juice

Ingredients for 1 serving

1 large sweet apple, unpeeled
    and organically grown if
    possible

2 sticks celery

1 bunch parsley

5 cm/2 inch segment of mooli
    radish

Small piece of lemon, including
    peel*

*Optional - you may find that it helps the
flavour

Instructions

Wash the ingredients, cut them into chunks and put them through a juice extractor. Stir and leave to stand for 20 minutes to break down the peppery taste of the radish before drinking.

Special Equipment

A juice extractor

What It's Good For

It would be hard to find a drink more rich in health-giving nutrients. This drink is: Rich in vitamin C. Helps to alkalinize your body. Fights fluid retention, which causes pain and swellings in nerves, joints and breasts, as well as migraine and headaches. Helps fight arthritis. If you have a cold the radish component will help to eliminate congestion. Radish juice also helps balance the thyroid gland.

Beetroot, Celery And Lemon Juice

Prepare quantities of ingredients according to how many people you are catering for

Bottled beetroot (beet) juice (or juice from raw beetroot made with a juice extractor)

Home-made celery juice

Fresh lemon juice

Instructions

Combine equal quantities of bottled beetroot juice and home-made celery juice made from fresh celery with a juice extractor, or use the proportions you prefer. Flavour with a little fresh lemon juice to taste.

If you juice your own raw beetroot, it will be very strong and only a little is required. It must be left to stand for 20 minutes before drinking or else it will have a very peppery taste.

Special Equipment

A juice extractor

What It's Good For

Beetroot juice is a powerful aid to your liver. Celery juice helps to alkalinize the body, thus combating the acidity that often leads to arthritis. It also contains coumarin, a substance which fights fluid retention by keeping your blood vessels strong and stimulating your lymphatic system. Fluid retention can simulate arthritis by pressing on joints and causing pain and swelling. Beetroot is one of the best plant sources of iron, needed for energy and for oxygen transport in your body.

Home-Made Broccoli Stem And Sharp Apple Juice

Prepare quantities of ingredients according to how many people you are catering for

Equal quantities of

Broccoli stems

Sharp apples such as Granny Smiths

Instructions

Broccoli juice is very sweet, which is why it is good mixed with a fairly sharp apple juice. Simply cut the broccoli stems and apples into chunks and feed into your juice extractor in the proportions you prefer. You may need to experiment a little. If necessary, add a little lemon juice to disguise the broccoli flavour.

Special Equipment

A juice extractor

What It's Good For

Save your broccoli heads for eating and the thick stems for juicing, especially if you have any female troubles linked to poor oestrogen metabolism, such as: breast cysts or lumps, endometriosis, fibroids, family history of breast cancer. Broccoli is a superb liver food and contains substances which help your liver to break down excess oestradiol, the form of oestrogen which in excess can encourage these problems.

Carrot And Orange Juice

Prepare quantities of ingredients according to how many people you are catering for

<u>Carrots</u>

<u>Fresh oranges</u>

Try to get organic oranges, or at least unwaxed ones. If you cannot obtain them, scrub ordinary oranges carefully in very hot water with detergent to remove the thin layer of pesticide-treated wax coating the skin, and then rinse.

Instructions

This is a lovely sweet combination. Juice your carrots in the juice-extractor together with some of the orange flesh and peel. Then juice the rest of the orange with a normal citrus juicer.

Mix together in the proportions you prefer and drink straight away.

If you do not have a juice extractor, use commercial juices and use your liquidizer to whizz in a piece of orange with the pith and peel still attached.

Special Equipment

<u>A juice extractor</u>

What It's Good For

Carrots are rich in beta carotene and other carotenes (a type of antioxidant) as well as in many minerals. Beta carotene can also be converted into vitamin A, although if you have an underactive thyroid this process may not be as efficient as it should be. Any beta carotene that your body cannot handle is stored in your skin. Fresh oranges are rich in the important B vitamin folic acid. The pith and peel is an excellent source of a type of antioxidant known as flavonoids, which can fight fluid retention.

Flavonoid-Rich Orange Juice

Ingredients

<u>Ready-made orange juice, plus</u>

<u>Fresh oranges</u>

Try to get organic oranges, or at least unwaxed ones. If you cannot obtain them, scrub ordinary oranges carefully in very hot water with detergent to remove the thin layer of pesticide-treated wax coating the skin, and then rinse.

Instructions

Liquidize a piece of fresh orange with pith and peel into a glass of normal orange juice. This will contain a far larger quantity of flavonoids than you could get in a flavonoid supplement pill!

What It's Good For

Fresh orange juice is rich in folic acid, one of the nutrients most likely to be in short supply in our diet. It is now known that one of the biggest causes of the high blood cholesterol levels that lead to heart attacks is a folic acid deficiency, which can be detected by measuring levels of a substance known as homocysteine in your blood. People with high homocysteine levels are at the highest risk of heart attacks. Levels can often be brought down by consuming more folic acid and vitamins B_6 and B_{12}.

Home-Made Ginger Tea With Lemon Zest

Ingredients to make one cup or mugful

Ingredients to make one cup or mugful

One tsp fresh grated ginger

One tsp fresh, finely shredded lemon zest*

*Try to get organic lemons, or at least unwaxed ones. If you cannot obtain them, scrub ordinary lemons carefully in very hot water with detergent to remove the thin layer of pesticide-treated wax coating the skin, and then rinse.

Instructions

Pour a cupful of boiling water on to a teaspoon of grated fresh ginger and a teaspoon of fresh lemon zest shreds. Leave to infuse for five minutes, then strain and drink.

What It's Good For

Ginger is known as a "hot bitter" herb, which helps your stomach to produce digestive juices and so aids digestion. Much research has been carried out into its benefits, especially against rheumatoid arthritis and travel sickness. In Chinese medicine, ginger is considered to warm and stimulate the circulation and to remove catarrh and combat bronchitis. Lemon zest is rich in flavonoids—anti-cancer antioxidants which also help the circulation by keeping blood vessels walls strong.

Almond Milk

Ingredients for 2 servings

<u>570 ml/1 pint/2 cups water</u>

<u>55 g/2 ounces/scant ½ cup chopped almonds*</u>

*Can be made by whizzing blanched almonds in a food processor

Instructions

Soak the chopped almonds in the water overnight in the goblet of your liquidizer.

In the morning whizz them together until the almonds have turned into a fine pulp, and strain the milk through a fine sieve.

This delicious milk is naturally sweet and excellent for drinking. The pulp can be added to rice pudding.

Try the same method with other nuts or seeds, such as brazils, cashews and sunflower seeds. You could also use oatmeal to make oat milk.

What It's Good For

While not as rich in protein as cow's milk, soya milk and nut milks do contain a good range of nutrients, especially calcium and magnesium, essential polyunsaturated oils, zinc and vitamin E. But if you have a young baby these alternative milks are not a suitable substitute for formula milks. Although almonds are calorie-rich (about 600 Calories per 100 grams) feeding nut milk too early, before the baby's digestion has matured, could result in developing an allergy.

Soda Pop

Ingredients

Equal quantities of sparkling mineral water and any combination of:

Red or white grape juice

Apple juice

Orange juice

Mango, passion fruit, peach, pineapple or raspberry juices

Use either ready-made juices or make your own with a juice extractor

Instructions

Just mix your favourite combinations together and drink immediately. Try for some interesting colours such as mixing raspberry and orange juice.

You could also liquidize small amounts of soft fruit into the juice before mixing it with the mineral water.

What It's Good For

These drinks are especially good for hyperactive children, who often react badly to the colourings and sugar in canned fizzy drinks. Commercial drinks can also contain large amounts of phosphorus. Although we all need phosphorus, if it gets out of balance with the other minerals in your body it can make calcium leach from your bones, encouraging bone softness and osteoporosis (brittle bone disease). Fresh fruit juices are of course rich in vitamin C and in flavonoid and carotene antioxidants.

Appendices

Appendix I: Superfoods—Their medicinal properties and health benefits

Food	Health benefits
Aubergine	Regarded in Ayurvedic medicine as a prime treatment for female hormonal complaints.
Beans and peas	Good sources of plant protein and one of the few rich plant sources of the amino acid lysine, needed to make carnitine. Lysine helps combat herpes[2,3]
Blue & purple fruits	Rich in the antioxidant anthocyanin which fights inflammation[147], keeps blood vessel walls strong[229] and helps prevent damage from pollutants.
Brown rice	Consumed daily, can help prevent hot flushes of menopause. Good source of B vitamins.
Beetroot	Contains betaine which stimulates liver cell function. Good source of iron.
Brassicas (broccoli etc)	Contain antioxidant indoles which help the liver break down excess oestrogen[40]. Also contain anti-carcinogenic sulphoraphane which stimulates the production of liver detox enzymes[251].
Carrots	Raw grated carrot taken daily helps to prevent roundworm infestations. Good source of the antioxidant beta carotene.
Celery	Celery juice and celery seed extract help alkalinize the body. Contains coumarin, which helps the body release fluid retention[74]. Can be an effective treatment for arthritis caused by inflammatory fluid pressure on joints.
Chilli pepper	Aids the microcirculation, opening up all tissues to a greater flow of blood and increasing the supply of oxygen and nutrients. Digestive stimulant. Helps prevent intestinal gas.
Coconut oil	Contains lauric acid, which combats lipid-coated viruses such as Epstein-Barr and others of the herpesvirus family[92].
Comfrey leaf	Eaten as a vegetable, very helpful against arthritis or any type of chronic pain. Helps to regenerate tissues. Comfrey tea helps repair the digestive system, healing ulcers and soothing inflammation.
Coriander leaf	Can greatly accelerate excretion of the heavy metals mercury, lead and aluminium. One researcher has reported that viral infections like herpes simplex and cytomegalovirus can only be eliminated for good when coriander leaf is used together with other treatments. He theorizes that perhaps viruses are more easily able to hide and flourish in areas with concentrations of heavy metals[252].
Cucumber	The ground or liquidized seeds can be used to treat tapeworm. The juice is a natural diuretic and soothing for urinary irritations such as cystitis.
Fenugreek seeds	In clinical trials, these have shown an insulin-like effect in the treatment of adult-onset diabetes[116]. Like slippery elm, they can be made into a soothing tea to create a protective coating for an irritated digestive system, and help to lubricate the large intestine.
Garlic	Taken raw, combats many bacteria and parasites. Can help treat bronchitis, dysentery, food poisoning, worm infestations, candidiasis and AIDS-related diarrhoea[212]. Lowers cholesterol and blood pressure.
Ginger	Warming digestive stimulant. Helps prevent flatulence. Often used as a remedy for nausea.
Leafy greens	Rich in lutein, a carotene which is now being used as a treatment for macular degeneration—a leading cause of blindness[253].

Lettuce	Very good source of silicon, needed for bones and joints. Wild lettuce was once used as a substitute for opium. The milky juice from the stems of cultivated lettuce also contains natural sedatives.
Mint	Peppermint tea acts as a balm for the digestive system, helping to prevent flatulence and relieving spasms and nausea. Stimulates the flow of bile.
Nuts, sunflower, sesame seeds	Rich in magnesium and essential polyunsaturated oils. Good sources of protein often providing, weight for weight, more protein than animalproducts
Onions	One of the richest sources of quercetin, a natural anti-histamine with a similar structure to the anti-allergy drug disodium chromoglycate. Quercetin has the most anti-viral activity of all the flavonoids[145,250]. Onions stimulate the flow of bile, help to reduce cholesterol and may help treat insulin resistance by reducing blood sugar.
Parsley leaf	One oaf the few good sources of the trace element vanadium, which has similar anti-diabetic properties to chromium. Like celery, parsley is rich in coumarin, which helps eliminate fluid retention and so can reduce the pain of inflammation.
Pumpkin seeds	Rich in zinc and essential polyunsaturated oils, pumpkin seeds are a good aid to the treatment of enlarged prostate.
Radishes	Radishes help treat the symptoms of the common cold, and also stimulate bile flow. Contain the sulphur compound raphanin, which regulates thyroxine production by the thyroid gland. Contributes to the treatment of both hypo- and hyperthyroidism.
Seaweed	E.g. nori, wakame, hijiki, arame. Rich in iodine, needed to maintain normal levels of female hormones and thyroid hormones.
Soya foods	Help to balance oestrogen[80]. Anti prostate cancer[227]. Reduce cholesterol[284].
Tomatoes	Rich in lycopene, which helps prevent breast and prostate cancer[79].
Turmeric	Contains powerful antioxidant curcumin. Anti-arthritis[68], reduces liver inflammation, assists liver drainage and repair. Boosts glutathione[213]. May help in treatment of cancer by inhibiting blood supply to tumours[214].

Once upon a time we had to take it on trust that eating good foods like these could actually help our health. Naturopathy books used obscure old-fashioned terms such as "blood cleansing and purifying", "blood building" and "strengthening the body". Now research has shown us that all these properties really do exist. The difference is that now we understand the workings of the body, and can use more scientific language. For instance we now know that the "blood building" properties of beetroot refer to its rich iron content. We know that the "detoxifying" effects of broccoli and cabbage refer to their indoles, which assist the liver's cells to do their job. We know that the "blood cleansing" effects of celery refer to its coumarin content, which helps "strengthen" the blood capillaries (make them less permeable) so that they can drain excess fluid and impurities out of the tissue spaces between the cells. "Improved oxygenation" means better transport of oxygen to cells by stimulating the blood flow, using cayenne pepper for example.

In fact, the more we know about the human body, the better we can understand the medicinal value of food.

Appendix II: The Vitamins and Minerals

Name	Key Words	Good Sources	Therapeutic Uses (according to research)
Vitamin A (Retinol)	Eyesight, growth, immune system, mucous membranes, normal development of tissues, protein synthesis	Butter, cheese, fish liver oils, liver, margarine. Beta carotene in green and yellow vegetables can be converted to vitamin A in the body.	Helps acne, psoriasis, gastric ulcers. Helps prevent the common cold. Reduces complications from measles. Improves eyesight.
Vitamin B$_1$ (Thiamine)	Conversion of carbohydrate to energy. Energy production. Brain, heart, muscle and nerve function. Release of acetylcholine from nerve cells. Inhibits oxidation of dopamine.	Beans, brown rice, lentils, pork, whole grains	Has been used as a painkiller for headaches and joint pain. Helps improve nerve function in epilepsy. Helps trigeminal neuralgia. Helps optic neuritis. Reduces nerve damage in diabetics.
Vitamin B$_2$ (Riboflavin)	Growth. Metabolism of fats, protein and carbohydrate. Activates vitamin B$_6$. Conversion of carbohydrate to energy and tryptophan to vitamin B$_3$.	Dairy products, eggs, liver, meat, soya flour, whole grains	May help acne rosacea, carpal tunnel syndrome, cataracts, mitochondria, some types of anaemia.
Vitamin B$_3$ (Niacin)	Conversion of carbohydrate to energy. DNA synthesis. Health of skin, nerves, brain and digestive system. Synthesis of fatty acids and steroids.	Beef liver, chicken, meat, nuts, peanuts, salmon and other oily fish, sunflower seeds, whole grains	May act as a mild anti-histamine. May help relieve tinnitis, reduce cholesterol, reduce insulin requirements in some diabetics, reduce period (menstrual) pains, reduce schizophrenia (in megadoses), wheezing in asthmatics.
Vitamin B$_5$ (Pantothenic acid)	Conversion of carbohydrate to energy. Growth and development. Health of nervous system. Production of anti-stress bormones.	Eggs, liver, meat, nuts, whole grains, yeast	May alleviate allergic reactions and help stress, rheumatoid arthritis, anaemia.
Vitamin B$_6$ (Pyridoxine)	Metabolism of protein, carbohydrate, fat, calcium, magnesium, selenium, homocysteine, histamine, energy. Blood and haemoglobin formation. Conversion of glycogen to glucose, and tryptophan to	Avocado pears, bananas, fish, meat, nuts, seeds, whole grains	May help childhood autism, asthma, carpal tunnel syndrome, morning sickness of pregnancy, Parkinson's disease, premenstrual acne, premenstrual syndrome, insulin resistance, fluid retention, Tourette syndrome, anaemia (including sickle .

	Function	Sources	Benefits
	vitamin B$_3$ or serotonin. Selenium transportation. Synthesis of prostaglandins from essential fatty acids. Zinc absorption		cell anaemia). May reduce sensitivity to monosodium glutamate
Vitamin B$_{12}$ (Cobalamin)	Detoxification of cyanide (found in tobacco smoke and in some foods). DNA synthesis. Growth and development. Healthy nerve cells.	Cheese, eggs, fish, liver, meat, yoghurt. Found only in animal foods, although some vegan products are fortified with extra B$_{12}$ by the manufacturers.	May help chronic pain, fatigue, mental confusion, multiple sclerosis, numbness of the extremities, some cases of mental illness, some cases of tinnitus.
Biotin	Metabolism of carbohydrate, protein, fat, energy. Formation of prostaglandins from essential fatty acids and glucose from amino acids, lactate and glycerol. Growth. Health of skin, hair, nerves, sweat glands, sex glands, bone marrow.	Widely distributed in meats, dairy produce and whole grains. Liver and egg yolk are particularly rich sources. Egg white inhibits absorption of biotin.	May help some cases of hair loss and scalp disease seborrhoeic dermatitis and other skin complaints, diabetic nerve damage. May reduce blood sugar in sume diabetics.
Folic acid (Folate)	Blood formation. Protein, RNA and DNA, glycine and methionine synthesis.	Leafy green vegetables, especially raw spinach. Liver, freshly squeezed orange juice, soya flour, whole grains, yeast extract.	Prevents spina bifida in the unborn. Treats anaemia if folic acid is deficient. Reduces homocysteine. May help reverse precancerous conditions of the cervix, depression and schizophrenia.
Vitamin C (Ascorbate)	Aids absorption of iron from vegetables. Antioxidant. Collagen formation. Immune system. Tyrosine and stress hormone production. Wound healing.	Broccoli, brussels sprouts, cabbage, fresh fruit (especially citrus), sweet (bell) peppers, kiwi fruit, raw leafy vegetables, tomatoes	Anti-histamine effect. Can control and cure the common cold. May help cancer and idiopathic thrombocytopenic purpura (blood disease), asthma, blood sugar control in diabetics, manic depression (bipolar disorder), Parkinson's disease (with vitamin E), wound healing, clearance of toxic chemicals. Enhances number, size and motility of white blood cells. Inhibits adrenochrome formation in schizophrenia. Lowers blood cholesterol. Protects eye lens against oxidative damage. Reverses pre-cancerous conditions.
Vitamin D (Calciferol)	Absorption of magnesium, iron, calcium, zinc and other minerals. Bone health, calcium and kidney metabolism, cell differentiation (anti-cancer action).	Butter, cod liver oil, halibut liver oil, herrings, kippers, mackerel, salmon, sardines, tuna	Can clear psoriasis when applied to the skin in the D$_3$ form. Improves osteoporosis, calcium absorption in the elderly. Inhibits the growth of some tumours. Reverses some cases of hearing loss. Together with calcium, can help treat migraine.

Vitamin E (Tocopherol)	Antioxidant, especially combating peroxidation of unsaturated fats in cell membranes. Development and maintenance of nerve and muscle function. Fertility, immunity, prostaglandin control, red cell membrane stability, reduces oxygen needs of muscles, spares vitamin A.	Almonds, butter, leafy green vegetables, oats, peanuts, soya oil, sunflower oil and seeds, wheatgerm and wheatgerm oil, whole grains	Can help Parkinson's disease, epilepsy, muscular dystrophy (with selenium), macular degeneration, osteoarthritis, neuropathy, premenstrual syndrome, cystic breast disease, hearing loss (with vitamin A), hepatitis, precancerous breast conditions, menopausal symptoms, systemic lupus erythematosus, sickle cell anaemia, complications of diabetes (and enhances insulin action). Reduces liver damage from carbon tetrachloride, pain from shingles and other chronic pain. Reduces scars when applied to skin, harmful effects of inhaling ozone, nitrogen oxide, and other constituents of smog or cigarette smoke. Enhances immune system. Increases HDL ("good") cholesterol. Inhibits platelet adhesiveness (blood "stickiness"). Halves risk of heart attack in those with heart disease. Heals sunburn when applied to the skin. Helps reduce side effects of anti-schizophrenic drugs. Prevents cataracts.
Vitamin K (phylloquinone or menaquinone)	Production of four proteins involved in blood clotting. Bone calcification and mineralization.	Alfalfa, broccoli, brussels sprouts, cabbage, leafy green vegetables, cauliflower, green tea, liver, meats, soybean, rapeseed and olive oils, tomatoes, whole grains	Can accelerate healing of bone fractures, increase bone formation in post-menopausal osteoporotic woman, reduce calcium losses in urine.
Calcium	Acetylcholine synthesis, action of many hormones, activation of saliva and many enzymes, blood clotting, blood pressure regulation, conversion of glycogen to glucose, muscle contractions, nerve impulses, structure of cells, bones and teeth, vitamin B12 absorption	Broccoli, cheese (especially hard cheeses) canned fish (if bones are consumed), cow's milk, leafy green vegetables, nuts, pulses, root vegetables, yoghurt, sunflower and sesame seeds	Can help muscle cramps, oestoporosis, high blood pressure, allergic symptoms, period (menstrual) pains, premenstrual emotional symptoms and fluid retention, migraine and hearing loss (with vitamin D), clearance of lead, mercury, aluminium and cadmium.
Chromium	Promotes good blood sugar balance and enhances the effectiveness of insulin	Liver, mushrooms, whole grains, yeast	Can increase the density of insulin receptors (thus aiding the function of insulin). Helps reduce high blood cholesterol, hypoglycaemia, hyperinsulinaemia, especially when given with magnesium.

	Functions	Sources	Benefits
Copper	Assists iron absorption and transport. Maintenance of connective tissues, blood vessels and myelin sheath around nerve fibres. Cholesterol regulation. Production of energy, haemoglobinadrenal hormones, pigments in skin and hair, ceruloplasmin and detoxifying enzymes SOD and cytochrome oxidase. Histamine inactivation.	Avocado pears, liver, molasses, nuts, olives, pulses, shellfish, whole grains	Helps anaemia, rheumatism, rheumatoid arthritis.
Iodine	Thyroid hormone production. Iodine is also actively concentrated from the blood by the stomach mucosa, salivary glands, choroid plexus of the brain and the lactating mammary glands, suggesting further functions as yet unknown.	Dairy products, fish and seafood, pineapple, raisins, seaweed (e.g. kelp). Very large amounts of iodine are found in the artificial food additive erythrosine (E127), used as a red colouring for cocktail and glace cherries. A high consumption of these foods is not advised if they contain this additive.	Can treat goitre. Can improve fibrocystic breast disease (certain specific forms of iodine only).
Iron	Needed for cell proliferation, function of white blood cells, liver cytochrome detoxification enzymes, oxygen supply to cells, energy production in cells, catalase enzyme which combats generation of free radicals by peroxides. Component of many enzymes.	Black sausage, cocoa powder and dark chocolate, liver, molasses, parsley, pulses, red meat, shellfish, some types of cheap wine, some green vegetables	Can improve detoxification ability in some individuals, and some forms of hearing loss. Can help period (menstrual) pains in some women, anaemia, restless leg syndrome.
Magnesium	Anti-diabetic. Balance and control of calcium, potassium and sodium ions, vitamins B_1, B_6 and methionine. Bone development. Energy production. Helps bind calcium to tooth enamel. Nerve transmission, muscle contraction and relaxation, protein synthesis, growth and repair. Removal of excess ammonia and acid from body.	Bitter chocolate, leafy green vegetables, nuts, sunflower and sesame seeds, soya beans, whole grains (particularly oats)	Can enhance strength gains during athletic training. Can help chronic fatigue, circulation, fibromyalgia, glaucoma, insulin resistance, mood, anxiety, stress-related symptoms, osteoporosis, asthma, insomnia, migraine, gum disease. Can prevent asthma attacks, kidney stones, eclampsia of pregnancy. Can reduce noise-induced hearing loss, high blood pressure, premenstrual symptoms and period (menstrual) pains, hypoglycaemia, hyperinsulinaemia, cholesterol.

Manganese	Needed for the antioxidant enzyme SOD, calcium metabolism, building and breaking down of proteins and nucleic acids, urea production, connective tissue and bone, dopamine production, fatty acid synthesis, melanin production. Involved in many enzymes in energy metabolism.	Leafy vegetables, nuts (especially pecans), pulses, tea, whole grains	May reduce epileptic seizures. May enhance action of white blood cells known as natural killer cells and macrophages.
Molybdenum	Detoxification of aldehydes. Haemoglobin, sulphate, taurine and uric acid production. DNA, iron, methionine and cysteine metabolism. Sulphite inactivation.	Beans (especially butterbeans). Buckwheat, lentils, liver and other organ meats, split peas, whole grains.	Very little research appears to have been carried out. Has mostly been used to treat Wilson's disease—a copper overload condition.
Selenium	Anti-cancer action. DNA repair. Needed for production of antioxidant enzyme glutathione peroxidase and prostaglandins, immune system, activation of thyroid hormone. Spares vitamin E.	Brazil nuts, fish and shellfish, meat, offal, whole grains	May bring clinical improvement in AIDS, enhance immune function, help asthma, pancreatitis, acne, muscular dystrophy (with vitamin E), rheumatoid– and osteoarthritis, prevent liver cancer, improve sperm motility, improve function of thyroid and kidneys, reduce risk of contracting viral hepatitis.
Zinc	Acid/alkaline balance, alcohol detoxification, carbon dioxide transport, collagen synthesis, energy metabolism, growth, haemoglobin, hormones, immunity, insulin storage, male fertility, nucleic acid synthesis, numerous enzymes, prostaglandin function, protein digesting enzymes, protein synthesis, SOD (antioxidant enzyme), vitamin A metabolism and distribution.	Eggs, leafy green vegetables, meat, nuts, seafood, seeds, whole grains	May improve abnormally low testosterone in men, sperm count and motility. May help acne, anorexia, birthweight and growth in at-risk babies, healing rate of gastric ulcers, mouth ulcers, management of sickle cell anaemia, thyroid function, tinnitus, white blood cell function, wound healing, enlarged prostate, common cold. May inhibit herpes virus, histamine release, disease activity in rheumatoid arthritis, visual loss in macular degeneration.

Scientific References

The scientific references for the information in this table have been omitted because they are too numerous for a book of this type. They are not difficult to find, and many specialist compilations or databases can supply them. Good sources are (1) *Nutritional Influences on Illness* by Melvyn Werbach MD, Third Line Press, Tarzana, USA 1993, ISBN 0961855037. (2) *Clinical Pearls* products from ITServices, Sacramento, USA, ISSN 1058-4595 www.prescription2000. com. (3) *Nutritional Health Bible* by Linda Lazarides, Thorsons, London, 1997 ISBN 0722534248. (4) PUBMED http://www.ncbi.nlm.nih.gov/entrez/query.fcgi

Appendix III: Protein and the Amino Acids

Protein in your food is broken down by your digestive juices into peptides and then into individual amino acids. Amino acids are able to cross through the walls of your intestines into your bloodstream. From here they are picked up and "knitted" into different types of protein: hormones, enzymes, bone or muscle tissue and so on. After eating a meal high in protein, your body works overtime to manufacture proteins, especially those for the liver and muscles, and serum albumin, a type of blood protein.

Any excess amino acids which cannot be used to make protein are broken down ready to be converted to glucose or to acetyl-CoA for making energy. They can also be stored as glycogen (stored carbohydrate) and triglyceride (stored fat).

If your glycogen stores are used up before you eat again, your muscles begin to release amino acids as fuel for energy production. This is why when you go on a low-calorie diet you lose lean tissue at the same time as body fat. But if you stay on a low-calorie diet for a long time, your metabolism will eventually slow down in order to reduce muscle loss.

As amino acids are broken down, ammonia is formed. This is a toxin and must be converted by your liver to urea which can be excreted in your urine. Your liver needs magnesium and several other nutrients to do this. If there is a shortage of these nutrients ammonia builds up and interferes with your glucose metabolism, causing fatigue and weakness. Excess ammonia also causes headaches, lethargy, irritability, and allergy-like reactions when you eat foods high in protein.

Therapeutic uses

The most outstanding uses for the amino acids are in

- Detoxification
- Mental health
- Athletics and body building
- Energy and chronic fatigue
- The heart and circulation

It is not always necessary to take supplements—some amino acids are found in large amounts in food. For example eating 100 grams of Brazil nuts will yield 1,000 mg of methionine, which aids the detoxification of excess oestrogen. This is double the amount of methionine you can get from meat, eggs and fish. Many people fail to get enough of certain amino acids because of faulty digestion. This can be helped by taking a digestive enzyme supplement such as bromelain.

The Amino Acids

Name	Key Words	Good Sources	Therapeutic Uses (according to research)
Alanine	Preventing ketosis. Can be converted to glucose. Can trigger glucagon release. Inhibitory neurotransmitter. Production of white blood cells.	Gelatine, meat, fish, sunflower seeds, almonds, peanuts, oats	Ketosis is an acidic condition caused by low-calorie diets. Eating these foods when dieting may help your body to cope better.
Arginine	Making tissues, hormones, sperm. Wound healing. Stimulating insulin release. Ammonia removal. Thymus stimulation. Making nitric oxide. Neutralizing superoxide free radical.	Gelatine, peanuts, almonds, sunflower seeds, Brazil nuts, meat, fish, oats and other grains	Artery occlusion problems such as angina, intermittent claudication and male impotence. High blood pressure. Glaucoma. Kidney disease. Alzheimer's and senility. Body-building.
Aspartates	Removing excess ammonia and converting to urea. DNA metabolism. Energy production. Excitatory neurotransmitter. Stimulates thymus gland, bone marrow, spleen. Helps stimulate glucagon secretion.	Gelatine, peanuts, almonds, sunflower seeds, meat fish, walnuts	Helping red blood cell-producing organs to regenerate after radiation.
BCAAs: Isoleucine Leucine, valine	Major components of collagen. Stimulating synthesis of muscle and other protein. Wound healing. Leucine can be used directly as an energy source instead of glucose.	Cheese, gelatine, sunflower seeds, peanuts, almonds, meat, fish, oats	Intensive physical stress. Preventing breakdown of body tissues after severe injuries or surgery. May benefit chronic fatigue syndrome.
Carnitine	Releasing energy from fat. Production of body heat. Turning amino acids into fuel for energy. Controlling ketone levels. Elimination of xenobiotics.	Red meat and liver, dairy products, yeast	Angina, intermittent claudication, congestive heart failure, Alzheimer's and senility, weight loss.
Cysteine	Making taurine and glutathione. Protein linkage. Can be converted to glucose. Fatty acid synthesis. Helps make lipoic acid. Helps make fingernails, hair, outer skin layer. Antioxidant. Detoxifies heavy metals.	Sunflower seeds, oats, Brazil nuts, wheat flour, peanuts, eggs	As NAC supplements, can treat paracetamol overdose, heavy metal poisoning, residues of drugs after cancer chemotherapy. May help in diabetes, otitis media and prevent damage to kidney function. Dissolves thick mucus.
Glutamic acid	Excitatory neurotransmitter. Removal of excess ammonia. Making other amino acids. Making folate.	Gelatine, cheese, sunflower seeds, almonds, peanuts, wheat flour	No therapeutic uses. Large amounts are found in food.

Glutamine	Can be turned into glucose. Source of energy for the brain and for cells lining intestines. Making GABA, glutamate and glutathione. Making vitamin B$_3$. DNA synthesis. Breaking down uric acid. Ammonia transport.	Mainly made in the body, but possibly found in potatoes and cabbage. Also found in germinated barley foodstuff.	Body-building. Critical illness. Intestinal healing. May help make tumours more sensitive to the cancer drug methotrexate while protecting normal cells. May help improve brain alertness. May help combat alcoholism.
Glutathione	Detoxification. Making glutathione peroxidase. Breaks down excessive insulin. Amino acid transport. Helps chronic inflammation. Control of hormones and prostaglandins. Vitamin C recycling.	Found in many foods, but broken down by our digestive system. Boost levels with cysteine-rich diet plus lipoic acid and silymarin.	Combating viruses. Treating chemical sensitivity. Detoxification. Preventing degenerative diseases. Extending natural life span.
Glycine	Inhibitory neurotransmitter. Growth and DNA metabolism. Forming collagen and phospholipids. Wound healing. Blood sugar control. Energy production. Making glutathione. Making bile salts. Building up glycogen. Detoxification.	Gelatine, almonds, sunflower seeds, peanuts, meat, fish, buckwheat flour, walnuts	May help gout. May help schizophrenia, manic depression and epilepsy. Gelatine may help osteoarthritis.
Histidine	Making histamine. Tissue maintenance and growth. Copper transport. Antioxidant.	Fish, meat, dairy products, gelatine, peanuts, sunflower seeds	May help rheumatoid arthritis. May protect against gastric inflammation when taking NSAIDS (aspirin-like drugs)
Lysine	Constituent of hormones and structural tissues. Regulation of calcium absorption. Collagen production. Carnitine production.	Dairy products, meat, fish, tofu, beans and lentils, broccoli, potatoes	Herpes infections, chronic fatigue syndrome, heart disease, high cholesterol
Methionine	Making cysteine and taurine. Making encephalins and endorphins. Metabolizing homocysteine. Detoxification.	Brazil nuts, meat, fish, sunflower and sesame seeds, dairy products, oats	Antihistamine. May help produce adrenal hormones. May help clinical depression, parkinsonism, schizophrenia. As SAM may help osteoarthritis, fibromyalgia, Alzheimer's.
Ornithine	Mostly the same as arginine.	See arginine	
Phenylalanine	Making tyrosine, cholecystokinin, phenylethylamine	Gelatine, cheese, peanuts, sunflower seeds, almonds, oats	Appetite control. Clinical depression. As DLPA may help chronic pain
Proline	Major constituent of collagen. Wound healing	Gelatine, cheese, wheat	May help gyrate atrophy of the eyes

	Functions	Food sources	Uses
Serine	Neurotransmitter, protein synthesis, methionine metabolism, glycoproteins, energy production, DNA	Gelatine, cheese, peanuts, sunflower seeds, almonds, eggs	As phosphatidylserine, may help age-related memory loss and health of nerve cell membranes
Taurine	Inhibitory neurotransmitter, stabilizing calcium, eye health, detoxification, antioxidant, stabilizing cell membranes, forming bile salts, controlling renin, promoting lactation, enhancing insulin action	Meat and organ meats, fish, milk (including human breast milk)	Congestive heart failure, abnormal heart rhythms, epilepsy, dementia, gall-stones, detoxification, cystic fibrosis
Threonine	Making serine and glycine. Can be converted to glucose. Copper transport. Making glycoproteins	Gelatine, meat, fish, cheese, sunflower seeds, peanuts, almonds	May help clinical depression. May help spasticity.
Tryptophan	Making serotonin, melatonin, vitamin B$_3$. Zinc absorption	Sunflower seeds, cheese, meat, fish, oats, Brazil nuts, peanuts	Clinical depression. May help schizophrenia, mania, aggression, Parkinson's disease, pain, appetite control
Tyrosine	Making thyroid and adrenal hormones, encephalins and amino sugars	Cheese, peanuts, fish, meat, sunflower seeds, almonds, oats, eggs	Adrenal insufficiency, hypothyroidism, chronic fatigue, parkinsonism, depression, brain function

Scientific References

The scientific references for the information in this table have been omitted because they are too numerous for a book of this type. They can be found by searching in medical and nutritional databases, or obtained from the *Amino Acid Report* by Linda Lazarides, published in 2002 by Waterfall 2000, ISBN 0953804623.

Appendix IV

Supernutrient supplements and their uses

Algae	Simple plants which grow in water. Rich in chlorophyll, DHA, GLA. Can contain up to 8% beta-carotene. Good source of protein if consumed in large amounts.
Blue-green algae (scientific name is cyanobacteria)	Contains pigment C-phycocyanin which can neutralize the hydroxyl (OH) free radical. Can produce health-damaging cyanobacterial toxins. Spirulina is a type of blue-green alga low in toxins. May help suppress appetite if consumed in large amounts.
Chlorella	Popular in Japan as a detoxification aid. Grown in man-made freshwater ponds. Richer in chlorophyll than blue-green algae.
CAROTENOIDS	Yellow, orange and red plant pigments. They have various antioxidant properties.
Beta-carotene	Found in carrots and leafy greens. Good quencher of singlet oxygen, which is similar to a free radical.
Lycopene	Found in tomatoes. Now thought to be a better quencher of singlet oxygen than beta-carotene.
FATTY ACIDS	
CLA	Conjugated linoleic acid. Anti-catabolic, anti bodyfat gain. Breast cancer prevention. Helps remove cholesterol deposits from artery walls.[124,125,254-256]
EPA	Omega 3 fatty acid. Found in the flesh of "oily" fish: salmon, herrings etc. Anti-inflammatory and anti-clotting effects[182]. May help schizophrenia[238].
Flax seed oil	Good source of omega 3 fatty acids. Found in linseeds (flax seeds).
GLA	Gamma linolenic acid. Found in seeds of evening primrose, blackcurrant and borage. Used against chronic fatigue syndrome, PMS, MS, eczema, osteoarthritis, hyperactivity[29].
Lauric acid	Found in coconut fat. Anti-viral, anti-bacterial, especially "stealth" bacteria and lipid-coated bacteria such as Epstein-Barr and other herpesviruses[92].
FLAVONOIDS	Often colourful, a family of antioxidants found in plants. Anti-inflammatory. Prevent excess leakiness of blood vessels. Used against varicose veins, fluid retention, circulation problems, heavy periods. Anti-bruising.
Bilberry extract	Good for gut infections. Many eye benefits. Improves flexibility of red cell membranes, thus helping the microcirculation to brain, eyes, ears, gums etc.
Ginkgo biloba	Contains quercetin and other flavonoids. Good for circulation generally: Raynaud's, tinnitus, eye diseases. Medical studies show great improvement in microcirculation of the brain[46].
Quercetin	Found in onions, apple peel, tea, red wine. Anti-allergy, anti-viral[145,250]. Stabilizes mast cell membranes, inhibits histamine release[146,147].

FOOD EXTRACTS	
Bromelain	An extract from pineapple stems, used as an aid to protein digestion. Has been successfully used after pancreatectomy. Acid-resistant so can begin working in the stomach. Anti blood-clotting, anti-inflammatory, anti-tumour. Breaks down fibrinous plaques in arteries. Rapidly clears bruising, pain and swelling after injury. Increases the permeability of organs and tissues to drugs such as chemotherapy and antibiotics, producing greater response. Reduces mucus viscosity.[10]
Green-lipped mussel extract	Anti-arthritic. May help rehydrate shortened tendons.
Lecithin (phosphatidyl-choline)	Type of phospholipid synthesized by the liver. Both water– and fat-soluble so aids entry and exit of many substances through cell membranes. Increases solubility of bile and dissolves gall-stones[219]. Best choline and inositol supplement. Helps liver cell membranes to excrete toxins which could damage them. Boosts carnitine by reducing carnitine excretion in urine.
Octacosanol	May help nerve repair and myelin regeneration. May help combat MS and parkinsonism, cerebral palsy, brain damage. May improve oxygen utilization. May be beneficial in endurance sports.
Shark cartilage and bovine tracheal cartilage	May benefit arthritis due to glucosamine content, but glucosamine is better absorbed[64]. Inhibits blood supply to tumours. Studies show taken orally bovine tracheal cartilage is far more anti-tumour than shark cartilage.
Shark liver oil	Contains alkylglycerols—oil-based chelating agents found in human bone marrow and breast milk. Can help detoxify heavy metals. May protect white blood cells from radiation.
Soy isoflavones	Also known as "phyto-oestrogens". Include genistein and daidzein. Highly concentrated so may promote hypothyroidism and raise oestrogen levels in children. Safety of high soya concentrate intake not proven.
Tocotrienols	Found in association with vitamin E in palm oil and barley oil. Similar to vitamin E. Cholesterol-lowering properties.[257]
Whey protein concentrate	Rich in cysteine. Used to raise glutathione levels.
NUTRITIONAL HERBS	Plant foods and concentrates used for their contribution to nutritional therapy
Broccoli extract	Contains antioxidant indoles which help liver enzymes to detoxify oestrogen[40]. Good for fibroids, breast and ovarian cysts, preventing breast cancer. Also contains anti-carcinogenic agent sulphoraphane which stimulates production of liver detox enzymes.
Cabbage	Juice and extract have powerful gut-healing and anti-ulcer action[258]
Carrot	Raw grated carrot helps prevent roundworm infestations.
Celery seed extract	Helps alkalinize the body and combats fluid retention. Very good for inflammation and arthritis.
Comfrey	Gut healer, wound healer, bone mender. Anti-arthritis. Anti-pain.

Garcinia cambogia	Tamarind extract. Contains hydroxycitrate, which partially inhibits an enzyme required for conversion of blood sugar to fat. Results in higher glycogen levels instead, which results in early satiety when sugar is consumed. Used as a weight loss aid.
Garlic	Anti-bacterial, anti-parasitic (when raw). Anti-blood-clotting, cholesterol-lowering, triglyceride-lowering, blood-pressure-lowering. If the smell is reduced, so is the medicinal action. Can help treat bronchial infections, dysentery, typhoid, cholera, bacterial food poisoning, worm infestations, candidiasis, AIDS-related diarrhoea[212].
Ginger	Warm circulatory stimulant. Promotes gastric acidity, aids digestion. May ease nausea[259] and travel sickness, treat catarrh, bronchitic conditions and prevent period pains. May help rheumatoid arthritis[260].
Grapefruit (citrus) seed extract	Has broad spectrum anti-bacterial and anti-parasitic properties[262]. Used to treat dysbiosis.
Kelp	Dried seaweed used as an iodine supplement.
Oregano oil	Anti-bacterial, anti-fungal. Used as a systemic treatment for candidiasis.
Pumpkin seeds	Important remedy to treat tapeworm and enlarged prostate. Rich in zinc, protein and essential fatty acids.
Slippery elm	The bark of Ulmus fulva. Rich in mucilage and tannin. Soothes digestive system and reduces irritation. Promotes gut healing.
Turmeric	Contains powerful antioxidant curcumin. Anti-arthritis[68], reduces liver inflammation, assists liver drainage and repair. Boosts glutathione[213]. Used as part of cancer therapy may inhibit blood supply to tumours[214].
MEDICINAL HERBS	Herbs used in nutritional therapy to enhance digestive, liver and gall-bladder function and for gut ecology
Artemisia annua (sweet wormwood)	A traditional Chinese herb used against malaria[261]. Has powerful anti-parasitic properties[262].
Gentian	Stimulates stomach acid production.
Golden seal	Very versatile. Contains berberine. Anti-bacterial, anti-parasitic, anti-fungal, anti-fever, anti-tumour. Drying, anti-catarrhal, gentle laxative and astringent, good for intestinal conditions involving excess mucus and inflammation. Used to treat mucus colitis, dysbiosis, gut inflammation, leaky gut syndrome, diarrhoea, poor appetite. (Berberine is as effective against food poisoning bacteria as conventional antibiotics.) Stimulates bile secretion and eases gallbladder congestion. Increases blood supply to the spleen. Activates macrophages.
Milk thistle (silymarin)	Contains powerful antioxidants. Prevents liver damage from carbon tetrachloride, paracetamol, death cap mushroom etc. Used to treat chronic hepatitis, cirrhosis. Stabilizes membranes of liver cells, preventing entry of toxic compounds. Inhibits iron-induced liver toxicity. Stimulates bile flow. Stimulates growth of new liver cells to repair liver. Stimulates milk flow in nursing mothers.
Uva ursi (bearberry)	Antiseptic effect on the urinary tract (urine must be alkaline—avoid consuming acidic foods). Used to combat cystitis, urinary infections, prostatitis. Effective against Klebsiella, Enterobacter and Streptococcus.

MISCELLANEOUS NUTRICEUTICALS	Substances synthesized in the body, which can be supplemented to enhance specific metabolic functions
Butyric acid	Formed by colonic fermentation of dietary fibre. Most important energy source for growth and repair of colonic mucosa.
Chondroitin sulphate	A mucopolysaccharide similar to those found in shark cartilage and green-lipped mussel. May help arthritis, but glucosamine sulphate is now thought more effective.
Coenzyme Q10	Made during the body's energy-production processes. Vital for oxygen and energy transfer between cell components and between blood and tissues. Important antioxidant. Used to treat chronic fatigue, congestive heart disease, gum disease, breast cancer. Production in body is dependent on adequate vitamin E.
Glucosamine sulphate	Good osteoarthritis treatment. Taken up by joint tissue, it stimulates the production of glycoaminoglycans (building blocks of cartilage) and reduces joint pain, tenderness and swelling.[63]
Lipoic acid	A sulphur-containing fatty acid involved in the chemistry of energy production. Important antioxidant. Neutralizes superoxide, hydroxyl and peroxyl free radicals, hypochlorous acid and singlet oxygen. Protects cell membranes. Anti-diabetic[263]. Supplementation increases glutathione levels.
N-acetyl glucosamine (NAG)	Amino sugar. Helps repair superficial layers of gut mucosa. Important in the renewal of all structures which depend on collagen.
"POWER" MUSHROOMS	Standardized extracts are better than whole mushrooms as lignin is hard to break down
Coriolus versicolor	Stimulates immune system. Boosts natural killer (NK) cells. Enhances T-cell reproduction. Helps clear dampness and phlegm found in post-viral fatigue. Anti-herpes, anti hepatitis-C.[264]
Cordyceps	Enhances sports performance[267].
Maitake	Helps blood sugar regulation, pre-diabetic states, hypoglycaemia, hepatitis.[285]
Reishi	Contains lentinan. Calms the spirit. Good for anxiety. Anti-allergy, anti-cancer, anti-bronchitis.[267]
Shiitake	Contains lentinan. Significant anti-viral effect. Anti hepatitis C. Anti-cancer. Source of vitamin D.[264]
PRO– AND PRE-BIOTICS	
Lactobacilli and Bifidobacteria	Help to prevent dysbiosis. Cholesterol– and/or triglyceride-reducing, anti breast and colon cancer, immune-stimulating (by triggering the gut-associated lymphoid tissue—GALT), increase vitamin production, improve lactose digestion. Effective treatment for infant diarrhoea. May be able to treat urinary and genital infections.[265-266,293]
Fructo-oligosaccharides	Vegetable inulin—a type of dietary fibre which stimulates the growth and reproduction of probiotics. May also have the same effect on certain undesirable bacteria such as Klebsiella.

Appendix V

Conventional nutrition versus nutritional therapy

The nutrition advice given by doctors, nurses and dieticians is usually nothing like the advice you have found in this book. If you have received conflicting advice, or if you have been told that you do not need food supplements, then you may find this section helpful.

Nutrition as currently taught at most universities is the study of fats, protein, carbohydrates and other components of food, as well as food production methods. It also covers the nutritional needs of animals and humans in general.

Diets designed by dieticians meet the Dietary Reference Values for vitamins and minerals set by the Government. Dieticians also plan diets for hospital patients or other people in residential settings. They give advice to people whose doctor wants them to follow a special low-sugar diet for diabetes or perhaps an iron-rich diet for anaemia or a calcium-rich diet for osteoporosis. Some dieticians design diets for specialist purposes such as patients undergoing kidney dialysis. Generally speaking dieticians are not trained as practitioners whose job it is to cure a health problem. In the orthodox medical setting, that is the doctor's job. But as you know by now, your doctor's knowledge may cover very little of the information in this book, because it does not form part of his or her training.

So who is trained in giving the type of health promoting advice described here? The answer is, no-one in the medical establishment, unless they decide to join the ranks of alternative medicine practitioners. This is rare, although beginning to grow in popularity.

But as you can see from the many scientific references on pages 295 to 304, the information in this book is far from "alternative". It comes from research reported in some of the most prestigious scientific journals in the world, such as the *Lancet, British Medical Journal, American Journal of Clinical Nutrition,* and *Journal of the American Medical Association.* The big problem is that this research is not being read, understood or interpreted in a way that will really help people. Mostly it is not read at all. The average GP has little knowledge of what lies between the covers of *Archives of Neurology* or the *Australian Paediatric Journal,* and assumes that any facts really worth knowing will reach him or her via the usual channels.

Generally speaking, nutritional therapy starts where conventional nutrition and dietetics leaves off, and treats a very wide range of problems with the aim of reversing them and restoring health wherever possible.

The safety of nutritional therapy

The potential dangers of taking too many vitamins seem to make good news headlines; scare stories pop up at regular intervals, usually warning us that:

- We do not need supplements; we only need a healthy diet.
- Just because something is natural doesn't mean it's safe.
- It is easy, and dangerous, to overdose on vitamins A or D.
- Vitamin C supplements can give you cancer.
- Iron supplements have poisoned children.
- High-dose vitamin B6 supplements have been banned from health food shops.
- Food supplements do not have to be safety-tested and are therefore not as safe as prescription medicines.
- The people who take food supplements are usually those who least need them.
- People may rely on self-medication with food supplements and endanger their lives by missing out on vital medical treatments.

In fact UK law allows for the instant banning of any food product that really is suspected to be unsafe. Mainly thanks to the media, we live in one of the most safety-conscious countries in the world, and the Government does not hesitate for one moment to ban any product where there is actual *evidence* of harm. On the contrary, as far as food supplements are concerned, it has not been able to come up with any evidence, despite funding a research study carried out in 1994-1996 by the Medical Toxicology Unit at Guy's and St Thomas' Hospital in London[286]. High dose vitamin B_6 supplements have *not* been banned from health food shops.

The health food industry simply does not sell supplements at the levels which have been found to cause overdosing problems in medical research studies. The researchers do not use products from the shelves of your local health food shop, they use specialist medical supplies which can be thousands of times more potent and are purely for research purposes. When I researched the shelves of my local health food shop some years ago, the strongest vitamin A or D supplement I could find was cod liver oil—something quite difficult to seriously overdose on.

Naturally you should never abuse any consumer product nor seriously disregard the directions on the label.

Prescription iron pills mistaken for sweets

On the other hand, two of the concerns listed above are valid. Very strong iron supplements are widely prescribed by doctors for anaemia, and there are cases where young children have found them and mistaken them for sweets. This can cause overdosing. Doctors used to prescribe the ferrous sulphate form of iron supplement because it was cheap. This was potentially harmful as it could corrode a child's stomach and digestive system. Any concentrated nutritional or herbal product which is not in a child-proof pack should be kept out of children's reach.

Secondly, nutritional therapy is not a substitute for necessary medical care. You should pay attention to the various warnings in this book about consulting a doctor if you have any persistent symptoms.

You can help to educate your doctor!

If you have been helped by nutritional therapy, *tell your doctor*. Time and time again people tell me that they have just thrown their doctor's prescription medicines away and used nutritional therapy instead, leaving the doctor to believe that the medicines must have solved the problem. Doctors need feedback on what works for you. If they hear good reports from several different patients on the benefits of nutritional therapy they will eventually want to use it in their practice. Give your doctor a copy of the instructions you followed to get well. Offer to give a talk to the practice staff. Write up the story of exactly what you did and tell your doctor he is welcome to send it to a medical journal. It could actually be published. The medical article referred to in this book, about a woman who purchased bromelain capsules and cured herself of ulcerative colitis, was written by her doctor, who was so astounded at her success that he wanted other doctors to know. Ulcerative colitis is considered an incurable condition, and the drugs usually prescribed to help control the symptoms cost the NHS thousands of pounds per patient per year.

You could also send your story to a newspaper. Doctors read newspapers too, and if your doctor sees several stories that people have been cured by nutritional therapy, he will want to use it in his practice.

Please fill in the questionnaire

At the back of this book you will find a feedback questionnaire which asks you about your success with nutritional therapy. It would be very helpful if you could fill this in so that the results of readers using this book can be compiled and used to assist medical research.

If you believe that, to help other people like you, the effectiveness of nutritional therapy should have more publicity, it would also be very helpful if you could give a contact phone number and tick the box giving permission for a health writer or medical journalist to contact you with a view to writing up your story.

RESOURCES

Further reading

Murray M, Pizzorno J. *Encyclopaedia of Natural Medicine*. Little Brown & Co, London, 1998.
Bartram T. *Bartram's Encyclopedia of Herbal Medicine*. Robinson Publishing Ltd, London, 1998.
Erasmus U. *Fats that Heal, Fats that Kill*. Alive Books, Burnaby, Canada, 1993.
Packer L, Colman C. *The Antioxidant Miracle*. John Wiley & Sons, New York and Chichester (UK), 1999.
Lazarides L. *The Amino Acid Report*. Waterfall 2000, London, 2002.
Gaby AR. *Preventing and Reversing Osteoporosis*. Prima Publishing, Rocklin, California, 1994.
Gerson M. *A Cancer Therapy: Results of 50 Cases*. Gerson Institute, Bonita, California, 1986.
Jochems R. *Dr Moerman's Anti-cancer Diet*. Avery Publishing, New York, 1990.

Websites

Society for the Promotion of Nutritional Therapy
www.nutrition-therapy.org
Linus Pauling Institute
http://osu.orst.edu/dept/lpi
Dr Abram Hoffer
www.islandnet.com/~hoffer/hofferhp.htm
Dr Jonathan Wright
www.tahoma-clinic.com
Medicinal mushrooms information
www.gmushrooms.com/Healthref.html
Scientific articles on the use of vitamin C megadoses
www.orthomed.com/publications1.html
New approaches to autism
http://osiris.sunderland.ac.uk/autism/durham95.html
Linda Lazarides
www.waterfall2000.com

Product suppliers (UK)

The Nutri Centre
International mail order suppliers of all available food supplements in UK
7 Park Crescent, London W1N 3HE.
For Supplement Orders & Professional Advice
Tel: 020 7436 5122
Book Orders & Library Services
Tel: 0207 323 2382
Online ordering
www.nutricentre.com

Biocare Ltd
Food supplements
Lakeside, 180 Lifford Lane, King's Norton, Birmingham B30 3NU.
Tel: +44 (0)121 433 3727
Email biocare@biocare.co.uk
www.biocare.co.uk

Lamberts Healthcare Ltd
Food supplements
1 Lamberts Rd, Tunbridge Wells, Kent TN2 3EH. Tel: 01892 554313

Clearspring Ltd
Health and macrobiotic foods, rice milk, seaweed products, agar
Unit 19A Acton Park Estate, London W3 7QE. Tel: +44 (0) 20 8746 0152
E-mail: mailorder@clearspring.co.uk
www.clearspring.co.uk

Infinity Foods Co-operative Limited
Health food wholesalers. Phone to find stockists of chestnut flour & sweet rice
67 Norway Street, Portslade, East Sussex BN41 1AE. Tel: +44 (0)1273 424060
Email: info@infinityfoods.co.uk

KTC (Edibles) Ltd
Coconut oil wholesalers
JS House, Moorcroft Drive, Wednesbury, W Midlands WS10 7DE
Tel: 0121 505 9200
www.ktc-edibles.co.uk

Magnetic Therapy Ltd
Suppliers of therapeutic magnets and books on magnet therapy
Ellesmere Centre, Walkden, Worsley, Manchester M28 3ZH. Tel: 0161 793 5110
www.magnetictherapy.co.uk

Source Foods
Suppliers of quality miso products
9 Cwm Business Centre, Marine St, Cwm, Ebbw Vale, Gwent NP3 6TB. Tel: 01495 371 698

Windmill Organics
Suppliers of chestnut flour to the UK market.
Phone to find local stockists
Tel: 0207 924 2300.

Ardovries Shearway Ltd
Suppliers of frozen blueberries to supermarkets.
Phone to find stockists.
Tel: 01622 891199.

Simply Organic
Nationwide deliveries of organic fruit & veg,
meat & fish, groceries, wine, beer and baby care.
Tel: 0845 1000 444
www.simplyorganic.net

The Fresh Food Company
Nationwide deliveries of fresh organic fruit,
salads, vegetables, herbs, breads, meat, Cornish
fish, wine and beer etc.
www.freshfood.co.uk

Burns Pet Nutrition
Health foods for cats and dogs
4 Avalon Court, Kidwelly, SA17 5EJ
Tel: 08000 18 18 90
www.burns-pet-nutrition.co.uk

The Healthy House
Paints etc. for people with allergic illness and
chemical sensitivities
Cold Harbour, Ruscombe, Stroud Glos GL6 6DA
Tel: +44 (0)1453 752216
Email: info@healthy-house.co.uk
www.healthy-house.co.uk

(International)

Life Extension Foundation
International internet suppliers of books and
supplements
www.lef.org

Practitioners (UK)

British Association of Nutritional Therapists
27 Old Gloucester St, London WC1N 3XX.
Tel: 08706 061284
Email: theadministrator@bant.org.uk
www.bant.org.uk
Send large sae and £2 for a list of practitioners.

British Society for Allergy, Environmental and Nutritional Medicine
Doctors specializing in nutritional medicine

PO Box 7, Knighton, Powys LD7 1WT.
Information line: 0906 3020 010
www.bsaenm.org.

Breakspear Hospital for Allergy and Environmental Medicine
Hertfordshire House, Wood Lane, Hemel
Hempstead, Herts HP2 4FD, UK.
Tel: 01442 261333
Email: info@breakspearmedical.com
www.breakspearmedical.com/
breakspear_hospital.htm

(Overseas)

American Academy of Environmental Medicine
7701 East Kellogg, Suite 625, Wichita, KS
67207, USA. Tel: (316) 684 5500

Australasian College of Nutritional and Environmental Medicine
13 Hilton St, Beaumaris, Vic 3193, Australia.
Tel: +61 3 9589 6088. www.acnem.org
Email mail@acnem.org

International Society for Orthomolecular Medicine
www.orthomed.org

Training (UK)

University of Westminster
BSc Degree in Nutritional Therapy
School of Integrated Health
Admissions Office
115 New Cavendish Street
London W1W 6UW, UK
Tel: +44 (0)20 7911 5883
Email cav-admissions@wmin.ac.uk
www.wmin.ac.uk/

University of Surrey
Postgraduate training in Nutritional Medicine
School of Biomedical and Life Sciences
Guildford, Surrey, GU2 7XH, UK
Tel: 01483 259730
Email m.rayman@surrey.ac.uk

(USA)

Bastyr University
Centre for the training of naturopathic physicians
14500 Juanita Drive Northeast, Bothell,
Washington 98011, USA.
Tel: +1 (425) 823 1300
www.bastyr.edu

Resources for practitioners

Books

Werbach MR. *Nutritional Influences on Illness.*
Third Line Press, Tarzana, California, 1993.
www.healthy.net/thirdline/
Anthony H, Birtwistle S, Eaton K, Maberly J.
Environmental Medicine in Clinical Practice.
BSAENM Publications 1997.

Periodicals

Clinical Pearls News
I.T.Services, 3301 Alta Arden #2, Sacramento,
CA 95825, USA.
Email office@clinicalpearls.com.
www.clinicalpearls.com.
Journal of Nutritional Medicine
Taylor & Francis Ltd, Rankine Rd, Basingstoke
RG24 8PR.
Tel: +44 (0)1256 813002 (UK)
+1 800 354 1420 (USA & Canada)
Email: enquiry@tandf.co.uk
Functional Medicine Update
Healthcomm International Inc., Gig Harbor,
Washington, USA.
www.healthcomm.com
Townsend Letter for Doctors and Patients
www.tldp.com
Alternative Medicine Review
www.thorne.com/altmedrev/index.html
Journal of Orthomolecular Medicine
www.orthomed.org/jom/jomlist.htm

Laboratory services (UK)

Biolab Medical Unit
(For doctors only)
The Stone House, 9 Weymouth Street, London
W1W 6DB, UK
Tel: +44 (0)207 636 5959/5905
E-mail: info@biolab.co.uk
www.biolab.co.uk

Health Interlink Ltd
(Welcomes all practitioners)
Unit B Ashfordby Business Park, Welby, Melton
Mowbray, Leics LE14 3JL. Tel: 01664 810011.

(International)

Great Smokies Diagnostic Laboratory
63 Zillicoa Street
Asheville, NC 28801, USA
Tel: 1-800-522-4762
Email: cs@gsdl.com
www.gsdl.com

The Great Plains Laboratory
11813 West 77th
Lenexa, KS 66214
Phone 913-341-8949 Fax 913-341-6207 Email
gpl4u@aol.com
www.greatplainslaboratory.com

International seminars

Institute for Functional Medicine
www.fxmed.com

REFERENCES

1. Steventon, GB et al. Xenobiotic Metabolism in Alzheimer's Disease.Neurology 1990;40:1095-1098.

2. Steventon, GB et al. Xenobiotic Metabolism in Parkinson's Disease. Neurology 1989;39:883-887.

3. Smithells RW et al. Apparent prevention of neural tube defects by periconceptional vitamin supplementation. Arch Dis Child 1981;56:911.

4. Pregnant women advised to take folic acid. The Times 18/12/1992, p 6.

5. Hurrell RF, Reddy M, Cook JD. Inhibition of non-haem iron absorption in man by polyphenolic-containing beverages. Br J Nutr 1999 Apr;81(4):289-95.

6. Dr Jonathan Wright's Guide to Healing with Nutrition. Keats, New Canaan, 1990.

7. Allison JR. The relation of hydrochloric acid and vitamin B complex deficiency in certain skin diseases. South Med J 1945;38:235-241.

8. Saltzman JR, Kowdley, KV. Bacterial overgrowth in the elderly. Facts and Research in Gerontology 1996;73-85.

9. Saltzman JR and Russell RM. The aging gut: nutritional issues. Gastroenterology Clinics of North America, June 1998;27(2):309-324.

10. Kelly GS. Bromelain: a literature review and discussion of its therapeutic applications. Alt Med Rev 1996;1(4):243-257.

11. Karnaze DS et al: Neurologic and evoked potential abnormalities in subtle cobalamin deficiency states, including deficiency without anemia and with normal absorption of free cobalamin. Arch Neurol 1990;47(9):1008-12.

12. Collipp PJ et al: Pyridoxine treatment of childhood bronchial asthma. Ann Allergy 1975;35(2):93-7.

13. Cox IM et al. Red blood cell magnesium and chronic fatigue syndrome. Lancet 1991;337 (8744):757-60.

14. Natta CL et al. Apparent vitamin B6 deficiency in sickle cell anaemia. Am J Clin Nutr 1984;40(2):235-9.

15. Abraham GE. The importance of magesium in the management of primary postmenopausal osteoporosis. J Nutr Med 1991;2:165-178.

16. Mertz W. Chromium in human nutrition: a review. J Nutr 1993;123(4):626-33.

17. Schwartz RA et al: Transketolase activity in psychiatric patients. J Clin Psychiatry 1979;40 (10):427-9.

18. Cefalu W. Data presented at the 57th Annual Scientific Session of the American Diabetes Association meeting in Boston, 23 June 1997.

19. Stadel BV. Dietary iodine and risk of breast, endometrial and ovarian cancer. Lancet 1976; 24 April:890-891.

20. Gao H, Li J, Wang E. Iodine deficiency and perceptive nerve deafness [Article in Chinese]. Lin Chuang Er Bi Yan Hou Ke Za Zhi 1998 May;12(5):228-30.

21. Lozoff B. Iron and learning potential in childhood. Bull NY Acad Med 1989;65 (10):1050-66.

22. Sun AH et al. Idiopathic sudden hearing los and disturbance of iron metabolism. A clinical survey of 426 cases. ORL J Otorhinolaryngol Relat Spec 1992;54(2):66-70.

23. Seelig MS. Consequences of magnesium deficiency on the enhancement of stress reactions; preventive and therapeutic implications [a review]. J Am Coll Nutr 1994;13(5):429-46.

24. Guidi GC et al. Selenium supplementation increases renal glomerular filtration rate. J Trace Elem Electrolytes Health Dis 1990;4(3):157-161.

25. Williamson D. Selenium deficiency causes flu virus to mutate into more dangerous forms. FASEB J 2001 June 8.

26. Tikkiwal M et al. Effect of zinc administration on seminal zinc and fertility of oligospermic males. Indian J Physiol Pharmacol 1987;31(1):30-34

27. Abbasi AA, Prasad AS, et al. Experimental zinc deficiency in man: effect on testicular function. J Lab Clin Med 1980 Sept;96(3):544-550.

28. Mitchell EA, Aman MG et al. Clinical characteristics and serum essential fatty acid levels in hyperactive children. Clin Pediatr 1987 Aug;26(8):406-411.

29. Gibson RA. The effect of dietary supplementation with evening primrose oil on hyperkinetic children. Proc Nutr Soc Aust 1985;10:196.

30. Stevens LJ et al. Omega-3 fatty acids in boys with behavior, learning and health problems. Physiol Behav 1996;59(4-5):915-20.

31. http://doctoryourself.com/hoffer_niacin.html.

32. Lazarides L. Schizophrenia. Nutritional Therapy Today 1996;3:6-8.

33. Randolph T, Moss RW. An Alternative Approach to Allergies (revised edition).Harper & Row, New York, 1989.

34. Marinkovich VA. The Immunology of Food Allergy. Personal Monograph 1999;1-7.

(Address: Allergy and Immunology, 801 Brewster Avenue, Suite 220 Redwood City, CA 94063, USA).

35. Monro J. Data presented at the New developments in ME research conference, Society for the Promotion of Nutritional Therapy UK, March 1995.

36. Report from the National Task Force on Chronic Fatigue Syndrome, Post Viral Fatigue Syndrome, Myalgic Encephalomyelitis. Westcare, 155 Whiteladies Road, Clifton, Bristol BS8 2RF, UK, 1994.

37. Packer L, Colman C. The Antioxidant Miracle. John Wiley & Sons, Chichester, 1999.

38. Biskind, MS. Nutritional therapy of endocrine disturbances. In Vitamins and Hormones Vol IV. Academic Press, New York, 1946, pp 147-180.

39. Fowke JH, Longcope C, Hebert JR. Brassica vegetable consumption shifts estrogen metabolism in healthy postmenopausal women. Cancer Epidemiol Biomarkers Prev 2000 August;9:773-779.

40. Kall MA et al. Effects of dietary broccoli on human in vivo drug metabolizing enzymes: evaluation of caffeine, oestrone and chlorzoxazone metabolism. Carcinogenesis 1996;17(4):793-9.

41. Rose DP et al: High-fibre diet reduces serum estrogen concentrations in premenopausal women. Am J Clin Nutr 1991;54(3):520-5.

42. Grundman M. Vitamin E and Alzheimer disease: the basis for additional clinical trials. Am J Clin Nutr 2000;71(Suppl):630S-636S.

43. Heuser G et al. Candida albicans and migraine headaches: a possible link. Journal of the Advancement in Medicine 1992 Fall;5 (3):177-187.

44. McGeer PL, McGeer EG. Inflammation of the brain in Alzheimer's disease: implications for therapy. J Leukoc Biol 1999 April;65:409-415.

45. Ohtsuka Y, Nakaya J. Effect of oral administration of L-arginine on senile dementia. Am J Med 2000 April 1;108:439.

46. Oken BS et al. The efficacy of Ginkgo biloba on cognitive function in Alzheimer disease. Arch Neurol 1998 Nov;55:1409-1415.

47. Reynolds EH, Preece JM, Bailey J, Coppen A. folate deficiency in depressive illness. Br J Psychiatr 1970;117:287-292.

48. Pettegrew JW, Levine J, McClure RJ. Acetyl-L-carnitine physical-chemical, metabolic, and therapeutic properties: relevance for its mode of action in Alzheimer's disease and geriatric depression. Mol Psychiatry 2000 Nov;5(6):616-32.

49. Crook TH et al. Effects of phosphatidylserine in age-associated memory impairment. Neurology 1991;24:42-48.

50. Crook T, Petrie W et al. Effects of phosphatidylserine in Alzheimer's disease. Psychopharmacol Bull 1992;28(1):61-66.

51. Broe GA, Grayson DA, Creasey HM et al. Anti-Inflammatory drugs protect against Alzheimer disease at low doses. Arch Neurol 2000 Nov;57:1586-1591.

52. Conklin KA. Dietary antioxidants during cancer chemotherapy: impact on chemotherapeutic effectiveness and development of side effects. Nutr Cancer 2000;37(1):1-18.

53. Hadjivassiliou M et al. Headache and CNS white matter abnormalities associated with gluten sensitivity. Neurol 2001;56:385-388.

54. Sano M et al. A Controlled trial of selegiline, alpha-tocopherol, or both as treatment for Alzheimer's disease. New England Journal of Medicine 1997 April 24;336(17):1216-1222.

55. Gold M et al. Plasma and red blood cell thiamine deficiency in patients with dementia of the Alzheimer's type. Archives of Neurology 1995, Nov;52:1081-1085.

56. Diaz-Arrastia R. Hyperhomocysteinemia: a new risk factor for Alzheimer disease? Arch Neurol 1998 Nov;55:1407-1408.

57. Hock C et al. Increased blood mercury levels in patients with Alzheimer's disease. Journal of Neural Transmission 1998;105:59-68.

58. Good PF, Perl DP et al. Selective accumulation of aluminum and iron in the neurofibrillary tangles of Alzheimer's disease: a laser microprobe (LAMMA) study. Ann Neurol 1992 March;31(3):286-292.

59. Terano T et al. Docosahexaenoic acid supplementation improves the moderately severe dementia from thrombotic cerebrovascular diseases. Lipids 1999;34(Suppl):S345-S346.

60. Vasquez A. Muskuloskeletal disorders and iron overload disease: comment on the American College of Rheumatology guidelines for the initial evaluation of the adult patient with acute musculoskeletal symptoms. Arthritis Rheum 1996 Oct;39(10):1767-8.

61. Chavez M. SAMe: S-Adenosylmethionine. Am J Health-Syst Pharm 2000 Jan 1;57:119-123.

62. Cenacchi T, Bertoldin T et al. Cognitive decline in the elderly: a double-blind, placebo-controlled multicenter study on efficacy of phosphatidylserine administration. Aging (Milano) 1993 April;5(2):123-133.

63. Reginster JY, Deroisy R et al. Long-term effects of glucosamine sulphate on osteoarthritis progression: a randomised, placebo-controlled clinical trial. Lancet 2001;357:251-256.

64. Prudden JF, Balassa LL. The biological activity of bovine cartilage preparations. Seminars in Arthritis and Rheumatism 1974 Summer;3(4):287-320.

65. Russell AL, McCarty MF. DL-phenylalanine markedly potentiates opiate analgesia-an example of nutrient/pharmaceutical up-regulation of the endogenous analgesia system. Med Hypotheses 2000;55(4):283- 288.

66. Ehrenpreis S, Balagot RC, Myles S et al. Further studies on the analgesic activity of D-phenylalanine in mice and humans. Way EL (Ed). Proceedings of the International Narcotic Research Club Convention 1979;379-82.

67. Horger I. Enzyme therapy in multiple rheumatic diseases. Therapiewoche 1983;33:3948-57 (in German).

68. Landis R, Khalsa KPS. Herbal Defence Against Illness and Ageing. Thorsons, London 1998, pp 381-2.

69. Britton J et al: Dietary magnesium, lung function, wheezing and airway hyperreactivity in a random adult population sample. Lancet 1994;344(8919):357-62.

70. Collipp PJ et al: Pyridoxine treatment of childhood bronchial asthma. Ann Allergy 1975;35(2):93-7.

71. Neuman I, Nahum H, Ben-Amotz A. Reduction of exercise-induced asthma oxidative stress by lycopene, a natural antioxidant. Allergy 2000;55:1184-1189.

72. Hasselmark L et al: Selenium supplementation in intrinsic asthma. Allergy 1993;48(1):30-6.

73. Misso NLA, Powers KA, Gillon RL et al. Reduced platelet glutathione peroxidase activity and serum selenium concentration in atopic asthmatic patients. Clin Exp Allergy 1996;26:838-847.

74. Casley-Smith J. High Protein Oedemas And The Benzo-pyrones. Reported in Lazarides L. The Waterfall Diet. Piatkus Books, London, 1999.

75. Rea W. Chemical Sensitivity Vol I. Reported in Lazarides L. The Waterfall Diet. Piatkus Books, London, 1999.

76. Vojdani A et al. Immunological cross reactivity between Candida albicans and human tissue. Journal of Clinical and Laboratory Immunology 1996;48:1-15.

77. Carlyle IP. Multiple sclerosis: a geographical hypothesis. Medical Hypotheses 1997;49:477-486.

78. Robson B. Conferences point to growing concern about possible links between breast cancer, environment. Canadian Medical Association Journal 1996 April 15;154(8):1253-1255.

79. Agarwal S, Rao AV. Tomato lycopene and its role in human health and chronic diseases. CMAJ 2000 Sept 19;163(6):739-744.

80. Lu L-JW, Anderson KE, Grady JJ, et al. Decreased ovarian hormones during a soya diet: implications for breast cancer prevention. Cancer Res 2000 Aug 1;60:4112-4121.

81. Reddy BS. Role of dietary fiber in colon cancer: an overview. Am J Med 1999 Jan 25;106 (1A):16S-19S.

82. Slattery ML et al. Eating patterns and risk of colon cancer. American Journal of Epidemiology 1998;148(1):4-16.

83. Cameron E, Pauling L. Supplemental ascorbate in the supportive treatment of cancer: prolongation of survival times in terminal human cancer. Proc Natl Acad Sci USA 1976;73 (10):3685-9.

84. Cameron E, Pauling L. Supplemental ascorbate in the supportive treatment of cancer: reevaluation of prolongation of survival times in terminal human cancer. Proc Natl Acad Sci USA 1978;75:4538-42.

85. Philpott W. Biomagnetic Handbook. ISBN 0963696408

86. Natelson B. Paper presented at the Fatigue 2000 conference, London, April 1999. Conference sponsored by the National ME Centre in conjunction with Essex Neurosciences Unit and South Bank University, England.

87. Nylander M et al. Mercury concentrations in the human brain and kidneys in relation to exposure from dental amalgam fillings. Swed Dent J 1987;11(5):179-87.

88. Demitrack MA et al. Evidence for impaired activation of the hypothalamic pituitary-adrenal axis in patients with chronic fatigue syndrome. Journal of Clinical Endocrinology and Metabolism 1991;73:1224-1234.

98. Cleare AJ, Wessely SC. Chronic fatigue syndrome: a stress disorder? British Journal of Hospital Medicine 1996;55(9):571-574.

90. Cheney P. Clinical management of chronic fatigue syndrome. Transcription on internet website of lecture dated 5-7 February 1999. http://www.nutritionadvisor.com/cheneymd.html.

91. Rayman MP. Dietary selenium: time to act. British Medical Journal 1997 Feb 8;314:387-388.

92. Isaacs CE, Kim KS, Thormar H. Inactivation of enveloped viruses in human bodily fluids by purified lipids. Annals of the New York Academy of Sciences 1994;724:457-464.

93. Griffith RS, Norins AL, Kagan C. A multicentered study of lysine therapy in Herpes

simplex infection. Dermatologica (SWITZERLAND) 1978;156(5):257-67.

94. Deale A et al. Cognitive behavior therapy for chronic fatigue syndrome: a randomized controlled trial. American Journal of Psychiatry 1997 March;154:3:408-414.

95. Hanck A. Vitamin C and cancer. Int J Vit Nutr Res 1983;Suppl 24: Vitamins in Medicine: Recent Therapeutic Aspects. Hanck A (Ed), pp 87-104.

96. Pinnock CB et al: Vitamin A status in children who are prone to respiratory tract infections. Aust Paediatr J 1986;22(2):95-9.

97. Houston DK, Johnson MA, Nozza RJ et al. Age-related hearing loss, vitamin B-12, and folate in elderly women. American Journal of Clinical Nutrition 1999 March;69(3):564-571.

98. Strome M et al. Hyperlipidemia in association with childhood sensorineural hearing loss. Laryngoscope 1988;98(2):165-9.

99. Mouret J et al. L-tyrosine cures, immediate and long term, dopamine-dependent depressions. Clinical and polygraphic studies. C R Acad Sci III 1988;306(3):9308 (in French).

100. Beckmann H, Athen D, Olteanu M, Zimmer R. DL-phenylalanine versus imipramine: a double-blind controlled study. Arch Psychiatr Nervenkr 1979 July 4;227(1):49-58.

101. Vahora SA et al. S-adenosylmethionine in the treatment of depression. Neurosci Biobehav Rev 1988;12(2):139-41.

102. Lietha R et al. Neuropsychiatric disorders associated with functional folate deficiency in the presence of elevated serum and erythrocyte folate: a preliminary report. J Nutr Med 1994;4:441-447.

103. Hawkes WC et al. Effects of dietary selenium on mood in healthy men living in a metabolic research unit. Biol Psychiatry 1996;39 (2):121-8.

104. Abou-Saleh MT et al. Serum and red blood cell folate in depression. Acta Psychiatr Scand 1989;80(1):78-82.

105. Bermond P. Therapy of side effects of oral contraceptive agents with vitamin B6. Acta Vitaminol Enzymol 1982;4(1-2):45-54.

106. Levine J, Barak Y, Gonzalves M et al. Double-blind, controlled trial of inositol treatment of depression. Am J Psychiatry 1995 May;152(5):792-794.

107. Sherman C. St. John's Wort Used in Severe Depression. Family Practice News 1998 April 15;17.

108. Pfeiffer CC, Braverman ER. Folic acid and vitamin B12 therapy for the low-histamine, high-copper biotype of schizophrenia. In Botez MI,

Reynolds EN (Eds). Folic Acid in Neurology, Psychiatry, and Internal Medicine. Raven Press, New York 1979, pp 483-7.

109. Jaffe R, Kruesi O. The biological-immunology window: a molecular view of psychiatric management. International Clinical Nutrition Review 1992 January;12(1):9-26.

110. Pfeiffer CC. Mental and Elemental Nutrients. Keats Publishing, New Canaan, CT, 1975.

111. Natali A et al. Relationship between insulin release, antinatriuresis and hypokalaemia after glucose ingestion in normal and hypertensive man. Clin Sci (Colch) 1993;85(3):327-35.

112. Sozen I, Arici A. Hyperinsulinism and its interaction with hyperandrogenism in polycystic ovary syndrome. Obstet Gynecol Survey 2000;55 (5):321-328.

113. Fritz T, Rosenqvist U. Walking for exercise - immediate effect on blood glucose levels in type 2 diabetes. Scand J Prim Health Care 2001;19:31-33.

114. Kubo K, Nanba H. Antidiabetic mechanism of maitake (Grifola frondosa). In: Royse DJ (Ed). Mushroom Biology and Mushroom Products. University Park, PA: Penn State University 1996;215-221.

115. Reaven G. Clinician of the month. Functional Medicine Update June 2001. HealthComm International, Gig Harbor, Washington USA.

116. Sharma RD et al. Effect of fenugreek seed on blood glucose and serum lipids in type I diabetes. European Journal of Clinical Nutrition, 1990;44:301-306.

117. Pfeiffer CC, Iliev V. Blood histamine decreasing and CNS effect in man. Fed Proc 1972;31:250.

118. Okayama H et al. Treatment of status asthmaticus with intravenous magnesium sulfate. Journal of Asthma 1991;28(1):11-17.

119. Nandi BK et al. Effect of ascorbic acid on detoxification of histamine under stress conditions. Biochem Pharm 1974;23:643-647.

120. Siani A, Guglielmucci F, Farinaro E, Strazzullo P. Increasing evidence for the role of salt and salt-sensitivity in hypertension. Nutr Metab Cardiovasc Dis 2000;10:93-100.

121. Anand IS, Chandrashekhar Y, Ferrari R et al. Pathogenesis of oedema in chronic severe anaemia: studies of body water and sodium, renal function, haemodynamic variables, and plasma hormones. Br Heart J 1993 Oct;70(4):357-62.

122. Borok G. Nutritional aspects of hypertension. South African Medical Journal 1989 August 5;76:125-126.

123. Rath M. The process of eradicating heart disease has become irreversible. Journal of Applied Nutrition 1996;48(1 & 2):22-33.

124. Kritchevsky D. Antimutagenic and some other effects of conjugated linoleic acid. Br J Nutr 2000;83(5):459-465.

125. Kritchevsky D, Tepper SA et al. Influence of conjugated linoleic acid (CLA) on establishment and progression of atherosclerosis in rabbits. J Am Coll Nutr 2000;19(4):472S-477S.

126. Goodwin J- K and Strickland KN. The role of dietary modification and nondrug therapy in dogs and cats with congestive heart failure. Vet Med 1998 October;919-926.

127. http://www.vaccineinfo.net/autismHg.htm Vaccinations, Mercury and Autism: Waters Kraus Press Release.

128. Megson M. Clinician of the month. FMU September 1999. HealthComm International, Gig Harbor, Washington USA.

129. Shaw W. September 1998. Health Interlink Seminar, St Albans, UK.

130. Lelord G et al. Clinical and biological effects of high doses of vitamin B6 and magnesium on autistic children. Acta Vitaminol Enzymol 1982;4(1-2):27-44.

131. Rimland H. Controversies in the treatment of autistic children: vitamin and drug therapy. J Child Neurol 1988;3 Suppl:S68-72. 132. Reichelt K-L, Ekrem J, Scott H. Gluten, milk proteins and autism: dietary intervention effects on behavior and peptide secretion. J App Nutr 1990;42(1):1-11.

133. Edelson SB, Cantor D. The neurotoxic etiology of the autistic spectrum disorders: a replication study. Toxicol Ind Health, 2000;16 (6):239-247.

134. Shaw W, Kassen E, Chaves E. Assessment of antifungal drug therapy in autism by measurement of suspected microbial metabolites in urine with gas chromatography-mass spectrometry. Clin Pract Altern Med, 2000 Spring;1(1):15-26.

135. Autism-vaccination link in United Kingdom? Autism Research Review International 1996;10(4):1.

136. Rimland B. Vitamin B6 in autism: the safety issue. Autism Research Review International 1996;10(3):3.

137. Kubo K, Nanba H. Modification of cellular immune responses in experimental autoimmune hepatitis in mice by maitake (Grifola frondosa). Mycoscience 1998;39:351-360.

138. Wu S, Zou D, Han SH et al. Therapeutic effect of Grifola polysaccharides in chronic hepatitis B [abstract P-18]. In: International Symposium on Production and Products of Lentinus Mushroom, Programme and Abstract, Qingyuan, Zhejiang Province, China: International Society for Mushroom Science, Committee on Science, Asian Region, Qingyuan County Government, Zhejiang Province, China, 1994.

139. Yu SY et al. A low selenium intake is associated with a high regional incidence of hepatitis B virus infections in China. Chemoprevention trial of human hepatitis with selenium supplementation in China. Biol Trace Elem Res 1989;20(15):15-22.

140. Andreone P et al. Vitamin E for chronic hepatitis B. Annals of Internal Medicine 1998 Jan 15;128(2):156-157.

141. von Herbay A et al. Vitamin E improves the aminotransferase status of patients suffering from viral hepatitis C: a randomized, double-blind, placebo-controlled study. Free Radical Research 1997;27:599-605.

142. Berkson BM. A triple antioxidant approach to the treatment of hepatitis C using alpha-lipoic acid (thioctic acid) silymarin, selenium, and other fundamental nutraceuticals. Clin Pract Altern Med 2000 Spring;1(1):27-33.

143. Wallace AE, Weeks WB. Thiamine treatment of chronic hepatitis B infection. Am J Gastroenterol 2001 March;96(3):864-868.

144. Schuppan D, Jia J-D, Brinkhaus B, Hahn EG. Herbal products for liver diseases: a therapeutic challenge for the new millennium. Hepatology 1999 October;30(4):1099-1104.

145. Spedding G, Ratty A, Middleton E Jr. Inhibition of reverse transcriptases by flavonoids. Antiviral Res 1989 Sep;12(2):99-110.

146. Middleton E Jr, Drzewiecki G. Flavonoid inhibition of human basophil histamine release stimulated by various agents. Biochem Pharmacol 1984 Nov 1;33(21):3333-8.

147. Middleton E Jr, Drzewiecki G. Effects of flavonoids and transitional metal cations on antigen-induced histamine release from human basophils. Biochem Pharmacol 1982 Apr 1;31 (7):1449-53.

148. Houglum K et al. A pilot study of the effects of d-alpha-tocopherol on hepatic stellate cell activation in chronic hepatitis C. Gastroenterology 1997;113:1069-1073.

149. Zametkin AJ. Cerebral glucose metabolism in adults with hyperactivity of childhood onset. New England Journal of Medicine 1990 Nov 15;323(20):1361-1366.

150. Egger J et al: Controlled trial of oligoantigenic treatment in the hyperkinetic syndrome. Lancet 1985;1:540-5.

151. Kaplan BJ, McNicol J, Conte RA et al. Dietary replacement in preschool-aged hyperactive boys. Pediatrics 1989;83:7-17.

152. The Shipley Project, National Society for Research into Allergy, West Yorkshire, UK, 1992.

153. Boris M, Mandel FS. Foods and additives are common causes of the attention deficit hyperactive disorder in children. Ann Allergy 1994;72:462-7.

154. Howard JMH. Clinical import of small increases in serum aluminum,", Clin Chem 1984;30(10):1722-1723.

155. Benton D. Vitamin and mineral intake and cognitive function. In Micronutrients in Health and in Disease Prevention. Bendich A and Butterworth CE (Eds). Marcell Dekker Inc., New York, 1991.

156. Longenecker J et al. Effects of prolonged sub-clinical dietary deficiencies on behavior. Fed Proc 1987;46:903.

157. Bekaroglu M, Aslan Y, Gedik Y et al. Relationships between serum free fatty acids and zinc, and attention deficit hyperactivity disorder: a research note. J Child Psychol Psychiatr 1996;37(2):225-227.

158. McCarty MF. Fish oil and other nutritional adjuvants for treatment of congestive heart failure. Med Hypotheses 1996 Apr;46(4):400-6.

159. Scheller S, Dworniczak S, Pogorzelska T et al. Effect of quercetin, caffeic acid and caffeic acid phenylethyl ester, solubilized in non-ionic surfactants, on histamine release in vivo and in vitro. Arzneimittelforschung 2000 Jan;50(1):72-6.

160. Reported in Wynn A & M: The Case For Preconception Care Of Men And Women. AB Academic Publishers, Bicester, 1991 p 20.

161. Whittaker P. Iron and zinc interactions in humans. Am J Clin Nutr 1998 Aug; 68(2 Suppl):442S-446S.

162. When Zinc Stores are Low, Folic Acid is a No No. International Medical Tribune Syndicate 1989 May 29;4/Research Briefs.

163. Luck MR et al. Ascorbic acid and fertility. Biology of Reproduction 1995;52:262-266.

164. Krsnjavi H et al. Selenium and fertility in men. Trace Elements in Medicine 1992;9(2):107-108.

165. Hatch EE, Bracken MB. Association of delayed conception with caffeine consumption. American Journal of Epidemiology 1993;138 (12):1082-1092.

166. Dlugosz L, Bracken MB. Reproductive effects of caffeine: a review and theoretical analysis. Epidemiologic Reviews 1992;14:83-100.

167. Anderson RA Jr et al. Alcohol and male fertility. Br J Alcohol Alcohol 1981;16(4):179-185.

168. Environment and infertility. Environmental Health Prospectives 1996 Feb;104(2):136-137.

169. Brandes JW et al. Sugar- free diet: a new perspective in the treatment of Crohn's disease? Randomised, controlled study. Z Gastroentereol 1981;19(1):1-12 (in German).

170. Thornton JR et al: Diet and Crohn's disease: characteristics of the pre-illness diet. Br Med J 1979;2(6193): 762-4.

171. Swaminathan R. Nutritional factors in osteoporosis. Int J Clin Pract 1999 Oct/Nov;53 (7):540- 548.

172. Vermeer C et al. Effects of vitamin K on bone mass and bone metabolism. J Nutr 1996;126 (4 Suppl):1187S-91S.

173. Nelson ME et al. Effects of high-intensity strength training on multiple risk factors for osteoporotic fractures: a randomized controlled trial. JAMA 1994 Dec 28;272(24):1909-1914.

174. Prasad AS. Zinc deficiency in women, infants and children. J Am Coll Nutr 1996;15 (2):113-20.

175. Favier A et al. Effects of zinc deficiency in pregnancy on the mother and the newborn infant. Rev Fr Gynecol Obstet 1990;85(1):13-27.

176. Shaw GM et al. Risks of orofacial clefts in children born to women using multivitamins containing folic acid periconceptionally. Lancet 1995;346(8972):393-6.

177. Habib FK et al. Metal-androgen interrelationships in carcinoma and hyperplasia of the human prostate. J Endocr 1976;71:133-141.

178. Lowe FC, Ku JC. Phytotherapy in treatment of benign prostatic hyperplasia: a critical review. Urology 1996;48:12-20.

179. DeMott K. Herbal/antioxidant agents reduce symptoms of BPH. Family Practice News 1999 November 15;29(22):24.

180. Webber MM. Selenium prevents the growth stimulatory effects of cadmium on human prostatic epithelium. Biochem Biophys Res Commun 1985127(3): 871-7.

181. Beard JL et al. Impaired thermoregulation and thyroid function in iron-deficiency anemia. American Journal of Clinical Nutrition 1990;52:813-9.

182. Davis DR et al. Omega-3 fatty acids in clinical practice. Journal of the Advancement of Medicine 1995;Spring;8(1):5-35.

183. Abraham GE. Nutritional factors in the etiology of the premenstrual tension syndromes. J Reprod Med 1983;28(7):446-64.

184. Williams MJ, Harris RI, Dean BC. Controlled trial of pyridoxine in the premenstrual syndrome. J Int Med Res 1985;13:174-9.

185. Stewart A. Clinical and biochemical effects of nutritional supplementation on the premenstrual syndrome. J Reprod Med 1987;32 (6):435-41.

186. Doll H et al. Pyridoxine (vitamin B6) and the premenstrual syndrome: a randomized crossover trial. J R Coll Gen Pract 1989;39 (326):364-8.

187. Michnovicz J, Bradlow HL. Vegetables from the Brassica genus, whether raw or lightly cooked, contain a chemical that promotes the inactivation of estrogen. Institute for Hormone Research, New York City. Reported in Science News 1990 June 16.

188. Berman M, Krutan MS, et al. Vitamin B-6 in premenstrual syndrome. Journal of The American Dietetic Association 1990 June;90(6):859-861.

189. Brush MG, Perry M. Pyridoxine and the premenstrual syndrome. Lancet 1985 June 15;1399.

190. Colborn T, Clement C (Eds). Chemically-Induced Alterations In Sexual And Functional Development: The Wildlife/Human Connection. Princeton, 1992.

191. Carlsen et al. Evidence for decreasing quality of semen during past 50 years. BMJ 1992 Sept 12;305.

192. Important new animal colony available for endometriosis research Endometriosis Association public statement, 1992). Also article by Mary Lou Ballweg in their newsletter Vol 13 No 2, 1992. Endometriosis Association, International Headquarters, Milwaukee, USA.

193. Bider D, Mashiach S et al. Endocrinological basis of hot flushes. Obstetrical & Gynecological Survey. 1989;44(7):495-499.

194. Genton C, Frei PC, Pecoud A. Value of oral provocation tests to aspirin and food additives in the routine investigation of asthma and chronic urticaria. J Allergy Clin Immunol 1985 July;76 (1):40-45.

195. Tarlo SM, Sussman GL. Asthma and anaphylactoid reactions to food additives. Canadian Family Physician 1993;May;39:1119-1123. Am J Obstet Gynecol 1987 May;156 (5):1284-8

196. Rebar RW, Spitzer IB. The physiology and measurement of hot flushes. Am J Obstet Gynecol 1987 May;156(5):1284-8.

197. Dupont E, Klug T, McCann C et al. Women with breast cancer have markedly decreased metabolic conversion of exogenous oestrogen to 2-hydroxyoestrogens. These differences may account for why some women get breast cancer on HRT and others do not. The prognostic value of altered estrogen metabolism in breast cancer. Ann Surgical Oncol. 2000;7(1):Supplement.

198. Reaven G. Clinician of the Month. FMU June 2001. HealthComm International, Gig Harbor, Washington USA.

199. Nelson ME, Fiatarone MA et al. Effects of high-intensity strength training on multiple risk factors for osteoporotic fractures. A randomized controlled trial. JAMA 1994;272(24):1909-1914.

200. Hudgins LC. Effect of high-carbohydrate feeding on triglyceride and saturated fatty acid synthesis. Proc Soc Exp Biol Med 2000;225:178-183.

201. NIH Guide: Health And Safety/Medical Sciences/Biomedical Vol. 18, No. 16, 1989 May 5, p 7. National Institutes of Health USA.

202. Cerniglia CE, Freeman JP, Franklin W, Pack LD. Metabolism of azo dyes derived from benzidine, 3,3'-dimethylbenzidine and 3,3'-dimethoxybenzidine to potentially carcinogenic aromatic amines by intestinal bacteria. Carcinogenesis (Lond) 1982;3(11):1255-1260.

203. Simon G, Gorbach S. Azoreductase promotes the reduction of azo food dyes to substituted phenyl and naphthyl amines, which are potent carcinogens. 5. The human intestinal microflora. Dig Dis Sci 1986;31:1475-1425.

204. Chung K-T, Stevens SE Jr, Cerniglia CE. The reduction of azo dyes by the intestinal microflora. Crit Rev Microbiol 1992;18 (3):175-190.

205. Norrman J. The Swedish Association of Local Authorities http://www.ceec-logon.net/download/norrman.doc

206. Mark D. Gold, Director, Aspartame Toxicity Information Center, 35 Inman St, Cambridge, MA 02139, USA.

www.holisticmed.com/aspartame/

207. Enig MG. Health and nutritional benefits from coconut oil and its advantages over competing oils. Price-Pottenger Nutrition Foundation 1996 Spring;20(1):3-5.

208. Wilcox AJ, Weinberg CR. Tea and fertility. Lancet 1991 May 11;337:1159-1160.

209. Burney PGJ, Neild JE, Twort CHC et al. Effect of changing dietary sodium on the airway response to histamine. Thorax 1989;44:36-41.

210. Greden JF. Anxiety or caffeinism: a diagnostic dilemma. Am J Psychiatry 1974 Oct;131(10):1089-1092.

211. Virtanen SM et al. Is children's or parents' coffee or tea consumption associated with the risk for type I diabetes mellitus in children? Eur J Clin Nutr 1994;47(4):279-85.

212. Abdullah TH et al. Enhancement of natural killer cell activity in AIDS with garlic. Deutsche Zeitschrift Fur Onkologie 1989; 21:52-53. (Address: Tariq H. Abdullah, Akbar Clinic and Research Foundation, Panama City, Florida 32404, USA.)

213. Julius M. Morbidity in the elderly and glutathione. The Experts Speak,Clinical Pearls 1996. (Address: Dr Mara Julius, School of Public Health University of Michigan 109 Observatory St. Ann Arbor, MI 48109-2029 USA.)

214. Arbiser JL et al. Curcumin Is an In Vivo Inhibitor of Angiogenesis, Mol Med 1998;4:376-383.

215. Lockwood K et al: Partial and complete regression of breast cancer in patients in relation to dosage of coenzyme Q10. Biochem Biophys Res Commun 1994;199(3):1504-8.

216. Tosiello L. Hypomagnesemia and diabetes mellitus. Archives of Internal Medicine 1996 June 10;156:1143-1148.

217. Anderson RA et al. Effects of supplemental chromium on patients with symptoms of reactive hypoglycaemia. Metabolism 1987;36(4):351-5.

218. Stebbing JB et al. Reactive hypoglycaemia and magnesium. Magnes Bull 1982;4(2):131-4.

219. Toouli J, Jablonski P, Watts JMK. Gallstone dissolution in man using cholic acid and lecithin. Lancet 1975 Dec 6:1124-1126.

220. Preventive Medicine Update, April 1996. HealthComm International, Gig Harbor, Washington, USA.

221. Sole MJ, Jeejeebhoy KN. Conditioned nutritional requirements and the pathogenesis and treatment of myocardial failure. Curr Opin Clin Nutr Metab Care 2000 Nov;3(6):417-24.

222. Chapman RA et al. Taurine and the Heart. Cardiovascular Research 1993:27:358-363.

223. Azuma J, Sawamura A, Awata N et al. Double-blind randomized crossover trial of taurine in congestive heart failure. Curr Ther Res 1983;34:543-557.

224. Klenner FR. Observations on the dose and administration of ascorbic acid when employed beyond the range of a vitamin in human pathology. Journal of Orthomolecular Medicine 1998;13(4):198-210.

225. Merkel RL. the use of menadione bisulfite and ascorbic acid in the treatment of nausea and vomiting of pregnancy. Am J Obstet Gynec 1952 August;64(2)416-418. Reported in Dr Jonathan Wright's Guide to Healing with Nutrition. Keats, New Canaan, 1990.

226. Berman E, Nourkayhan S et al. Zinc: a key urological element. Poster presentation, American Urological Association annual meeting, Chicago, 1974.

227. Kolonel LN, Hankin JH, Whittemore AS et al. Vegetables, fruits, legumes and prostate cancer: a multiethnic case-control study. Cancer Epidemiol Biomarkers Prev 2000 August;9:795-804.

228. Lagrue G et al: Idiopathic cyclic edema. The role of capillary hyperpermeability and its correction by Ginkgo biloba extract. Presse Med 1986;15(31):1550-3 (in French).

229. Hughes RE, Wilson HK. Flavonoids: some physiological and nutritional considerations. Progress and Medicinal Chemistry 1977;14:285-301.

230. Dr Ellen Grant. Sexual Chemistry. Cedar, London 1994. ISBN 0749313633.

231. Carney MW et al: Thiamine, riboflavin and pyridoxine deficiency in psychiatric in-patients. Br J Psychiatry 1982;141:271-2.

232. Schwartz RA et al: Transketolase activity in psychiatric patients. J Clin Psychiatry 1979;40 (10):427-9.

233. Donnelly S et al: Subacute combined degeneration of the spinal cord due to folate deficiency in association with a psychotic illness. Ir Med J 1990;83(2):73-4.

234. Kanofsky JD: Vitamin C and schizophrenia. Nutrition Report 1990;8(9):65-72.

235. Srinivasan DP: Trace elements in psychiatric illness. Br J Hosp Med 1984;32(2):77-9.

236. Horrobin DF: The relationship between schizophrenia and essential fatty acid and eicosanoid metabolism. Prostaglandins Leukot Essent Fatty Acids 1992;46(1):71-7.

237. Vaddadi KS: Use of gamma-linolenic acid in the treatment of schizophrenia and tardive dyskinesia. Prostaglandins Leukot Essent Fatty Acids 1992;46(1):67-70.

238. Laugharne JD et al: Fatty acids and schizophrenia. Lipids 1996;31 Suppl:S163-5.

239. Andrews RC: Unification of findings in schizophrenia by reference to the effects of gestational zinc deficiency. Med Hypotheses 1990;31(2):141-53.

240. Brown AS et al: Neurobiological plausibility of prenatal nutritional deprivation as a risk factor for schizophrenia. J Nerv Ment Dis 1996;184 (2):71-85.

241. Susser E et al: Schizophrenia after prenatal famine. Further evidence. Arch Gen Psychiatry 1996;53(1):25-31.

242. Siblerud RL: The relationship between mercury from dental amalgam and mental health. Am J Psychother 1989;43(4):575-87.

243. Thomson GOB, Raab GM, Hepburn WS et

al. Blood-lead levels and children's behaviour - results from the Edinburgh lead study. J Child Psychol Psychiat 1989;30(4):515-528.

244. Detre Z, Jellinek H, Miskulin M, Robert AM. Studies on vascular permeability in hypertension: action of anthocyanosides. Clin Physiol Biochem 1986;4(2):143-9.

245. Ernst E. Ginkgo biloba for tinnitus: a review. Clin Otolaryngol 1999;24:164-167.

246. Schuschke DA. Dietary copper in the physiology of the microcirculation. Journal of Nutrition 1997;127:2274-2281.

247. Bartolo M, Antignani PL. Drug therapy of venous insufficiency. Phlebologie 1985 Apr-Jun;38(2):353-7 (in French).

248. Jarvill-Taylor KJ et al. A hydroxychalcone derived from cinnamon functions as a mimetic for insulin in 3T3-L1 adipocytes. J AM Coll Nutr 2001;20(4): 327-336.

249. Kane S, Goldberg MJ. Use of bromelain for mild ulcerative colitis. Ann Intern Med 2000 April 18;132(8):680.

250. Kaul TN, Middleton E Jr, Ogra PL. Antiviral effect of flavonoids on human viruses. J Med Virol 1985 Jan;15(1):71-9.

251. Fahey JW, Talalay P. Antioxidant functions of sulforaphane: a potent inducer of phase ii detoxication enzymes. Food Chem Toxicol 1999;37:973-979.

252. Omura Y, Beckman St. Role of mercury (Hg) in resistant infections & effective treatment of Chlamydia trachomatis and Herpes family viral infections (and potential treatment for cancer) by removing localized Hg deposits with Chinese parsley and delivering effective antibiotics using various drug uptake enhancement methods. Acupuncture & Electro-Theraputics Research 1995 Aug-Dec;20(3-4):195-229.

253. Landrum JT et al. A one year study of the macular pigment: the effect of 140 days of a lutein supplement. Exp Eye Res, 1997;65:57-62.

254. Ip C. Review of the effects of trans fatty acids, oleic acid, n-3 polyunsaturated fatty acids, and conjugated linoleic acid on mammary carcinogenesis in animals. American Journal of Clinical Nutrition 1997;66(Suppl.):1523S-1529S.

255. Dyck DJ. Dietary fat intake, supplements, and weight loss. Can J Appl Physiol 2000 Dec;25 (6):495-523.

256. Pariza MW, Park Y, Cook ME. conjugated linoleic acid and the control of cancer and obesity. Toxicol Sci 1999;52(Suppl.):107-110.

257. Theriault A et al. Tocotrienol: a review of its therapeutic potential. Clin Biochem 1999;32 (5):309-319.

258. Cheney G, Waxler SH, Miller IJ. vitamin U therapy of peptic ulcer. California Med 1956 Jan;84(1):39-42.

259. Vutyavanich T, Kraisarin T, Ruangsri R-A. Ginger for nausea and vomiting in pregnancy: randomized, double-masked, placebo-controlled trial. Obstet Gynecol 2001;97:577-582.

260. Srivastava KC. Effect of onion and ginger consumption on platelet thromboxane production in humans. Prostaglandins, Leukotrienes and Essential Fatty Acids 1989;35:183-185.

261. Ashton M et al. Artemisinin kinetics and dynamics during oral and rectal treatment of uncomplicated malaria. Clinical Pharmacology and Therapeutics 1998;63(4):482-492.

262. Galland L et al. Giardia lamblia infection as a cause of chronic fatigue. Journal of Nutritional Medicine 1990;1:27-31.

263. Konrad T et al. Alpha-lipoic acid treatment decreases serum lactate and pyruvate concentrations and improves glucose effectiveness in lean and obese patients with type 2 diabetes. Diabetes Care1999 February;22 (2):280-287.

264. Christopher Hobbs. Lecture on medicinal mushrooms July 2000, University of Middlesex, UK.

265. Marteau PR, de Vrese M, Cellier CJ, Schrezenmeir J. Protection from gastrointestinal diseases with the use of probiotics. Am J Clin Nutr 2001;73(Suppl.):430S-436S.

266. Vanderhoof JA. Probiotics: future directions. Am J Clin Nutr 2001;73 (Suppl.):1152S-1155S.

267. Bucci LR. Selected herbals and human exercise performance. Am J Clin Nutr 2000;72 (Suppl):624S-636S.

268. Cox C, Sutherland W, Mann J, de Jong S, Chisholm A, Skeaff M. Effects of dietary coconut oil, butter and safflower oil on plasma lipids, lipoproteins and lathosterol levels. Eur J Clin Nutr 1998 Sep;52(9):650-4.

269. Ludwig DS et al. Starchy foods may trigger overeating. Pediatrics 1999;103:e26.

270. Cannon, G. The Politics of Food. Century, London 1988.

271. KeyNote and Mintel market research polls, 1991-1992.

272. Steventon GB, Sturman S, Waring RH, Williams AC. A review of xenobiotic metabolism enzymes in Parkinson's disease and motor neuron disease. Drug Metabol Drug Interact 2001;18 (2):79-98.

273. Masson M. Bromelain in the treatment of blunt injuries to the musculoskeletal system. A case observation study by an orthopaedic surgeon

in private practice. Fortschritte Der Medizin 1995;113 (19):30346. Reported in HerbalGram (www.herbalgram. org) Issue No 39.

274. Oral enzyme therapy in osteoarthritis of the knee. Proteolytic enzymes are effective with few risks. MMW Fortschr Med 2001 Jun 7;143 (23):44-6 (in German).

275. Klein G, Kullich W. Reducing pain by oral enzyme therapy in rheumatic diseases. Wien Med Wochenschr 1999;149(21-22):577-80(in German).

276. Arons I, Freeman J, Sokoloff B, Eddy WH. Bioflavonoids in radiation injury. 1. The effect of ionizing radiation on capillaries. Brit J Radio 1954;27:583-585.

277. Lorscheider FL et al. Mercury exposure from "silver" tooth fillings: emerging evidence questions a traditional dental paradigm. FASEB Journal 1995;9:504-508.

278. Thorley-Lawson DA, Babcock GJ. A model for persistent infection with Epstein-Barr virus: the stealth virus of human B cells. Life Sci 1999;65(14):1433-53

279. Wiertz EJ, Mukherjee S, Ploegh HL. Viruses use stealth technology to escape from the host immune system. Mol Med Today 1997 Mar;3(3):116-23.

280. Utiger RD. Estrogen, thyroxine binding in serum, and thyroxine therapy. NEJM 2001;344(23):1784-5.

281. Vincent A, Fitzpatrick LA. Soy isoflavones: are they useful in menopause? Mayo Clinic Proc 2000;75:1174-1184.

282. Theriault A et al. Tocotrienol: a review of its therapeutic potential. Clin Biochem 1999;32(5):309-319.

283. Willett WC et al. Intake of trans fatty acids and risk of coronary heart disease among women. Lancet 1993;341(8845)

581-5.

284. Erdman JW Jr. Soy protein and cardiovascular disease: a statement for healthcare professionals from the nutrition commitee of the AHA. Circulation 2000;102:2555-2561.

285. Mayell M. Maitake extracts and their therapeutic potential -- a review. Alternative Medicine Review Feb 2001.

286. Shaw D, Kolev S, Leon C, Bell G et al. Toxicological problems resulting from exposure to traditional medicines and food supplements. MAFF R&D and Surveillance Report 170, 1996.

287. Fleet JC. New support for a folk remedy: cranberry juice reduces bacteriuria and pyuria in elderly women. Nutr Rev 1994;52(5):168- 70.

288. Wheeler MA et al. Effect of long-term oral L-arginine on the nitric oxide synthase pathway in the urine from patients with interstitial cystitis. Journal of Urology 1997 Dec;158:2045-2050.

289. Rattan V et al. Effect of combined supplementation of magnesium oxide and pyridoxine in calcium-oxalate stone formers. Urol Res 1994;22 (3):161- 5.

290. Blacklock NJ et al. Sucrose and idiopathic renal stone. Nutr Health 1987;5(1):9- 17.

291. Laurent J, Lagrue G. Dietary manipulation for idiopathic nephrotic syndrome: a new approach to therapy. Allergy 1989;44:599-603.

292. Reyes AA, Karl IE, Klahr S. Role of arginine in health and in renal disease. Am J Physiol 1994 Sept;267(3Pt2):F331-46.

293. Reid G et al. Vaginal flora and urinary tract infections. Current Opinion in Infectious Disease 1991;4:37-41.

294. Yee S, Choi BH. Oxidative stress and neurotoxic effects of methylmercury poisoning.

Neurotoxicology 1996;17(1):17-26.

295. Masai M et al. Effect of dietary intake on urinary oxalate excretion in calcium renal stone formers. Br J Urol 1995;76 (6):692-6.

296. Jones D. Data presented at the New developments in ME research conference, Society for the Promotion of Nutritional Therapy UK, March 1995.

RECIPE INDEX

GENERAL INDEX

FEEDBACK QUESTIONNAIRE

If you believe that Nutritional Therapy should be available through your doctor, you can help to make this possible by completing this questionnaire. The results achieved by readers using this book will be compiled and used to assist medical research. Only by such research does the face of medicine change.

You do not have to complete the last section, which ask for your name and contact details, but it will help the author if you do.

1. Did you have a health problem before using this book? .... YES/NO

2. If so, what was it? ....

3. Has this health problem improved? .... YES/NO

4. How long did you apply nutritional therapy to your problem as described in this book? (Delete as appropriate)
LESS THAN 1 MONTH/1-2 MONTHS/3-6 MONTHS/6-12 MONTHS

5. During this period, how closely did you follow the instructions and recipes in this book? (Delete as appropriate)
HARDLY AT ALL/OCCASIONALLY/REGULARLY
QUITE CLOSELY/VERY CLOSELY

6. Please list your symptoms and indicate their severity on a score of 1 (mild) to 5 (severe) both before and after self-treatment

Symptom	Score before	Score after
(1)	....	....
(2)	....	....
(3)	....	....
(4)	....	....
(5)	....	....
(6)	....	....

(Continued overleaf)

7. Did you find nutritional therapy (as applied using this book)
VERY DIFFICULT/DIFFICULT/DIFFICULT AT FIRST BUT BECOMING
EASIER/FAIRLY EASY FROM THE START/VERY EASY

8. If you have any comments on the usefulness of this book, please indicate them
here

....

....

....

....

....

....

....

....

....

9. If you believe that, to help other people like you, the effectiveness of nutritional
therapy should have more publicity, it would be very helpful if you could give your
name and a contact phone number, and tick and sign the box giving permission for
a health writer or medical journalist to contact you with a view to writing up your
story

Your name ....

Address ....

....

Phone (daytime)................................. (evenings) ....

❑ I give my permission for a health writer to contact me

Signature ....

Please send this page to Linda Lazarides
c/o Waterfall 2000, BCM Waterfall, London WC1N 3XX
Your help is much appreciated

The Amino Acid Report

by Linda Lazarides

Maximize the power of vegetarian protein

Protein is one of our most basic needs, but research into how its building blocks, the amino acids, can be combined in different ways to assist health is only just beginning. Linda Lazarides brings you a complete update on the amino acids, what the body uses them for, and the research into their effects on health. Contains much information not published elsewhere.

MEAT, FISH AND DAIRY PRODUCTS ARE NOT ALWAYS THE BEST SOURCES OF AMINO ACIDS

Read about new amino acid research in **chronic fatigue syndrome** (M.E.) ✦ Military research by the U.S. Government on amino acids to treat **stress** ✦ Which aminos are vital to liver **detoxification** ✦ A new theory about **multiple sclerosis** ✦ Research into powerful effects of methionine against **arthritis** and **fibromyalgia** ✦ How to raise levels of the weight loss aid **carnitine** with a different, cheaper supplement ✦ The most effective ways to **maximize glutathione**, which can protect you from Parkinson's disease, chronic fatigue, cancers and autoimmune diseases and can even extend your natural life span ✦ A **fallacy** exposed: find out why chocolate is not a high-risk food for **herpes** sufferers, and which really **are** the high-risk foods ✦ Learn about one of the hottest topics in medicine today—**nitric oxide** made from the amino acid arginine.

High blood pressure, low sex drive, glaucoma, gout, athletic endurance, depression, schizophrenia, pain, Alzheimer's disease and gall-bladder disease—we now know that all can respond to the right amino acid combinations.

The *Amino Acid Report* brings you the quality writing you have come to expect from Linda Lazarides. Comprehensive information on amino acids in seven meat and fish foods and 41 vegetarian foods, including yoghurt, mushrooms, beans, lentils, tofu, potatoes, rice, buckwheat and five different nuts and seeds. Full of charts and tables for you to compare information. The figures are derived from the most comprehensive source in the world—the Agricultural Research Service of the U.S. Department of Agriculture.

ISBN 0-9538046-2-3

Order now from any bookshop
or send a cheque for £11.99 payable to Waterfall 2000 to:
Waterfall 2000, BCM Waterfall, London WC1N 3XX

Please quote Reference "Amino Acid Report" and allow 28 days for delivery